Terrorism and Disaster
Individual and Community Mental Health Interventions

There is widespread belief amongst clinicians that terrorism (and torture) produce the highest rates of psychiatric sequelae of all the types of disaster and, further, that the traumatic effects of terrorism are not limited to the direct victims alone; they extend to families, helpers, communities, and even regions far from the affected site. This new book follows on from Ursano et al.'s earlier title *Individual and Community Responses to Trauma and Disaster* to expand the focus on terrorism as a particular type of disaster.

The authors and editors assembled here represent the world's experts in their respective fields, and together they examine the effects of terrorism, assessing lessons learned from recent atrocities such as 9/11, the Tokyo sarin attack, and the Omagh bombing. Issues of prevention, individual and organizational intervention, the effect of leadership, the effects of technological disasters, and bioterrorism/contamination are all examined in detail. This is essential reading for all professionals working in trauma and disaster planning.

Robert J. Ursano, Carol S. Fullerton, and **Ann E. Norwood** are all based in the Center for the Study of Traumatic Stress, Department of Psychiatry at the Uniformed Services University of the Health Sciences in Bethesda. This group of editors are internationally known and recognized for their long experience of clinical work and research in the area of posttraumatic stress disorder associated with disaster, terrorism, and bioterrorism.

From reviews of the previous book:

'Comprehensive, scholarly, gripping reading. This is a SUPERB book. This volume is the most comprehensive, scholarly and well-done book covering the entire range of traumata and disasters . . . Material never before presented in such a readable and definitive form.' Margaret T. Singer.

'A sterling compilation of authors and researches . . . this book will establish a new gold standard for mental health responses to traumatic effects.' Terence Keane.

Terrorism and Disaster

Individual and Community Mental Health Interventions

Edited by

Robert J. Ursano

Carol S. Fullerton

Ann E. Norwood

Uniformed Services University of the Health Sciences, F. Edward Hebert School of Medicine, Bethesda, USA

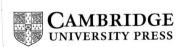

CAMBRIDGE
UNIVERSITY PRESS

PUBLISHED BY THE PRESS SYNDICATE OF THE UNIVERSITY OF CAMBRIDGE
The Pitt Building, Trumpington Street, Cambridge, United Kingdom

CAMBRIDGE UNIVERSITY PRESS
The Edinburgh Building, Cambridge CB2 2RU, UK
40 West 20th Street, New York, NY 10011–4211, USA
477 Williamstown Road, Port Melbourne, VIC 3207, Australia
Ruiz de Alarcón 13, 28014 Madrid, Spain
Dock House, The Waterfront, Cape Town 8001, South Africa

http://www.cambridge.org

First published 2003

Printed in the United Kingdom at the University Press, Cambridge

Typefaces Minion 10.5/14 pt., and Formata   *System* LATEX 2_ε [TB]

A catalog record for this book is available from the British Library

Library of Congress Cataloging in Publication data

ISBN 0 521 82606 3 hardback
ISBN 0 521 53345 7 paperback

The editors would like to credit the help of Lisa McCurry, Catherine Levinson, the Armed Forces Institute
of Pathology Video Taping Services WRAMC, and the AV Department of the Uniformed Services Universtiy.

Every effort has been made in preparing this book to provide accurate and up-to-date information that is in
accord with accepted standards and practice at the time of publication. Nevertheless, the authors, editors
and publisher can make no warranties that the information contained herein is totally free from error, not
least because clinical standards are constantly changing through research and regulation. The authors,
editors and publisher therefore disclaim all liability for direct or consequential damages resulting from the
use of material contained in this book. Readers are strongly advised to pay careful attention to information
provided by the manufacturer of any drugs or equipment that they plan to use.

Contents

**Part IV   The intersection of disasters and terrorism: Effects
            of contamination on individuals**

Contributors

Rhonda Adessky
Center for Traumatic Stress, Department
of Psychiatry, Hadassah University Hospital,
Jerusalem, Israel

Joyce Adkins, Ph.D.
Deployment Health Clinical Center, Walter
Reed Army Medical Center, Washington, DC

Ralph E. Bally, Ph.D.
Staff Psychologist, National Naval Medical
Center, Bethesda, MD

Neta Bargai
Center for Traumatic Stress, Department
of Psychiatry, Hadassah University Hospital,
Jerusalem, Israel

Ruth Boker
Center for Traumatic Stress, Department
of Psychiatry, Hadassah University Hospital,
Jerusalem, Israel

Ambassador Prudence Bushnell
Dean, Leadership and Management School,
Foreign Service Institute, Department
of State, Arlington, VA

Rina Cooper
Center for Traumatic Stress, Department
of Psychiatry, Hadassah University Hospital,
Jerusalem, Israel

David Cowan, Ph.D.
Deployment Health Clinical Center, Walter
Reed Army Medical Center, Washington, DC

Charles C. Engel, Jr, M.D., M.P.H.
Department of Psychiatry, Uniformed
Services University of the Health Sciences,
F. Edward Hebert School of Medicine,
Bethesda, MD; Deployment Health Clinical
Center, Walter Reed Army Medical Center,
Washington, DC

Sara Freedman
Center for Traumatic Stress, Department
of Psychiatry, Hadassah University Hospital,
Jerusalem, Israel

Carol S. Fullerton, Ph.D.
Associate Professor (Research), Department
of Psychiatry, Uniformed Services University
of the Health Sciences, F. Edward Hebert
School of Medicine, Bethesda, MD

Ellen T. Gerrity, Ph.D.
Associate Director for Aggression and
Trauma, National Institute of Mental Health,
Bethesda, MD

Mary C. Grace, M.Ed., M.S.
Senior Research Associate, University
of Cincinnati College of Medicine,
Cincinnati, OH

Thomas A. Grieger, M.D.
Associate Professor, Department of
Psychiatry, Uniformed Services
University of the Health Sciences,
F. Edward Hebert School of Medicine,
Bethesda, MD

Benjamin T. Griffeth, M.D.
Staff Psychiatrist, National Naval Medical
Center, Bethesda, MD

Bonnie L. Green, Ph.D.
Professor of Psychiatry, Georgetown
University, Washington, DC

Hilit Hadar
Center for Traumatic Stress, Department of
Psychiatry, Hadassah University Hospital,
Jerusalem, Israel

Jesse J. Harris, D.S.W.
Dean, School of Social Work, University
of Maryland, Baltimore, MD

Harry C. Holloway, M.D.
Professor of Psychiatry and
Neuroscience, Department of
Psychiatry, Uniformed Services
University of the Health Sciences,
F. Edward Hebert School of Medicine,
Bethesda, MD

Ambereen Jaffer, M.P.H.
Deployment Health Clinical Center,
Walter Reed Army Medical Center,
Washington, DC

Wayne J. Katon, M.D.
Professor, Department
of Psychiatry and Behavioral Sciences,
University of Washington School of
Medicine, Seattle, WA

John S. Kennedy, M.D.
Assistant Professor, Department of
Psychiatry, Uniformed Services University of
the Health Sciences, F. Edward Hebert School
of Medicine and Staff Psychiatrist, National
Naval Medical Center

Jacob D. Lindy, M.D.
Supervising and Training Analyst and
Director, Cincinnati Psychoanalytic Institute,
Cincinnati, OH

John L. Lyszczarz, M.D.
Assistant Professor, Department of
Psychiatry, Uniformed Services University of
the Health Sciences, F. Edward Hebert School
of Medicine and Staff Psychiatrist, National
Naval Medical Center, Bethesda, MD

James E. McCarroll, Ph.D.
Research Professor, Department of
Psychiatry, Uniformed Services University of
the Health Sciences, F. Edward Hebert School
of Medicine, Bethesda, MD

Carol S. North, M.D.
Professor, Department of Psychiatry,
Washington University, St Louis, MO

John Oldham, M.D.
Professor and Chairman, Medical University
of South Carolina, Charleston, SC

Tuvia Peri
Center for Traumatic Stress, Department of
Psychiatry, Hadassah University Hospital,
Jerusalem, Israel

**Beverley Raphael, A.M., M.B.B.S., M.D.,
F.R.A.N.Z.C.P., F.R.C.**
Centre for Mental Health, North Sydney,
New South Wales, Australia

James J. Reeves, M.D.
Assistant Professor, Department of
Psychiatry, Uniformed Services University of
the Health Sciences, F. Edward Hebert School
of Medicine and Staff Psychiatrist, National
Naval Medical Center, Bethesda, MD

Rivka Tuval-Mashiach
Center for Traumatic Stress, Department of
Psychiatry, Hadassah University Hospital,
Jerusalem, Israel

James Rundell, M.D.
Director, TRICARE Europe, Frankfurt,
Germany; Professor, Department of
Psychiatry, Uniformed Services University of
the Health Sciences, F. Edward Hebert School
of Medicine, Bethesda, MD

Arieh Y. Shalev, M.D.
Director, Center for Traumatic Stress,
Department of Psychiatry, Hadassah
University Hospital, Jerusalem, Israel

Jon A. Shaw, M.D.
Professor and Director, Division of Child and
Adolescent Psychiatry, University of Miami
School of Medicine, Miami, FL

Vivian Sheliga, D.S.W.
Deployment Health Clinical Center, Walter
Reed Army Medical Center, Washington, DC

Peter Steinglass, M.D.
Director, Ackerman Institute for Family
Therapy, New York

Arnfinn Tønnessen, Ph.D.
Division of Disaster Psychiatry, Medical
Faculty, University of Oslo, The Norwegian
Armed Forces Joint Medical Services,
Norway

Robert J. Ursano, M.D.
Professor and Chairman, Department
of Psychiatry, Uniformed Services
University of the Health Sciences,
F. Edward Hebert School of Medicine,
Bethesda, MD

Lars Weisaeth, M.D., Ph.D.
Professor and Head, Division of Disaster
Psychiatry, Medical Faculty, University
of Oslo; Head, Department of
Psychiatry, Joint Norwegian
Armed Forces Medical Services,
Oslo, Norway

Simon Wessely, M.D.
Professor, Department of Psychological
Medicine, King's College London and
Institute of Psychiatry, London, UK

Elizabeth Terry Westerhaus, M.A.
Department of Psychiatry, Washington
University, St Louis, MO

Douglas Zatzick, M.D.
Assistant Professor, Department of
Psychiatry, Research Faculty, Harborview
Injury Prevention and Research Center,
University of Washington School of
Medicine, Seattle, WA

Preface

This volume broadens the scope of *Trauma and Disaster: The Structure of Human Chaos* to include an expanded focus on a special type of disaster, terrorism. Terrorism seeks to achieve political, ideological, or theological goals through a threat or action that creates extreme fear or horror. Many believe that terrorism (and torture) produce the highest rates of psychiatric sequelae amongst all types of disasters. The Tokyo sarin attack, the 9/11 attacks on the Pentagon and World Trade Center, and the anthrax letters have raised the specter of unconventional weapons (chemical, biological, nuclear, radiological, and high-yield explosives: known as CBRNE) and the employment of the familiar such as airliners in novel and terrifying ways. While disasters often are extraordinary events, trauma is all too common throughout the world. The effects of trauma are not circumscribed to direct victims; they extend to families, helpers, communities, and even regions far removed from the affected site. They extend over time as well as space as secondary stressors such as relocation, job loss, and traumatic reminders occur.

Like its predecessor's, the goal of this book is to examine commonalities across disasters as well as to highlight important differences. Several selected chapters from the previous edition related to terrorism have been included and updated. Data and observational 'lessons learned' distilled from recent terrorist events – 9/11, USS *Cole*, Oklahoma City, the bombing of the US embassy in Nairobi – are presented from several perspectives. The section on acute interventions considers assessment and treatments of individuals and groups from a wide vantage point ranging from the molecular to health care delivery systems. The final section of the book explores the effects of contamination on individuals and communities. The belief in exposure to an invisible toxin or organism and its implications for psychological and social function is a critical interface between disasters and terrorism especially CBRNE.

Many people have supported our work and to them we owe our deepest gratitude. We thank Cambridge University Press for its early recognition of the importance of psychological and behavioral consequences of disasters and trauma. We are indebted to the superb authors who have shared their experience and knowledge in the chapters that follow. They represent the cutting edge of thinking in disasters and traumatic stress and its real world applications. We also greatly appreciate the support of Drs Harry Holloway, David Marlowe, James Zimble, Larry Laughlin, Val Hemming, and Jay Sanford. They have afforded us the vision and the opportunity for much of the work that is reflected in this volume. Finally, and most importantly, we thank those individuals, groups, and communities that have shared their experiences with traumatic events that we might better assist those affected by future tragedies.

Part I

Introduction

Trauma, terrorism, and disaster

Carol S. Fullerton, Robert J. Ursano, Ann E. Norwood,
and Harry H. Holloway

For us, this was something that did not compute. We could not keep up fast enough with the implications of what was going on. We could not accept it. We could not believe it . . .. That it could be damaged I could accept, but when I learned that the Towers had collapsed, I was just speechless. I could not believe it. I could not comprehend it because these are massive structures, and it was unbelievable to think that something like that could happen. You could not even begin to think about the human toll at first, inasmuch as you were trying to respond to the situation itself, which was so shocking . . .. It turned out that there was no need because there were no survivors of the magnitude we anticipated. That was both surprising and horrifying as we began to understand why.

John Oldham, M.D.
Former Director, New York State Psychiatric Institute
Chairman, Department of Psychiatry, Medical University of South Carolina

A traumatic event is defined by its capacity to evoke terror, fear, helplessness, or horror in the face of a threat to life or serious injury (American Psychiatric Association, 1994). A wide host of traumatic events can stun, terrify, and disrupt communities. Communities exposed to disasters experience multiple traumatic events including threat to life, loss of property, exposure to death, and often economic devastation. Disasters by definition overwhelm institutions, health care, and social resources and require from months to years for both individuals and communities to recover. Natural disasters can strike without much notice, as can human-made traumas such as transportation disasters, factory explosions, and school shootings which have become a seemingly common part of modern-day life.

Individual traumatic events such as motor vehicle accidents, sudden unexpected death of a close friend or relative, or witnessing violence and physical assault, put a huge demand on individuals and families but usually have little consequence for the larger community. In many Western cultures (but not all cultures), such individual traumas are seen as accidents that do not disrupt cultural assumptions about social values or destroy access to social processes. Surveys in the general population estimate that approximately 69 percent of the US population are exposed to disasters or individual traumatic events over their lifetime (Norris, 1992). Of those exposed, 15 to 24 percent develop posttraumatic stress disorder (PTSD) (Breslau *et al.*, 1991; Kessler *et al.*, 1995).

Large-scale terrorist attacks are a particular type of disaster. They are human-caused, intentional interpersonal violence. Terrorists have used bombings, contamination, and weapons of mass destruction including chemical agents. The sarin nerve gas release in Tokyo and the anthrax attacks in the United States demonstrate the particular ability of chemical and biological weapons to create fear and social disruption. In addition to injuries and killing victims, the anthrax attack also forced the desertion of commercial and public buildings, disrupted the distribution of mail, occasioned social conflict, and evoked considerable fear and concern despite the fact that these attacks produced fewer casualities than car accidents and probably no greater economic loss. Terrorist events such as the Tokyo subway sarin gas attack in 1995, the bomb that exploded on a busy shopping street in Omagh, Northern Ireland, the World Trade Center attack on September 11, the 1998 embassy bombing in Nairobi, Kenya, and the 1995 Oklahoma City bombing, vividly demonstrate the strong psychological and social responses engendered by terrorism (North *et al.*, 1999; Pfefferbaum, 1999; Murakami, 2000; Tucker *et al.*, 2000; Schuster *et al.*, 2001; Galea *et al.*, 2002; Koplewicz *et al.*, 2002; Luce *et al.*, 2002; North *et al.*, 2002) and their impact on our beliefs and values (Jernigan *et al.*, 2001; *Morbidity and Mortality Weekly Report*, 2001).

Whether the perpetrators of terrorist acts represent powerful nations attempting to exert social control or small revolutionary religious or political groups attempting to impose their will upon their opponents, the purpose of most terrorists is to change the behavior of others by frightening or terrifying them and to kill those 'who do not believe' (Benedek *et al.*, 2002). Terrorism destroys the sense of safety and creates terror in individuals, communities, and nations. How the psychological response to a terrorist attack is managed may be the defining factor in the ability of a community to recover (Holloway *et al.*, 1997).

The deliberate infliction of pain and suffering as occurs in a terrorist attack is a particularly potent psychological stressor. In a nationally representative survey in the United States conducted the week after the September 11 terrorist attack, 44 percent of the adults reported one or more substantial symptoms of stress, and 90 percent reported at least low levels of stress symptoms (Schuster *et al.*, 2001). In the area most directly affected by the September 11 attack, 17.3 percent of the population were estimated to have PTSD or depression 1–2 months after the attack (Galea *et al.*, 2002). In a national study 1–2 months after September 11, rates of probable PTSD were 11.2 percent in New York City, 2.7 percent in Washington DC,

3.6 percent in other metropolitan areas, and 4.0 percent in the rest of the United States (Schlenger *et al.*, 2002). Approximately 35 percent of those directly exposed to the Oklahoma City terrorist bombing developed PTSD by 6 months (North *et al.*, 1999). An ongoing threat of terrorist attacks affects both the severity and duration of posttraumatic stress responses (Shalev, 2000).

Preventive medicine, a familiar organizing structure for conceptualizing infectious outbreaks, can also organize our understanding and interventions for behavioral and psychological responses to disasters (Ursano *et al.*, 1995b; Pfefferbaum and Pfefferbaum, 1998). In this model one identifies the pathogen, its source, and those exposed. For the psychiatric consequences of disasters the stressful psychological, physiological, and social events of the disaster are the pathogens. Terrorist attacks differ from disasters in the prominence of terror as the agent of disease and disruption.

Primary (preevent), secondary (event), and tertiary (postevent) interventions can decrease the risk of maladaptive behaviors, distress, mental disorder and disrupted functioning (Sorenson, 2002). Importantly, preevent interventions to decrease exposure to the traumatic event (e.g., practice drills) or its severity (e.g., seat belts) are an important and often overlooked component of mental health disaster planning (Aguirre *et al.*, 1998; Ursano, 2002). Identifying the groups of people that are most highly exposed to these stressors is the critical second step in determining the community consequences of a disaster or terrorist attack.

Characteristics and dimensions of traumatic events, disasters, and terrorism

Traumatic events can be first characterized by who is exposed, individuals or communities/populations (e.g., rape versus tornado). Individually experienced traumatic events can be further classified as intentional (e.g., assault) or unintentional, i.e., 'accidental' such as motor vehicle accidents. Similarly, community/population based traumatic events (i.e., disasters) are broadly categorized as human-made (e.g., terrorism, war, industrial accidents) or natural (e.g., earthquakes, floods, hurricanes) (Fig. 1.1). Often human-made disasters have been shown to be more disturbing and disruptive than natural disasters (for review see Norris, 2002). However, this distinction is increasingly difficult to make. The etiology and consequences of natural disasters often are affected by human beings. For example, the damage and loss of life caused by an earthquake can be magnified by poor construction practices and high-density occupancy. Similarly, humans may cause or contribute to natural disasters through poor land-management practices that increase the probability of floods. Interpersonal violence between individuals (assault) or groups (war, terrorism) is perhaps the most disturbing traumatic experience. Disasters, as well as individual traumatic events, are also characterized by their severity as well

Table 1.1 Dimensions of traumatic events

Threat to life
Exposure to the grotesque (dead)
Physical harm or injury
Loss of significant others
Loss of property
Information stress

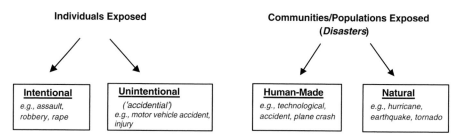

Figure 1.1   Characteristics of traumatic events.

as the nature of the stressful dimensions of the particular disaster (Green, 1990) such as: threat to life, exposure to the grotesque, physical harm or injury, loss of significant others, loss of property, or information stress (Table 1.1).

A major component of all traumatic events is disruption of the experience of safety. Some dimensions of traumatic events are more likely to engender psychiatric morbidity. High perceived threat, low controllability, lack of predictability, and high loss and injury are associated with the highest risk of psychiatric morbidity (American Psychiatric Association, 1994; Epstein *et al.*, 1997; Boudreaux *et al.*, 1998; North *et al.*, 1999; Schuster *et al.*, 2001; Zatzick *et al.*, 2001). For example, exposure to the dead and mutilated increases the risk of adverse psychiatric events (Ursano and McCarroll, 1990; Ursano *et al.*, 1995a; McCarroll *et al.*, 1996). Some groups such as first responders (firefighters, police, and Emergency Medical Technicians), hospital workers, and mortuary volunteers are routinely exposed to the dead and injured and therefore are nearly always at increased risk for a psychiatric illness and morbidity.

Increasingly, traumatic bereavement is recognized as posing special challenges to survivors (Raphael, 1977; Fullerton *et al.*, 1999; Prigerson *et al.*, 1999; Shear *et al.*, 2001). Interventions for bereavement are different than those for exposure to life threat both for adults and children (Pynoos *et al.*, 1987; Pynoos and Nader, 1993).

Table 1.2 Similarities and differences in terrorism, natural disaster, and technological disaster

Dimension	Terrorism[a]	Natural disaster[b]	Technological disaster[c]
Altered sense of safety	+++	+++	+++
Intentional	+++		
Unpredictable	+++	++	+++
Localized geographically		+++	++
Local fear	++	+++	+++
National fear	+++		
National bereavement	+++	+	+
Consequences spread over time	+++	++	++
Loss of confidence in institutions	+++	+	+++
Community disruption	+++	+++	+++
Target basic societal infrastructure	+++		
Overwhelm health care systems	+	+++	++
Hoaxes/copycats	+++		

[a]Terrorism, e.g., bombings, hostage-taking.
[b]Natural disaster, e.g., hurricanes, tornadoes, earthquakes.
[c]Technicological disasters, e.g., nuclear leaks, toxic spills.

In children traumatic play, a phenomenon similar to intrusive symptoms in adults, is both a sign of distress and an effort at mastery (Terr, 1981). While the death of loved ones is always painful, an unexpected and violent death can be more difficult. Even when not directly witnessing the death, family members may develop intrusive images based on information gleaned from authorities or the media.

Witnessing or learning of violence to a loved one increases vulnerability to psychiatric distress as well as does knowledge that one has been exposed to toxins (e.g., chemicals or radiation) (Baum *et al.*, 1983; Weisaeth, 1994). In this case, information itself is the primary stressor. Often times toxic exposures have the added stress of being clouded in uncertainty as to whether or not exposure has taken place and what the long-term health consequences may be. Living with the uncertainty can be exceedingly stressful. Typically uncertainty accompanies bioterrorism and is the focus of much concern in the medical community preparing for responses to terrorist attacks using biological, chemical, or nuclear agents (Holloway *et al.*, 1997; DiGiovanni, 1999; Benedek *et al.*, 2002).

Terrorism often can be distinguished from other natural and human-made disasters by the characteristic extensive fear, loss of confidence in institutions, unpredictability and pervasive experience of loss of safety (Table 1.2). In a longitudinal national study of reactions to September 11, 64.6 percent of people outside of New York City reported fears of future terrorism at 2 months and 37.5 percent at 6 months

(Silver *et al.*, 2002). In addition, 59.5 percent reported fear of harm to family at 2 months and 40.6 percent at 6 months. Terrorism is one of the most powerful and pervasive generators of psychiatric illness, distress, and disrupted community and social functioning (Holloway *et al.*, 1997; North *et al.*, 1999).

Health consequences of terrorism and disaster

The psychosocial, cognitive, and biologic effects of traumatic events are complex and interrelated (McEwan, 2001; Ursano, 2002; Yehuda, 2002). The behavioral and psychological responses seen in disasters are not random and frequently have a predictable structure and time course. For most individuals posttraumatic psychiatric symptoms are transitory. These early symptoms usually respond to education, obtaining enough rest, and maintaining biological rhythms (e.g., sleep at the same time, eat at the same time). Media exposure can be both reassuring and threatening. Limiting such exposure can minimize the disturbing effects especially in children (Pfefferbaum *et al.*, 2001). Educating spouses and significant others of those distressed can assist in treatment as well as in identifying the worsening or persistence of symptoms. At times, traumatic events and disasters also have beneficial effects serving as organizing events and providing a sense of purpose as well as an opportunity for positive growth experiences (Ursano, 1987; Foa *et al.*, 2000).

For some, however, the effects of disaster linger long after its occurrence, rekindled by new experiences that remind the person of the past traumatic event. PTSD is not uncommon following many traumatic events from terrorism to motor vehicle accidents to industrial explosions. In its acute form PTSD may be more like the common cold, experienced at some time in one's life by nearly all. If it persists, it can be debilitating and require psychotherapeutic and pharmacological intervention.

PTSD is not, however, the only trauma-related disorder, nor perhaps the most common (Fullerton and Ursano, 1997; North *et al.*, 1999; Norris, in press) (Table 1.3). People exposed to terrorism and disaster are at increased risk for depression, generalized anxiety disorder, panic disorder, and increased substance use (Breslau *et al.*, 1991; Kessler *et al.*, 1995; North *et al.*, 1999, 2002; Vlahov *et al.*, 2002). Forty-five percent of survivors of the Oklahoma City bombing had a postdisaster psychiatric disorder. Of these 34.3 percent had PTSD and 22.5 percent had major depression (North *et al.*, 1999). Nearly 40 percent of those with PTSD or depression had no previous history of psychiatric illness (North *et al.*, 1999). After a disaster or terrorist event the contribution of the psychological factors to medical illness can also be pervasive – from heart disease (Leor *et al.*, 1996) to diabetes (Jacobson, 1996). Importantly, injured survivors often have psychological factors affecting their physical condition (Shore *et al.*, 1989; Kulka *et al.*, 1990; Smith *et al.*, 1990; North *et al.*, 1999; Zatzick, 2001).

Table 1.3 Health outcomes

Psychiatric diagnoses
Posttraumatic stress disorder
Acute stress disorder
Major depression
Substance-use disorders
Generalized anxiety disorder
Adjustment disorder
Organic mental disorders secondary to head injury, toxic exposure, illness, and dehydration
Psychological factors affecting physical disease (in the injured)

Psychological/behavioral responses
Grief reactions and other normal responses to an abnormal event
Family conflict

Acute stress disorder (ASD) was introduced into the diagnostic nomenclature in *DSM-IV* (American Psychiatric Association, 1994). ASD is a constellation of symptoms very similar to PTSD but persists for a minimum of 2 days and a maximum of 4 weeks and occurs within 4 weeks of the trauma. The only difference in symptom requirements between the two diagnoses is that dissociative symptoms must be present in order to diagnose ASD. The dissociative symptoms can occur during the traumatic event itself or after it. A common early response to traumatic exposure appears to be a disturbance in our sense of time, our internal time clock, resulting in time distortion – time feeling speeded up or slowed down (Ursano and Fullerton, 2000). Along with other dissociative symptoms this time distortion indicates an over four times greater risk for chronic PTSD and may also be an accompaniment of depressive symptoms.

Traumatic bereavement (Prigerson *et al.*, 1999), unexplained somatic symptoms (Ford, 1997; McCarroll *et al.*, 2002), depression (Kessler *et al.*, 1999), sleep disturbance, increased alcohol, caffeine, and cigarette use (Shalev *et al.*, 1990), as well as family conflict and family violence are not uncommon following traumatic events. Anger, disbelief, sadness, anxiety, fear, and irritability are expected responses. In each, the role of exposure to the traumatic event may be easily overlooked by a primary-care physician. Anxiety and family conflict can accompany the fear and distress of new terrorist alerts, toxic contamination, and the economic impact of lost jobs and companies closed or moving. Medical evaluation which includes inquiring about family conflict can provide reassurance as well as begin a discussion for referral, and be a primary preventive intervention for children whose first experience of a disaster or terrorist attack is mediated through their parents.

Community effects of terrorism and disaster

While there are many definitions of terrorism and disaster, a common feature is that the event overwhelms local resources and threatens the function and safety of the community. With the advent of instantaneous communication and media coverage, word of terrorism or disaster is disseminated quickly, often in real time witnessed around the globe. The disaster community is soon flooded with outsiders: people offering assistance, curiosity-seekers, and the media. This sudden influx of strangers affects the community in many ways. The presence of large numbers of media representatives can be experienced as intrusive and insensitive. Hotel rooms have no vacancies, restaurants are crowded with unfamiliar faces, and the normal routine of the community is altered. At a time when, traditionally, communities turn inward to grieve and assist affected families, the normal social supports are strained and disrupted by outsiders.

Inevitably, after any major trauma, there are rumors circulated within the community about the circumstances leading up to the traumatic event and the government response. Sometimes there is a heightened state of fear. For example, a study of a school shooting in Illinois noted that a high level of anxiety continued for a week after the event, even after it was known that the perpetrator had committed suicide (Schwarz and Kowalski, 1991).

Outpourings of sympathy for the injured, dead, and their friends and families are common and expected. Impromptu memorials of flowers, photographs, and memorabilia are frequently erected. Churches, synagogues, temples, and mosques play an important role in assisting communities' search for meaning from such tragedy and in assisting in the grief process.

Over time, anger often emerges in the community. Typically, there is a focus on accountability, a search for someone who was responsible for a lack of preparation or inadequate response. Mayors, police and fire chiefs, and other community leaders are often targets of these strong feelings. Scapegoating can be an especially destructive process when leveled at those who already hold themselves responsible, even if, in reality, there was nothing they could have done to prevent adverse outcomes. In addition, nations and communities experience ongoing hypervigilance and a sense of lost safety while trying to establish a new normal in their lives.

There are many milestones of a disaster which both affect the community and may offer opportunities for recovery. There are the normal rituals associated with burying the dead. Later, energy is poured into creating appropriate memorials. Memorialization carries the potential to cause harm as well as to do good. There can be heated disagreement about what the monument should look like and where it should be placed. Special thought must be given to the placement of memorials. If the monument is situated too prominently so that community members cannot

Table 1.4 High-risk groups

Directly exposed to life threat
Injured
First responders
Bereaved
Single parents
Children
Elderly
Women
Individuals with:
   prior PTSD
   prior exposure to trauma
   prior or current psychiatric or medical illness
   lack of supportive relationships

avoid encountering it, the memorial may heighten intrusive recollections and inter-fere with the resolution of grief reactions. Anniversaries of the disaster (one week, one month, one year) often stimulate renewed grief.

High-risk groups

Posttraumatic stress is most often seen in those directly exposed to the threat to life and the horror of a traumatic event. The greater the 'dose' of traumatic stressors, the more likely a group is to develop high rates of psychiatric morbidity. Importantly, as noted earlier, psychiatric illness can develop even in those with no previous psychiatric history (North *et al.*, 1999). Therefore those needing treatment will not all have the usually expected accompanying risk factors and coping strategies of other mental health populations. While each disaster has its unique aspects, certain groups are routinely exposed to the dead and injured and, therefore, are at risk for psychiatric sequelae (Table 1.4). Adults, children, and the elderly in particular who were in physical danger and who directly witnessed the events are at risk. Traumatically bereaved parents of adult children are a group often forgotten as community programs and neighbors remember the spouse or partner and children of the deceased.

Those at greatest risk include the primary victims, those who have significant attachments with the primary victims, first responders, and support providers (Wright and Bartone, 1994). Those who were psychologically vulnerable before the terrorist attacks may also be buffeted by the fears and realities of job loses, unten-ably longer commutes, or eroded interpersonal and community support systems overtaxed now by increased demands.

Similarly, police, paramedics, and other first responders who assist the injured and evacuate them to medical care, and hospital personnel who care for the injured are all groups that need opportunities to process what happened, education on normal responses, and information on when to seek further help. Those who are charged with cleaning up the site of the tragedy are also vulnerable to persistent symptoms. Overidentification with the victims (e.g., 'It could have been me') and their pain and grief can perpetuate the fear response (Ursano *et al.*, 1999). This normally health and growth promoting mechanism of identification with victims and heroes can turn against us in this setting like an autoimmune disorder. Inevitably, each disaster situation will also contain individuals who are 'silent' victims and often overlooked. By paying close attention to the patterns and types of exposure, these individuals can be identified and be given proper care.

Risk communication

Multiple studies confirm that we assess risk and threat based on our feelings of control and our level of knowledge and familiarity with an event (for example, see MacGregor and Fleming, 1996). Therefore peanut butter is not recognized sufficiently as a risk to health and air travel is seen as overly risky (Slovic, 1987). Widespread fear, uncertainty, and stigmatization are common following terrorism and disasters. These fears require education about the actual risk and instruction in how to decrease risk whether the risk is falling buildings in an earthquake or infection from a biological weapon. Instruction in active coping techniques can increase feelings of control and efficacy. In particular, fears of biological contagion or other contaminants can decrease community cohesion and turn neighbor against neighbor as one tries to feel safe by identifying those who are exposed or ill as 'not me'.

The fear of exposure to toxic agents, including biological, chemical, and radiologic agents, can lead hundreds or even thousands to seek care, overwhelming our hospitals and health care system. Belief that one has been exposed to chemical and biological weapons leads individuals to seek health care and change life patterns regardless of actual exposure. After the Aum Shinrikyo attack in Tokyo in which 11 victims died, over 5000 people sought care for presumed exposure (Okumura *et al.*, 1998). In Israel, after a SCUD missile attack during the Gulf War, fear of chemical weapons exposure was the reason for nearly 700 of 1000 war-related emergency room visits (Karsenty *et al.*, 1991; Bleich *et al.*, 1992). The resources demanded by such events are large and made larger by the uncertainties associated with the event. Triage of anxious and distressed individuals is critical to being able to provide appropriate care to those who are physically injured.

Clear, accurate, and consistent information exchange is needed between health care professionals, government and local leaders, and the general public in times of a disaster. For medical and public health care professionals, explaining and describing risk is probably the most challenging situation for communicating with nonscientists. Difficulty translating scientific information, conflicting risks and messages, and disagreement on the extent of the risk and how to assess it presents key challenges. Physicians have the ear of their community in their medical office, at community functions and schools, and through the media and therefore, are an important natural network for educating about risk and prevention.

Medical and behavioral health personnel provide important expertise in development of public information plans. Information from official and unofficial sources before, during, and after a disaster will shape expectations, behaviors and emotional responses (Holloway *et al.*, 1997). The delivery of consistent, updated information across multiple channels by way of widely recognized and trusted sources diminishes the extent to which misinformation can shape public attribution (Peters *et al.*, 1997). It is critical that the information provided be truthful even if it is bad news. Trusted media representatives may fulfill a vital function by delivering simple, salient, and repeated messages regarding matters of concern to the public. These messages could educate the public concerning the nature of the threat and how to act to avoid harm and get help.

Intervention

The normal process of recovery involves talking with others about the event, learning coping strategies, and seeking help (Table 1.5). A number of treatment approaches for PTSD have been proposed to be helpful, including: psychodynamic therapy, group therapy, psychological debriefing, cognitive–behavioral therapy, pharmacotherapy, psychosocial rehabilitation, and marital and family therapy (for reviews, see Foa *et al.*, 2000; Yehuda, 2002). Early psychiatric interventions to disaster are directed to minimizing exposure to traumatic stressors and educating about normal responses to trauma and disasters. Consultations to other health care professionals who will see individuals seeking medical care for injuries and to community leaders who need assistance in identifying at risk groups and understanding the phases of recovery are also important early on. More traditional health care services such as advising people on when to seek professional treatment; assisting in the resolution of acute symptomatology occurring in the days and weeks after the initial exposure; identifying those who are at higher risk for the development of psychiatric disorders; and engaging them in treatment and support are important to the health of the community.

Early symptoms usually respond to a number of approaches, such as helping patients and their families identify the cause of the stress and limiting further exposure (e.g., by avoiding excessive news coverage of the traumatic event) and advising

Table 1.5 Early intervention with trauma survivors

1. *Basic needs*
   Safety/security/survival
   Food and shelter
   Orientation
   Communication with family, friends, and community
   Assessment of the environment for ongoing threat/toxin

2. *Psychological first aid*
   Protect survivors from further harm
   Reduce physiological arousal
   Mobilize support for those who are most distressed
   Keep families together and facilitate reunion with loved ones
   Provide information, foster communication and education
   Use effective risk-communication techniques

3. *Needs assessment*
   Assess current status, how well needs addressed, recovery environment, what
       additional interventions needed for:
           group
           population
           individual

4. *Monitoring the rescue and recovery environment*
   Observe and listen to those most affected
   Monitor the environment for toxins and stressors
   Monitor past and ongoing threats
   Monitor services that are being provided
   Monitor media coverage and rumors

5. *Outreach and information dissemination*
   'Therapy by walking around'
   Using established community structures
   Flyers
   Websites
   Media interviews, releases, and programs

6. *Technical assistance, consultation, and training*
   Consultation to emergency hospital personnel
   Establish outreach programs to provide community support and social intervention
       programs to decrease chronicity
   Educate medical personnel and community groups (media, schools, PTAs, hospitals,
       corporations) on normal responses to trauma and loss
   Educate of medical personnel on likely presentations of psychiatric disorders to
       primary care physicians: somatization, grief reactions, depression, substance abuse,
       family violence, spouse and child abuse

Table 1.5 (*cont.*)

Consultation, education, and training to other groups (e.g., clergy, teachers/schools, parenting groups, employment groups) and responders

Leaders

7. *Fostering resilience/recovery*

Social interactions

Coping skills training

Risk-assessment skills training

Education about stress response, traumatic reminders, coping, normal vs. abnormal functioning, risk factors, services

Group and family interventions

Fostering natural social support

Looking after the bereaved

Repair organizational fabric

8. *Triage*

Clinical assessment

Referral when indicated

Identify the vulnerable, high-risk individuals and groups

Emergency hospitalization

9. *Treatment*

Reduce or ameliorate symptoms or improve functioning via:

individual, family, and group psychotherapy

pharmacotherapy

spiritual support

short-term or long-term hospitalization

Adapted from Ursano *et al.* (1995b); National Institute of Mental Health (2002).

patients to get enough rest and maintain their biologic rhythms (e.g., by going to sleep at the same time each night and by eating at the same times each day). Key components of early intervention can be provided by mental health professionals and by other health care providers (National Institute of Mental Health, 2002). Early interventions include meeting basic needs (safety, food, and protection from the elements), psychological first aid, assessing needs, monitoring the rescue and recovery environment, outreach and information dissemination, technical assistance, consultation and training, fostering resilience/recovery; triage, and treatment (Table 1.5).

It is important to remember that one of the goals of psychiatric care is to facilitate the treatment of the injured by removing individuals who do not require emergency medical care from the patient flow. Designation of a location near the hospital but separate from the chaos is important for initial treatment and triage. Hospitals or other institutions serving as entry points for care can serve as locations where persons with psychologic symptoms can receive respite (Benedek *et al.*, 2002).

Educating patients and their families can also help them to identify worsening or persistent symptoms. Anxiety and family conflict can be triggered by the fear of new threats or by the economic impact of the loss of a job after a traumatic event.

Interpersonal withdrawal and social isolation are particularly difficult symptoms and often bode a complex trauma response. Social withdrawal tends to limit the normal recovery mechanisms, e.g., the 'natural debriefing process' (Ursano *et al.*, 2000), talking with others, active coping, and help-seeking. Depression may be a primary contribution to withdrawal and requires evaluation and treatment.

Increased somatic symptoms have been frequently reported after disasters, particularly toxic exposures (Engel and Katon, 1999) and exposure to the dead (McCarroll *et al.*, 2002) and can be an expression of anxiety or depression. In these individuals, conservative medical management with education and reassurance are the core of medical treatment. Discussion of specific worries and fears can decrease symptoms, initiate the normal metabolism and digestion of stress symptoms, and identify any need for further specific treatment.

Although group debriefing techniques and critical incident debriefings have often been used in the aftermath of natural disasters, school shootings, and terrorist events, there is no convincing evidence that such debriefings reduce the development of psychiatric illness or prevent the development of PTSD. Nonetheless open discussions among survivors of traumatic events and among disaster workers may foster better understanding of the traumatic experience and group cohesion. This may decrease individual isolation and stigma, and facilitate identification of individuals who may require further mental health attention (Raphael, 2000). Debriefing may have its beneficial effect by encouraging talking and limiting the disability and impairment associated with withdrawal and stigma. Debriefing of homogeneous groups and being careful to not mix people with widely differing exposures (which can increase traumatic exposure for some in the group) are helpful strategies.

Evidence from clinical trials suggests that cognitive–behavioral therapy facilitates recovery from PTSD following trauma. Cognitive–behavioral therapy involves education about the nature and universality of symptoms, examination of the precipitants of symptoms (particularly cognitive distortions), and development of reframing and interpretive techniques to minimize further symptoms. Clinical trials for the treatment of depression, anxiety, and PTSD suggest that even brief therapeutic interventions of this nature may reduce immediate symptoms and diminish the development of long-term morbidity (Bryant *et al.*, 1998; Foa *et al.*, 2000).

Table 1.6 Resources for terrorism and disaster intervention

American Psychiatric Association: http://www.psych.org
American Psychological Association: http://www.apa.org
Red Cross: http://www.redcross.org
Uniformed Services University of the Health Sciences (USUHS), Center for the Study of
   Traumatic Stress, Department of Psychiatry: http://www.usuhs.mil/psy/disasteresources.html
   (or go to USUHS home page: http://www.usuhs.mil and click on 'Disaster Care Resources')
Substance Abuse and Mental Health Services Administration (SAMHSA):
   http://www.samhsa.gov

Pharmacotherapy with selective serotonin reuptake inhibitor (SSRI) agents has been shown effective with PTSD (Foa *et al.*, 2000). Limited use of sleep stabilizing medications as well as antianxiety agents can also relieve symptoms and more rapidly return those distressed to baseline functioning.

Given that medical resources may be quickly overwhelmed in the aftermath of a traumatic event, nonphysicians trained in the delivery of various early interventions (e.g., social workers, psychiatric nurses, and specifically trained others such as Red Cross volunteers) can more effectively achieve delivery of care. In establishing priorities, delay in instituting mental health diagnosis and treatment may increase long-term morbidity. Employee assistance programs are an important resource when specific businesses or buildings, as can occur in a terrorist event, have been affected.

Conclusion

The chaos that occurs when lives are thrown into the turmoil of terrorism and disaster has a structure that is increasingly becoming evident through research, clinical work, and community concern. Further understanding of the consequences of terrorism and disaster will aid leaders and health care providers in planning for such events (see Table 1.6 for additional Internet resources). The chapters that follow highlight national and international responses to terrorism and disaster. They discuss and suggest interventions for leaders, health care providers, researchers, individuals, and communities. The development of community disaster plans, medical intervention and prevention plans to address the responses to traumatic events, and the training of leaders in the stresses of traumatic events can greatly help individuals and their communities. Education about the nature of terrorism and disaster is needed to increase the knowledge base for intervention and the resources for furthering our understanding. Consultation and mutually helpful relationships among clinicians, researchers, and community leaders are essential to these efforts.

REFERENCES

Aguirre, B. E., Wenger, D. and Vigo, G. (1998). A test of the emergent norm theory of collective behavior. *Sociological Forum*, **13**, 301–320.

American Psychiatric Association (1994). *Diagnostic and Statistical Manual of Mental Disorders*, 4th edn. Washington, DC: American Psychiatric Press.

Baum, A., Gatchel, R. J. and Schaeffer, M. A. (1983). Emotional, behavioral, and physiological effects of chronic stress at Three Mile Island. *Journal of Consulting and Clinical Psychology*, **51**, 565–572.

Benedek, D. M., Holloway, H. C. and Becker, S. M. (2002). Emergency mental health management in bioterrorism events. *Emergency Medicine Clinics of North America*, **20**, 393–407.

Bleich, A., Dycian, A., Koslowsky, M., Solomon, Z. and Wiener, M. (1992). Psychiatric implications of missile attacks on a civilian population. Israel: Lessons from the Persian Gulf War. *Journal of the American Medical Association*, **268**, 613–615.

Boudreaux, E., Kilpatrick, D. G., Resnick, H. S., Best, C. L. and Saunders, B. E. (1998). Criminal victimization, posttraumatic stress disorder, and comorbid psychopathology among a community sample of women. *Journal of Traumatic Stress*, **11**, 665–678.

Breslau, N., Davis, G. C., Andreski, P. and Peterson, E. L. (1991). Traumatic events and posttraumatic stress disorder in an urban population of young adults. *Archives of General Psychiatry*, **48**, 216–222.

Bryant, R. A., Harvey, A. G., Dang, S. T., Sackville, T. and Basten, C. (1998). Treatment of acute stress disorder: A comparison of cognitive–behavioral therapy and supportive counseling. *Journal of Consulting and Clinical Psychology*, **66**, 862–866.

DiGiovanni, J. (1999). Domestic terrorism with chemical or biological agents: Psychiatric aspects. *American Journal of Psychiatry*, **156**, 1500–1505.

Engel, C. C. and Katon, W. J. (1999). Population and need-based prevention of unexplained symptoms in the community. In *Institute of Medicine, Strategies to Protect the Health of Deployed US Forces: Medical Surveillance, Record Keeping, and Risk Reduction*, eds. L. M. Joellenbeck, P. K. Russell and S. B. Guze, pp. 173–212. Washington, DC: National Academy Press.

Epstein, J. N., Saunders, B. E. and Kilpatrick, D. G. (1997). Predicting PTSD in women with a history of childhood rape. *Journal of Traumatic Stress*, **10**, 573–588.

Foa, E. B., Keane, T. M. and Friedman, M. J. (eds.) (2000). *Effective Treatments for PTSD*. New York: Guilford Press.

Ford, C. V. (1997). Somatic symptoms, somatization, and traumatic stress: An overview. *Nordic Journal of Psychiatry*, **51**, 5–13.

Fullerton, C. S., Ursano, R. J., Kao, T. C. and Bharitya, V. R. (1999). Disaster-related bereavement: Acute symptoms and subsequent depression. *Aviation, Space, and Environmental Medicine*, **70**, 902–909.

Fullerton, C. S. and Ursano, R. J. (eds) (1997). *Posttraumatic Stress Disorder: Acute and Long-Term Responses to Trauma and Disaster*. Washington, DC: American Psychiatric Press.

Galea, S., Ahern, J., Resnick, H., *et al.* (2002). Psychological sequelae of the September 11 terrorist attacks in New York City. *New England Journal of Medicine*, **346**, 982–987.

Green, B. L. (1990). Defining trauma: Terminology and generic dimensions. *Journal of Applied Social Psychology*, **20**, 1632–1642.

Holloway, H. C., Norwood, A. E., Fullerton, C. S., Engel, C. C. and Ursano, R. J. (1997). The threat of biological weapons: Prophylaxis and mitigation of psychological and social consequences. *Journal of the American Medical Association*, **278**, 425–427.

Jacobson, A. M. (1996). The psychological care of patients with insulin-dependent diabetes mellitus. *New England Journal of Medicine*, **334**, 1249–1253.

Jernigan, J. A., Stephens, D. S., Ashford, D. A., *et al.* (2001). Bioterrorism-related inhalational anthrax: The first 10 cases reported in the United States. *Emergency Infectious Disease*, **7**, 933–946.

Karsenty, E., Shemer, J., Alshech, I., *et al.* (1991). Medical aspects of the Iraqi missile attacks on Israel. *Israel Journal of Medical Science*, **27**, 603–607.

Kessler, R. C., Barber, C., Birnbaum, H. G., *et al.* (1999). Depression in the work place: Effects of short-term disability. *Health Affairs*, **18**, 163–171.

Kessler, R. C., Sonnega, A., Bromet, E., Hughes, M. and Nelson, C. B. (1995). Posttraumatic stress disorder in the National Comorbidity Survey. *Archives of General Psychiatry*, **52**, 1048–1060.

Koplewicz, H. S., Vogel, J. M., Solanto, M. V., *et al.* (2002). Child and parent response to the 1993 World Trade Center bombing. *Journal of Traumatic Stress*, **15**, 77–85.

Kulka, R. A., Schlenger, W. E., Fairbank, J. A., *et al.* (1990). *Trauma and the Vietnam War Generation: Report of Findings from the National Vietnam Veterans Readjustment Study*. New York: Brunner/Mazel.

Leor, J., Poole, W. K. and Kloner, R. A. (1996). Sudden cardiac death triggered by an earthquake. *New England Journal of Medicine*, **334**, 413–419.

Luce, A., Firth-Cozens, J., Midgley, S. and Burges, C. (2002). After the Omagh bomb: Posttraumatic stress disorder in health service staff. *Journal of Traumatic Stress*, **15**, 27–30.

MacGregor, D. G. and Fleming, R. (1996). Risk perception and symptom reporting. *Risk Analysis*, **16**, 773–783.

McCarroll, J. E., Fullerton, C. S., Ursano, R. J. and Hermsen, J. M. (1996). Posttraumatic stress symptoms following forensic dental identification: Mt. Carmel, Waco, Texas. *American Journal of Psychiatry*, **153**, 778–782.

McCarroll, J. E., Ursano, R. J., Fullerton, C. S., Liu, X. and Lundy, A. (2002). Somatic symptoms in Gulf War mortuary workers. *Psychosomatic Medicine*, **64**, 29–33.

McEwan, B. S. (2001). From molecules to mind: Stress individual differences and the social environment. *Annals of the New York Academy of Science*, **935**, 42–49.

Morbidity and Mortality Weekly Report (2001). Update: Investigation of bioterrorism-related anthrax, Connecticut. *Morbidity and Mortality Weekly Report*, **50**, 1077–1079.

Murakami, H. (2000). *Underground: The Tokyo Gas Attack and the Japanese Psyche*. New York: Random House.

National Institute of Mental Health (2002). *Mental Health and Mass Violence: Evidence-Based Early Psychological Intervention For Victims / Survivors of Mass Violence: A Workshop to Reach Consensus on Best Practices*, NIH Publication No. 02–5138. Washington, DC: US Government Printing Office.

Norris, F. (1992). Epidemiology of trauma: Frequency and impact of different potentially traumatic events on different demographic groups. *Journal of Consulting and Clinical Psychology*, **60**, 409–418.

Norris, F. H. (in press). 50 000 disaster victims speak: An empirical review of the empirical literature, 1981–2001. *Psychiatry*.

North, C. S., Nixon, S. J., Shariat, S., *et al.* (1999). Psychiatric disorders among survivors of the Oklahoma City bombing. *Journal of the American Medical Association*, **282**, 755–762.

North, C. S., Tivis, L., McMillen, J. C., *et al.* (2002). Psychiatric disorders in rescue workers after the Oklahoma City bombing. *American Journal of Psychiatry*, **159**, 857–859.

Okumura, T., Suzuki, K., Fukuda, A., *et al.* (1998). The Tokyo Subway sarin attack: Disaster management. 2: Hospital response. *Academy of Emergency Medicine*, **5**, 618–624.

Peters, R. G., Covello, V. T. and McCallum, D. B. (1997). The determinants of trust and credibility in environmental risk communication: An empirical study. *Risk Analysis*, **17**, 43–54.

Pfefferbaum, B. (1999). Posttraumatic stress responses in bereaved children after the Oklahoma City bombing. *Journal of the American Academy of Child and Adolescent Psychiatry*, **38**, 1372–1379.

Pfefferbaum, B. and Pfefferbaum, R. L. (1998). Contagion in stress: An infectious disease model for posttraumatic stress in children. *Child and Adolescent Psychiatric Clinics of North America*, **7**, 183–194.

Pfefferbaum, B., Nixon, S. J., Tivis, R. D., *et al.* (2001). Television exposure in children after a terrorist incident. *Psychiatry*, **64**, 202–211.

Prigerson, H. G., Shear, M. K., Jacobs, S. C., *et al.* (1999). Consensus criteria for traumatic grief: A preliminary empirical test. *British Journal of Psychiatry*, **174**, 67–73.

Pynoos, R., Frederick, C., Nader, K., *et al.* (1987). Life threat and posttraumatic stress in school-age children. *Archives of General Psychiatry*, **44**, 1057–1063.

Pynoos, R. S. and Nader, K. (1993). Issues in the treatment of posttraumatic stress in children and adolescents. In *International Handbook of Traumatic Stress Syndromes*, eds. J. P. Wilson and B. Raphael, pp. 535–549. New York: Plenum Press.

Raphael, B. (1977). Preventive intervention with the recently bereaved. *Archives of General Psychiatry*, **34**, 1450–1454.

Raphael, B. (2000). Conclusion: Debriefing – science, belief and wisdom. In *Psychological Debriefing: Theory, Practice and Evidence*, eds. B. Raphael and J. P. Wilson, pp. 351–359. New York: Cambridge University Press.

Schlenger, W. E., Caddell, J. M., Ebert, L., *et al.* (2002). Psychological reactions to terrorist attacks. Findings from the national study of Americans' reactions to September 11. *Journal of the American Medical Association*, **288**, 581–588.

Schuster, M. A., Stein, B. D., Jaycox, L. H., *et al.* (2001). A national survey of stress reactions after the September 11, 2001, terrorist attack. *New England Journal of Medicine*, **345**, 1507–1512.

Schwarz, E. D. and Kowalski, J. M. (1991). Malignant memories: PTSD in children and adults after a school shooting. *Journal of the American Academy of Child and Adolescent Psychiatry*, **30**, 936–944.

Shalev, A. Y. (2000). Measuring outcome in posttraumatic stress disorder. *Journal of Clinical Psychiatry*, **61** (Suppl. 5), 33–39.

Shalev, A. Y., Bleich, A. and Ursano, R. J. (1990). Posttraumatic stress disorder: Somatic comorbidity and effort tolerance. *Psychosomatics*, **31**, 197–203.

Shear, M. K., Frank, E., Foa, E., *et al.* (2001). Traumatic grief treatment: A pilot study. *American Journal of Psychiatry*, **158**, 1506–1508.

Shore, J. H., Vollmer, W. M. and Tatum, E. L. (1989). Community patterns of posttraumatic stress disorders. *Journal of Nervous and Mental Disease*, **177**, 681–685.

Silver, R. C., Holman, E. A., McIntosh, D. N., Poulin, M. and Gil-Rivas, V. (2002). Nationwide longitudinal study of psychological responses to September 11. *Journal of the American Medical Association*, **288**, 1235–1244.

Slovic, P. (1987). Perception of risk. *Science*, **236**, 280–285.

Smith, E. M., North, C. S., McCool, R. E. and Shea J. M. (1990). Acute postdisaster psychiatric disorders: Identification of persons at risk. *American Journal of Psychiatry*, **147**, 202–206.

Sorenson, S. B. (2002). Preventing traumatic stress: Public health approaches. *Journal of Traumatic Stress*, **15**, 3–7.

Terr, L. C. (1981). 'Forbidden games': Post-traumatic child's play. *Journal of the American Academy of Child Psychiatry*, **20**, 741–760.

Tucker, P., Pfefferbaum, B., Nixon, S. J. and Dickson, W. (2000). Predictors of post-traumatic stress symptoms in Oklahoma City: Exposure, social support, peri-traumatic responses. *Journal of Behavioral Health Services and Research*, **27**, 406–416.

Ursano, R. J. (1987). Posttraumatic stress disorder: the stressor criterion. *Journal of Nervous and Mental Disease*, **175**, 273–275.

    (2002). Post-traumatic stress disorder. *New England Journal of Medicine*, **34**, 130–131.

Ursano, R. J. and Fullerton, C. S. (2000). Posttraumatic stress disorder: Cerebellar regulation of psychological, interpersonal and biological responses to trauma? *Psychiatry*, **62**, 325–328.

Ursano, R. J., Fullerton, C. S., Kao, T. C. and Bhartiya, V. R. (1995a). Longitudinal assessment of posttraumatic stress disorder and depression after exposure to traumatic death. *Journal of Nervous and Mental Disease*, **183**, 36–42.

Ursano, R. J., Fullerton, C. S. and Norwood, A. E. (1995b). Psychiatric dimensions of disaster: Patient care, community consultation, and preventive medicine. *Harvard Review of Psychiatry*, **3**, 196–209.

Ursano, R. J., Fullerton, C. S., Vance, K. and Kao, T. C. (1999). Posttraumatic stress disorder and identification in disaster workers. *American Journal of Psychiatry*, **156**, 353–359.

Ursano, R. J., Fullerton, C. S., Vance, K. and Wang, L. (2000). Debriefing: Does natural debriefing tell us a story? In *Psychological Debriefing: Theory, Practice and Evidence*, eds. B. Raphael and J. P. Wilson, pp. 32–42. New York: Cambridge University Press.

Ursano, R. J. and McCarroll, J. E. (1990). The nature of a traumatic stressor: Handling dead bodies. *Journal of Nervous and Mental Disease*, **178**, 396–398.

Vlahov, D., Galea, S., Resnick, H., *et al.* (2002). Increased use of cigarettes, alcohol, and marijuana among Manhattan, New York, residents after the September 11 terrorist attacks. *American Journal of Epidemiology*, **155**, 988–996.

Weisaeth, L. (1994). Psychological and psychiatric aspects of technological disasters. In *Individual and Community Responses to Trauma: The Structure of Human Chaos*, eds. R. J. Ursano, B. G. McCaughey and C. S. Fullerton, pp. 72–102. Cambridge: Cambridge University Press.

Wright, K. M. and Bartone, P. T. (1994). Community responses to disaster: The Gander plane crash. In *Individual and Community Responses to Trauma and Disaster: The Structure of Human Chaos*, eds. R. J. Ursano, B. G. McCaughey and C. S. Fullerton, pp. 267–284. Cambridge: Cambridge University Press.

Yehuda, R. (2002). Post-traumatic stress disorder. *New England Journal of Medicine*, **34**, 108–114.

Zatzick, D. F., Kang, S. M., Hinton, L., *et al.* (2001). Posttraumatic concerns: A patient-centered approach to outcome assessment after traumatic physical injury. *Medical Care*, **39**, 327–339.

Part II

Terrorism: National and international

September 11, 2001 and its aftermath, in New York City

John M. Oldham

September 11, 2001 is a day that will be embedded in our memories for the rest of our lives. I will describe some observations from my vantage point, recognizing that every New Yorker has his or her own very personal and powerful experience to tell.

At 8.00 a.m. on September 11, several of us convened for a regular meeting at the New York State Psychiatric Institute of the Executive Committee of the Columbia/Cornell Behavioral Health Service Line. Not long after the meeting got under way, we were interrupted to be told that the World Trade Center was 'being bombed.' We rushed to my office, from which there is a direct view to the south, down the Hudson River, and saw with horror the black billows of smoke pouring out of the World Trade Center. Disbelief, denial, shock, and outrage were among our emotions, as we watched the subsequent cascade of events, followed by grief, fear, and devastation as the extent of the disaster became clear.

In spite of the prior assault on the World Trade Center, the Oklahoma bombing disaster, the attack on the USS *Cole*, and the destruction of the American embassies in Kenya and Tanzania, there was no emotional or psychological preparation for this event. Ordinary minds had rejected the reality of those historical warnings, and the possibility of a 'clear and present danger' had, until September 11, seemed the stuff of fiction. But a new, brutal reality has been unavoidable ever since. Relentless media coverage hypnotized the nation with images of the collapsing towers, of individuals leaping to their deaths, of terrified survivors running for their lives, and of exhausted rescue workers, firemen, and policemen, working overtime at Ground Zero.

Once over the initial shock, the psychiatric community throughout the city mobilized with an outpouring of volunteers to help. At Columbia Presbyterian Medical Center, we immediately had an emergency meeting of the hospital leadership, with the expectation that there would be large numbers of physically wounded patients who would be brought our way once the Lower Manhattan medical facilities became saturated.

Table 2.1 Initial events

Disbelief
Lack of ambulance transport
Lack of wounded
Management of volunteers
Traffic

In the Psychiatric Emergency Room, prior to the attack, we already had 20 patients awaiting admission, since the autumn had been a busy time in New York, particularly in psychiatry. Ambulance transport was totally unavailable throughout the city, since all ambulances were deployed to the disaster site. Using state vans, we transported some of these patients to our satellite hospital in Northern Manhattan, and some to the New York Psychiatric Institute, to clear out the Psychiatric Emergency Room. It soon became apparent, however, that these arrangements had been unnecessary since the number of wounded survivors was far exceeded by the number who perished. We prepared information outlining common emotional reactions to a massive disaster, and this was widely distributed throughout the medical center, with four fully staffed information centers created where additional written materials were made available. A 24-hour hotline was organized to handle calls of any nature relating to the disaster, and a special station was established near the Emergency Room, where professional staff were posted to provide in-person assistance (Table 2.1). Volunteers abounded, with a generosity of spirit and concern that was remarkable.

On September 13, we held a 'Town Meeting' for all employees in the Department of Psychiatry and the New York Psychiatric Institute, and every seat was taken, with people sitting on the floor and standing in the aisles. Brief remarks were presented by experts in disaster psychiatry, and an open and active discussion helped us all think about what to expect, how to help each other, and how to identify and help those at risk for more extreme stress reactions. Training sessions were subsequently organized by professionals experienced in dealing with trauma; these sessions focused on what disaster experts have learned about appropriate help shortly after a disaster, and appropriate identification of long-term treatment needs and methods. In addition, outreach training was developed, to participate in the city-wide and state-wide ongoing disaster response (Table 2.2). Calls for help came from many quarters and took many forms. Individual counseling was provided by psychiatrists responding to needs identified by the New York State Office of Mental Health, by the New York County District Branch of the American Psychiatric Association, and by many other groups. Requests ranged from needs for counselors for companies whose offices had been in the World Trade Center, to

Table 2.2 Interventions

Information
Hotline
Outreach station
Town meetings
Training sessions

Table 2.3 Initial emotional responses

Anxiety over subways, bridges, tall buildings
Fear
Courage
Bravery
Strength
Grief
Resiliency
Decreased stigma

advice for physically unharmed but emotionally traumatized occupants of buildings near the site.

Our hospital held an emergency meeting of its medical board every day at 7.00 a.m., but attendance was difficult since travel to and from the city was extremely complicated. On September 11, all subways were closed, and all bridges and tunnels surrounding Manhattan were closed in both directions. Medical personnel worked double or triple shifts, to care for the regularly hospitalized patients. Bridges were initially reopened only outbound from the city, and employees living in the suburbs, anxious to reach home for family care responsibilities, were not sure they could get back the next day.

These concerns seem quite secondary to the devastation at Ground Zero and the tragic loss of so many lives, but they illustrate some of the many hidden and derivative aspects of this disaster. Police blockades and checkpoints were established all over the city, which remained in place for weeks. Traffic was snarled, and anxiety levels were quite high. Fear spread to include concerns about taking the subways, crossing any of the bridges or tunnels, or going up in tall buildings, fueled by the media and by predictions of a 'second wave' of attacks. As time elapsed, that initial state of intense fear was replaced with grief in response to the devastation itself, and to the magnitude of the disaster (Table 2.3).

I had an occasion to join several state and federal officials for a police-escorted, hard-hat walk around and into parts of the smoldering ruins at the Ground Zero site, and nothing in the media coverage adequately conveyed the impact of the magnitude of the destruction. Underground fires raged for, it turned out, months, and round-the-clock efforts to clear the wreckage site seemed to move at a snail's pace, given the size of the job. It was estimated that after the towers collapsed, the distance between the steel floors was about the width of one's finger. The psychological and emotional impact of merely viewing the scene in person was powerful, much less working on site as a fireman, policeman, or rescue worker. In addition, it came as a shock to realize that lower Manhattan had been transformed into a war zone. Military personnel in fatigues were everywhere, along with tight security, barriers, and police checkpoints.

Other than Ground Zero itself, perhaps the most overwhelming experience for those of us who did not directly suffer personal losses in the disaster was to pay a visit to the Family Center, originally located at the Lexington Avenue Armory and then moved to Pier 94. No one could walk down the seemingly endless wall of photographs of those lost, reading the handwritten personal messages from survivors to their lost loved ones, without a wrenching appreciation of the reality of their pain and suffering.

Consultation to government and business

In spite of, and in the face of, the enormous stress resulting from the events of September 11 and the ensuing war and bioterrorism, the strength and resilience of the citizens of New York were impressive. For a considerable period of time, the usual stigma that surrounds emotional or mental problems seemed to melt away. People at all levels sought help (Table 2.4). I was asked by the Commissioner of Mental Health to speak to a senior state banking official, since the headquarter offices of the New York State Banking Department were in a building adjacent to the Twin Towers. In the disaster, although they fortunately did not lose anyone, all 600 employees were evacuated and were on the street when one of the towers collapsed. They were covered with ash, ran for their lives, and all of them thought they were going to die. The banking official sought help because after only a few weeks they were now being told that their building was structurally sound and they were required to move back in, with a whole wall of windows facing the disaster site of tangled, smoking steel. We decided to arrange a meeting of the managers and supervisors of the banking department at the Psychiatric Institute. About 20 senior managers came, and Randall Marshall, one of our trauma experts, and I spent several hours with them. Mostly we gave them some facts, reviewing what were normal reactions in an abnormal situation, in a sense giving them permission to feel the way they were feeling. The group clearly had already bonded together subsequent to the tragedy, and they came up with a whole set of creative ideas of their own that turned out to be quite helpful. Again, this illustrated how unusual these times

Table 2.4 Consultation to business

Precipitated by loss or return to work
Information mastery
Facilitate creative solutions
Explain behavioral and emotional responses

were. Ordinarily, I believe that bank managers would not hug each other warmly and seek emotional support from each other, as they did, not to mention their unhesitating willingness to attend a meeting at a psychiatric facility. Several weeks later, I received information that the banking department's previously arranged two-day symposium would be held as scheduled, for about 800 people, at One Chase Plaza, just adjacent to Ground Zero, and that the employees had successfully moved back in to their building, illustrating the strength and determination of the citizens of New York.

Life in the city in those days constantly seemed to reflect extremes – from remarkable courage, bravery, and strength, to overwhelming stress and devastation. I was at a meeting with a group of lawyers, and one of the speakers was a very senior judge empowered to issue death certificates for the lost World Trade Center victims, and the burden of this responsibility was enormous. The judge reported that he had issued about 1500 death certificates so far, and one thing that surprised him was how few families had applied, compared to the total number of deaths, since this step was necessary for families to obtain death benefits. I pointed out to the judge that a common coping mechanism during times of severe stress is avoidance of situations that reactivate or intensify the stress, which was sure to be part of the reason. Also, when death occurs in most circumstances, families have to identify and claim the body and arrange a funeral, whether they want to or not. In this situation, in contrast, most victims were not recovered, so many families clung to a protracted hope that their relative might still be in a coma, in a hospital somewhere. Or, family member could just say, 'I can't deal with it yet.'

The judge mentioned another illustration of the complicated nature of his task, referring to one woman who came to see him to obtain death certificates for her three siblings (a brother and two sisters), all three of whom were killed. The brother was a freelance employee who happened to be working in the World Trade Center that day. One sister was self-employed, and the second sister was unemployed. The judge described that his impulse was just to sign them all, but he could not because he had been warned that there would be opportunists coming along, taking advantage of the situation to try to collect benefits that were not rightfully theirs. If he did not approve these requests until further checking was done (and it was not clear how that was going to be done), he might further traumatize this woman who seemed truly to be suffering from the loss of her three siblings. The wisdom and courage of this dedicated judge were striking. And, incidentally, several weeks later the local news reported that this woman claiming to have lost three siblings had been identified as a known con artist, and she had been arrested.

About two weeks after September 11, I received a phone call from a senior executive of one of the companies that had lost about 400 employees in the disaster, out of the 1900 employees in the company who worked in the Twin Towers. The company official described the overwhelming set of challenges they were dealing with, from massive grief of families and colleagues, to the logistical nightmare of relocating and supporting all 1500 employees who survived, either because they had not yet arrived for work on September 11, or because they had been successfully evacuated. The company had other offices in midtown and had been offered access to Radio City Music Hall for a memorial service on the following Tuesday, which they were considering, anticipating that they could have as many as 5000 people attending. But the company official wanted advice about the timing of the event, concerned that it might be too soon. One of the things that struck me about this call was how hard it was for all of us to make decisions and know what to do. This man was a world-class executive who, throughout his entire career, had made nothing but hard decisions, but nothing had prepared him for these circumstances. I advised him that I knew of no blueprint for this situation, so that there really were no right or wrong decisions. I shared with him my feeling at the time, that there is a difference between coping and remembering, and I felt it was too soon to be remembering. The executive was immediately relieved, because he had sensed that this might be the case, yet he had felt quite bewildered about how to proceed. He just needed an objective outside person to help put things in perspective.

These are but a few of the enormous numbers of anecdotes that we have all heard about individual experiences in the disaster, from catastrophic loss to acts of phenomenal heroism, and each of those stories is important. But let me focus on just three other areas: information dissemination and the role of the media, the challenge to coordinate the many bureaucratic systems involved in the relief effort, and the need for research and data collection.

Challenges

One of the challenges in the first few weeks after September 11 was how to determine what amount of information we needed to be told or how much we could tolerate. It was tempting to start referring to the disaster as a historical event that, however horrible, was over with and our task was to recover from it. Yet we had to face the fact that we could not resume 'business as usual'; rather, our world had changed, and our new reality needed to include the possibility of future attacks. Federal spokespersons repeatedly announced that 'credible evidence' existed indicating that other attacks might occur. In addition, in Washington and New York, reports of anthrax infection were emerging. It was important that the public be given good information, yet good information might not have been immediately available. So that when anthrax deaths began to occur, after federal officials categorized early cases as isolated and treatable, widespread mistrust of public pronouncements began to develop, with a widely heard belief that the government was withholding essential information. Yet how much information is the right amount?

One characteristic of our times is the universality of telecommunications, so that the instant nation-wide 'real-time' coverage of this disaster was unprecedented. Everyone remembers the miniaturized window in the upper right corner of all syndicated news channels, replaying over and over again the destruction of the towers. There was a hypnotic quality about those scenes, so that many of us advised our patients just to turn off the television deliberately for blocks of time. Eventually, public service announcements provided some balance, such as the one that said 'There has been one death from anthrax, and there were 20 000 deaths last year from the flu.' Part of the challenge that all of us have is to achieve, in any disaster, an appropriate 'managed message,' getting good, accurate, essential information out without overdosing ourselves with too much, or misleading each other with too little, or wrong, information.

Second, it is important to coordinate the multiple federal, state, and local health care and social service agencies that are crucially involved in any disaster of this magnitude. What we quickly learned was that there was no shortage of responders and volunteers seeking to help. As an example, I received an email at 4.00 p.m. on a Friday afternoon asking for volunteers in three categories (clinical, administrative, and clerical) to staff 24-hour shifts at an office of the State Emergency Management Organization being set up at Pier 90 in New York City. Within an hour after communicating this request, we had more volunteers in all categories than there was need for. Similar experiences were reported throughout the city. A small organized group of psychiatrists interested in the mental health aspects of disaster management and response assumed the task of obtaining and scheduling psychiatrists to be on site 24 hours a day at the Pier 94 Family Center, and the outpouring of volunteer time from the professionals for this emotionally draining duty was phenomenal.

At the same time, there can be confusion and miscommunication. For example, there was a widespread belief that the federal relief money applied for by the state mental health agency could only be used to train 'paraprofessionals' for crisis intervention. In fact, the funding was specified for the provision of outreach crisis intervention, but individuals eligible to receive training and to provide these outreach services could be either members of paraprofessional groups (e.g., clergy, teachers) or mental health professionals themselves. Another source of confusion arose when considering appropriate early response, generally consisting of grief counseling and crisis intervention, compared to later-stage identification of those with protracted stress reactions that might constitute psychiatric diagnoses such as posttraumatic stress disorder (PTSD) or major depressive disorder, who should be referred to mental health professionals for definitive treatment. Resources made available by the Federal Emergency Management Administration could be used for training in and provision of needs assessment and referral, in addition to ongoing outreach crisis intervention, but not to fund the direct provision of medical treatment for diagnosed psychiatric disorders. Repeatedly, these distinctions were unclear to people. Furthermore, in spite of estimates based on past disasters that significant percentages of survivors of the World Trade Center disaster would be at high risk to develop PTSD or other conditions, it was not clear who would provide the needed treatment to these individuals. Would the existing mental health professional community absorb the increased 'practice burden'? In addition, would professionals be deployed to New York from elsewhere in the country for this purpose, and if so, would other federal monies be available to support this temporary workforce? What about state licensing rules, hospital privileges, and the wide range of usual requirements for such professionals?

And finally, it is critical that systematic and reliable data be recorded that help us know what happened, what helped, and what did not help. Merely the use of the word 'research' in the context of trauma and disaster can raise legitimate concerns. Certainly, what is not helpful is a thoughtless process where a highly traumatized survivor of a disaster receives dozens of different telephone and mail surveys from all over the country, asking the same questions. Yet we need to learn as much as possible from every disaster, by careful documentation of individual experiences. New treatments have been developed for conditions like PTSD that promise good results and help people truly recover from massively stressful events, helping prevent patterns we have seen in the past, such as the emergence of large numbers of patients with chronic and refractory conditions.

The New York after September 11, 2001 will never be the same as the New York before September 11, 2001. The toll taken by this massive disaster, produced by malevolent human intent, has been enormous. But in many ways, the current New York is tougher and stronger than ever.

3

Leadership in the wake of disaster

Prudence Bushnell

On September 11, 2001, I was among the millions of people who watched in horror as our world changed with the impact of a terrorist massacre. Like many other Americans, I wept in sympathy for the victims and survivors, and I watched with admiration New York Mayor Giuliani's acts of leadership. I also found myself thrown back in time into the painful maelstrom of August 7, 1998 when, as US Ambassador to the Republic of Kenya, I too felt the effects of Osama bin Laden's hatred of Americans. The journey that confronts the survivors of September 11 and the challenges to their leaders are familiar to some Americans, including those in Oklahoma City and within our foreign-affairs community. The lessons I learned as a leader of a community that traveled from the rubble toward recovery are the subject of this article.

Mayor Giuliani may have acted more out of instinct than design in the aftermath of the bombings of the Twin Towers but the leadership qualities he demonstrated, including visibility, caring, and empathy, are critical elements to helping people cope. In a world where disasters, from airplane accidents to terrorist attacks, are increasingly part of our reality, understanding how ordinary people react to extraordinary events becomes more important to effective leadership. Information and experience that once belonged to mental health and disaster professionals need to enter mainstream management and leadership practice. What my colleagues, friends, and I learned as we muddled through the aftermath of the attack on our embassy will, I hope, be useful.

The bombing: Planned, unanticipated, and devastating

My story begins at the US Embassy in Nairobi, Kenya, on August 7, 1998. For two years, I had been Chief of Mission of an embassy that, like all others around the world, was an amalgam of different US government agencies. In our case, the activities ranged from supporting other embassies in Africa to helping Kenyans deepen their culture of democracy, enhance economic potential, provide humanitarian assistance, eradicate diseases like HIV/AIDS and malaria, and conserve a wonderful biodiversity. Nairobi was the second-largest post in sub-Saharan Africa with more than 700 employees, most of them Kenyan, working out of our embassy downtown and in other buildings around the city. Like most US ambassadors, I was concerned about the possibility of a terrorist attack. Our building, like more than 80 percent of US embassies, did not meet recommended security standards. I was not prepared, however, to be blown up.

Friday, August 7 was an ordinary day. People were working, cashing checks for the weekend, visiting the medical unit, or coming to shop at the commissary. One office was offering cake to celebrate all the birthdays that week. Only my absence from the weekly senior staff meeting was unusual. I was in the high-rise office building next door, meeting with the Kenyan Minister of Commerce to discuss an upcoming trade delegation. On the busy street corner outside the embassy building, Kenyans were also going about their business.

At 10.37 a.m., a truck entered the parking area at the rear of the embassy, which was sandwiched between a seven-story office building and the high-rise where I was in my meeting. The two occupants of the truck tried to gain entry to our basement parking lot. When our Kenyan security guard refused them, a man got out of the vehicle to argue, then threw what we later learned was a stun grenade. The noise brought people from blocks around to their windows – an instinctive reaction that would prove fatal for many.

Seconds later, the driver of the truck detonated the bomb. The blast left a crater 10 feet deep and 40 feet wide and registered at more than 4.0 on the Richter scale. The explosion ripped the back wall off the Embassy, pancaked the seven-story office building, and destroyed much of the interior of the building where I was meeting with the Commerce Minister. More than 5000 people were injured, mostly from flying glass hitting them in the face and chest, and 213 lay dead. Inside the embassy, the blast instantly killed 46 of the 120 occupants; it injured and trapped many more.

Within minutes, the normal Friday morning turned to chaos. Thousands of people rushed to our street corner, mixing with dazed and bleeding survivors, to help the injured and begin digging for people through the rubble of what was once a seven-story building. Inside the embassy, survivors grabbed wounded colleagues and struggled out of the building to regroup on the steps outside. There was no 911 to call, so our people organized themselves. Marine Guards and other security personnel set up a protective cordon outside. Volunteers, including young summer interns, re-entered what was now a death trap to rescue those who remained. Our doctor and three nurses set up triage on the sidewalk, commandeering private vehicles to get the badly injured to the hospital. An office manager began recording which of our casualties were being sent to what hospital, while another raced to the Agency for International Development building across town in order to contact Washington and set up a crisis control center.

In the building a few yards away, I was oblivious to what was happening outside. Initially knocked out by the bomb blast, I started down the 21 endless flights of rubble-strewn stairs with one of my Commerce Department colleagues and hundreds of other injured and bloodied people. It was only when we reached the street 45 minutes later and saw the carnage and the burning hulk of what was once our embassy that I realized what had happened. We were almost immediately spotted and pushed into a car that sped to a nearby hotel where we could receive medical help. As we were examined, I listened to the desperate conversations of my colleagues on the embassy radio net. Kenyan resources were clearly overwhelmed. We were on our own.

The response: Chaotic, courageous, and united

A few hours later I convoked the senior staff, who had miraculously survived the blast, to organize our 'to do' list. It was both compelling and endless: locate supplies, rescue people, dig through rubble for survivors, contact Washington, tend the wounded, find the missing, secure the embassy, assist the Kenyans, inform the community, see to the media, organize and anticipate future needs . . . and on and on and on.

No task was too heroic or too mundane and, ignoring pre-established job descriptions, we tackled each and every one with adrenaline-charged energy and accomplished amazing things. By the time I got home that night, we were into the second shift of our 24-hour operations center and our colleagues in Washington, seven hours behind Nairobi time, were frantically expediting search and rescue teams and supplies. Organized groups of Kenyans and Americans fanned out to morgues, hospitals, and homes to locate and identify colleagues. Other members of the community sought out families of those who had not been spared. Our most severely injured were getting necessary attention, and a medical evacuation aircraft was on its way. Downtown, the rescue efforts went on. News of a similar attack on our embassy in Tanzania left no doubt that this was an act of terrorism.

Our Chargé d'Affaires in Tanzania was John Lange. He later wrote about the performance of his multi-talented staff and underscored the fact that everyone mattered and everyone contributed. Never mind what the job descriptions said, people demonstrated their worth time and again by what they did, not what positions they may have held. I found the same to be true in Nairobi.

Our large and experienced staff needed only minimal direction to put their skills to work in the those first hours. Doing so – doing something, doing anything – provided a necessary comfort from feelings of helplessness and despair. As we became increasingly well organized, we even assumed a mask of normalcy. This had a thin veneer, however. Behind our bursts of energy and devotion to multiple tasks, visible and invisible wounds festered as the extent of our losses sank in.

The rescue: necessary, helpful, and resented

Over the next two days, hundreds of people arrived from the United States and other countries to help, including a plane full of FBI agents. Logistical support, like transport and lodging requirements, compounded our 'to do' list. 'Who's in charge?' and 'Who does what?' surfaced among the many issues arising from the influx of so many people. In those long hours after the bombing, the victims-turned-rescuers had become a tight, protective, and insular community. As utterly exhausted as we were, we would not relinquish control of what we thought of as 'our' tragedy. Former colleagues who had transferred from the embassy to new assignments only weeks earlier returned to help and found themselves treated as outsiders. A phenomenon of 'We-who-had-endured-the-unthinkable' and 'They-who-could-not-understand' emerged as a part of our culture. I was no more immune from this than others; this was still my embassy and I was determined to maintain a leadership role.

Even as we recognized the need for help, we resented its intrusion. We cast our rescuers into a supporting role, which thankfully, they assumed with grace. I know we were not an easy group to assist and, although with hindsight I regret that, I do not know how we could have behaved differently. As damaged as we were, the need to get back on our feet and take care of our own was insurmountable.

The lingering effects: Sorrow, anger, and fear

Within 48 hours of the attack, we held our first memorial service at my residence. Solemnly and gently we talked about our 12 fallen American colleagues as the vital, three-dimensional friends they were. Then we said goodbye to them and their families who accompanied the coffins home the next day. A few days later, we similarly honored our 32 Kenyan colleagues killed in the attack. These were just the first in a series of funerals and memorials held around the country over the next month. The rituals were important, not just to honor and show respect but also to begin resurrecting a community from the remains of what had been blown apart. No matter what relationships had existed with former colleagues, each death created a void that left us incomplete. Coming together again, even in mourning, was an essential step in re-creating ourselves.

For a long time we were a community of walking wounded, even if the scars were not always apparent. While many were physically injured, all of us had faced trauma. No matter how close or how far we had been from 'ground zero,' no one was unaffected. Within a week we put the entire embassy staff through psychological debriefing. The sessions helped, though they were by no means a cure. Ironically, few of us chose to take advantage of the option the State Department offered to be transferred out of Nairobi. Even most of those who had been medically evacuated returned, some with shards of glass still in them. People's motivations differed, but I think that instinctively many of us felt that remaining and rebuilding together would somehow help us heal. If we were handicapped as individuals, we could at least lean on one another as a community to trudge up the steep slope to normalcy that lay ahead.

In a few weeks, the rescue workers left, the Washington crisis task force disbanded, the press moved on, and we were working cheek to jowl in the poorly constructed Agency for International Development building surrounded by barbed wire, sandbags, sniffer dogs, and dozens of newly-assigned Marines in combat gear. Reminders of failure surrounded us. Phones and faxes did not work; computers, equipment, and files were missing; everything took forever to come together. We dearly missed former colleagues, and even though we greatly appreciated the people who joined us from different parts of the world, it was still difficult to integrate them into the community of bomb victims and survivors.

Our frustration mounted as, overwhelmed with real and emotional problems, we lacked a single point of contact with Washington colleagues, who were now dealing with other world crises. My own efforts to gain attention to our practical and emotional needs were clumsy, my effectiveness hampered by the diminished performance that scarred all of us. Later I read Colin Powell's observation that a leader should not be afraid to piss people off; unintentionally, I was already taking his advice.

Having initially acted with courage and solidarity, the bomb's victims moved into another phase. Anger permeated the culture, inside the embassy and out. According to estimates, Kenya lost 5 to 10 percent of its GDP as a result of the bombing. One hundred buildings and 250 businesses were wholly or partially damaged. Of the 5000 wounded, 400 people would remain severely disabled. Many Kenyans felt, understandably, that had it not been for the American presence, such death and destruction would not have assaulted their capital. Public and private criticism of our reactions in the hours after the blast rained on us. The security cordon we had set up immediately after the explosion was seen as an act of hostility, and our focus on saving people in the embassy as a sign of indifference to Kenyan needs. My effort to explain some of our actions by noting the presence of looters in our building enraged Kenyans even further. Some truths, I learned painfully, are best not told.

The Kenyans' display of anger and hatred hurt and frustrated us. All of a sudden, 'we' who were victims became 'they,' responsible for unspeakable damage to thousands of innocent people. Shoring up the frayed friendship the terrorists had sought to destroy took time and conscious effort. If our point of view was to be heard, we had to listen first. Outreach to the Kenyan community became even more important when subsequent FBI investigations led to terrorist networks buried in a marginalized, increasingly embittered, and utterly innocent Muslim community.

A lingering sense of vulnerability added fear to other emotions. A bomb threat a few weeks after the attack reignited the terror that had already left an imprint on many of us. Later, when an alert to all US embassies of possible terrorist attacks around Christmas forced us to close down and cancel holiday activities, I wondered whether my team and I would have the strength to cope.

We had held no stage-managed discussions of our feelings after the initial debriefing sessions. Instead, they emerged with unexpected bursts in otherwise normal discussions. A lot of problem-solving had to be done and many of us talked again and again about 'the event' – where we were, what we did, what we saw, what we said – as if oral reviews would somehow make sense of it. Distracting as it may have been to outsiders, it was both essential and irresistible to us. We understood each other's intensity of feelings and we never lost interest in the stories.

The progress: Uneven, inconsistent, and celebrated

Slowly, slowly, we moved forward, marking the milestones. We celebrated the purchase of a building we would later occupy as our temporary headquarters by saluting the American flag raised over the base that had stood in front of our old embassy. We welcomed 1999 with the traditional 'sun downer' at Nairobi game park. As 'Auld lang syne' played in the background, we shared hugs, tears, and a spectacular sunset. We had survived; we were a community. In the garden of the Ambassador's residence we inaugurated a memorial fountain, the lip of which held the names of our friends and colleagues who had perished in the embassy. We were joined in the ceremony by the family members of those who had died. I was frankly – and sadly – slow to recognize how the relatives of American victims, in particular, needed a reconnecting point as much as we. Some of them had been torn from the community and their way of life within 72 hours of the bombing. The change that had been imposed on their lives was far greater than what we faced.

When, in early 1999, we finally received a Congressionally mandated assistance package of $37 million we were at last able to tend to the needs of the many Kenyans physically and economically injured by the bomb. In the embassy, we hired and trained people to replace those we had lost and continued to address the untold complications of tending to the welfare of permanently disabled employees and survivors. Eventually, the Department of State created an Office of Casualty Affairs to assist; its work goes on to this day.

As we climbed that hill toward normalcy, I was constantly struck by the multitude of ways that members of the community were coping. We, Kenyans and Americans, were all over the place. Some were moving on, others still needed to mourn; some continued to talk about the bombing, others were silent. There were those who buried themselves in work and others who were establishing new priorities. One group followed what they facetiously called the 'RAD' method of survival – repression, alcohol, and denial. A few people took advantage of counseling, but most did not. Anything that smacked of mental health assistance offended many – Kenyans and Americans. We did not like being considered 'sick,' and we shunned labels as vigorously as we rebelled against the thought of references to counseling ending up in our personnel files.

How people responded over time had nothing to do with gender, race, culture, or proximity to the blast. I learned that ordinary reactions to extraordinary disasters, like a terrorist event, fill a very wide spectrum and no amount of wishful thinking will change the pace or substance of the reaction. Our challenge was to listen and understand behavioral cues, and the only way to do that was to reach out. Our medical staff, once they saw that people would not be coaxed into coming to them, took to office corridors to reach people where they worked. Later, a regional psychiatrist was assigned to the embassy to help people who are still piecing together body and soul.

The surprises: Unanticipated results, little closure

One component over which I did have control was the resurrection of our management systems. Work priorities were redirected; goals, however limited, reestablished; newcomers welcomed and integrated. The structures were familiar and comforting. Returning to 'business as usual' represented a triumph, but doing so sometimes had unexpected consequences.

Preparing awards for the traditional biannual ceremony should have been easy; after all, we had plenty of outstanding performances to recognize. As we began writing the justifications, however, Pandora's box opened. What type of award was most suitable for whom? How could we pat ourselves on the back for acts that stemmed from terrible tragedy? How could one action, injury, or sacrifice be compared to another? Enormous controversy ensued and raw feelings emerged as people disagreed over who would be recognized and why. Rather than bringing us together, the process was dividing us. We finally decided to establish arbitrary, defensible criteria to the selections, to forego any remuneration, and to focus the award ceremony on a dedication of the memorial fountain at my residence.

Integrating newcomers was another practice with which we had lots of experience. Embassies are accustomed to the steady arrivals and departures of American personnel in particular. We knew we needed to make a special effort to incorporate new staff into the community and were mindful to provide information about the unusual circumstances they would find. New Kenyan employees were welcomed, and incoming Americans were briefed both before and after arriving in Nairobi. There has been varied success in generating greater understanding and our Kenyan colleagues are now concerned about what will happen once the last of the Americans who experienced the bombing leaves. Who would be there to appreciate the enormity of the trauma that is still affecting a number of people?

Some of the Americans who left Nairobi during the normal rotation cycle to fill jobs in other posts also encountered difficulty. Were they being treated as 'damaged goods' or did they just feel like 'damaged goods?' The stiff upper lip culture of the foreign-affairs community does not encourage special treatment, and most of us would have rejected it had it been offered. Some cases merited special attention and almost inevitably, some mismatches were made, imposing additional strains.

Even the Department of State, long accustomed to dealing with civil wars, natural and human-made disasters, personnel evacuations, and the like, had much to learn about taking care of the survivors of terrorism. Changes have emerged from the lessons – guidance on how to help children deal with trauma, for example – others still need to be made.

Ten months after the bombing, my husband and I left Kenya to prepare for our assignment in Guatemala. The effects of the journey from victim to survivor are still unfolding, some of them positive, some not. Subsequent anniversaries, commemorative events, and contact with other survivors and family members have softened hard-edged grief. I was surprised by the comfort I found in returning to Nairobi last August to participate in the commemoration of a memorial park on the site of the old embassy. Instead of the raw pain I expected when I looked at the names of all those who died, inscribed on the wall in the center of the park, I experienced a far more gentle sadness. But intense anger resurfaced when I faced the perpetrators of the attack last winter as they stood trial for mass murder. The defendant who had thrown a stun grenade to lure people to the windows in order to suffer the greatest impact of the bomb repulsed me by his disinterest as he picked his teeth during my testimony. Watching Osama bin Laden's people strike again on September 11 brought much of the past into the present. As people in Oklahoma City have noted, there is no closure. There is, however, a possibility to move on as time helps knit memories and after-effects into one's life. What helps me to move on is to reflect and communicate what I have learned.

It is important to me that others who have had their lives shattered by terrorism (or other disasters) not have to muddle through for months in the same way we did. While we have yet to discover 'best practices' in helping people in the workplace overcome trauma, some lessons have already been learned.

Table 3.1 Leadership following catastrophe

Conceptualize as a process, not an event
Recreate normalcy, even if an illusion
Tolerate diminished results
Redirect priorities
Set and celebrate achievable goals
Use rituals
Resurrect community
Avoid 'we' and 'they' phenomenon
Reach out
Pay attention to behavioral cues
Listen
Model tone and behaviors
Take care of yourself

The lesson: learn how to take care of your people

As a leader of my community, I discovered what mental health and disaster professionals have already learned about people's behavior following a traumatic event.
Yes, as Diane Myers notes in her chapter in *Disaster Response and Recovery: A
Handbook for Mental Health Professionals*, everyone is touched by disaster, even if
the experience is not a direct one. And, yes, each individual does react differently
and many of us will not seek assistance to help resolve psychological effects. But
what does this mean for managers or leaders charged with getting results? It means
that unless you understand what your people are experiencing and assist them
appropriately, you are not going to get the results you seek.

Taking care of our people in Nairobi taught me the following:
- Remember you are dealing with a process, not an event;
- Recreate normalcy, even if an illusion, and tolerate diminished results;
- Redirect priorities, set and celebrate achievable goals, however small;
- Use rituals to allow individuals a chance to heal within the embrace of community;
- Resurrect community, carefully integrating those who replace absent colleagues
  and tending to the families of those who were lost;
- Beware the 'we' and 'they' phenomenon and try not to get sucked in;
- Pay attention to behavioral cues and reach out;
- Hold yourself to the tone and behaviors you seek in others;
- Listen, if you want to be heard;
- Take care of yourself, if you want to take care of your people.

Disasters and terrorism strike the innocent who do not deserve what has happened or the pain that ensues. Neither do they deserve to have their difficulties

compounded by organizations, practices, or leaders who do not know what to do. Preventing the unthinkable is our first order of business, and many people are now engaged in doing just that. Dealing with the unthinkable, should it happen, is our second responsibility and most of us in mainstream leadership functions have much to learn. The lessons are out there, gained through difficult journeys. If we can seize and build on those lessons, we give worth to the experience of those who have gone before and assist those who come after. Mayor Giuliani's leadership on September 11 provides some clues about what works. Let's use them.

4

Children of war and children at war: Child victims of terrorism in Mozambique

Jon A. Shaw and Jesse J. Harris

On the southeastern rim of Africa, northeast of South Africa, east of Zimbabwe, and bordered by the Indian Ocean lies the 'shattered land' of Mozambique. Mozambique has suffered the consequences of war, famine, and drought. Of the approximate 14.6 million inhabitants, it is estimated that 6.5 million require international food aid, with 3.2 million dependent on free emergency food. Robert Gersony, in his 1988 report to the Department of State, noted that approximately 2 million refugees have fled their homes. The Mozambique Red Cross estimates that the majority of these refugees are children. Fifty percent of the population is reported to be under 15 years of age (Uqueio, personal communication).

There is increasing awareness and sensitivity to the plight of 'children in a warring world.' In the last few decades there has been a significant change in the nature and intensity of war. Armed conflicts around the world have been increasingly characterized by low intensity and episodic conflict, the employment of guerrilla armies, and the victimization of the civilian population. Dyregrov *et al.* (1987) have suggested that 80–90 percent of all casualties in the current spectrum of armed conflicts are civilians.

In his monograph *Children of War*, Rosenblatt (1983) states that:

there are places in the world like Northern Ireland, Israel, Lebanon, Cambodia, and Vietnam that have been at war for the past twenty years or more...the children living in these places have known nothing but war in their experiences. The elements of war, explosions, destructions, dismemberments, eruptions, noises, fire, death, separation, torture, grief, which ought to be extraordinary and temporary for any life are for these children normal and constant.

Certainly, this is true of children living in Mozambique.

The war in Mozambique has raged since 1976, when the Mozambique National Resistance (RENAMO) was formed, initially at the behest of the Rhodesian Intelligence Agency and subsequently supported by the South Africa's Department of Military Intelligence. RENAMO has made little effort to win the hearts of the people or even to hold territory and is predominantly motivated to destabilize the government of Mozambique. By 1985, Isaacman, a professor of African history, estimated that 1800 schools and 25 percent of the health clinics were destroyed and that approximately 325 000 children had died as a result of the war (Isaacman, 1987). RENAMO has successfully waged a guerrilla war by attacking railroads, roads, and electricity lines. They initiated hit and run attacks on villages seizing arms, ammunition, uniforms, medicine, and, more recently, children. Children have been captured, used as porters, coerced into military training, and forced to participate in guerrilla attacks on other villages. Currently, RENAMO controls virtually 80 percent of the country with the exception of major cities and province capitals.

On December 31, 1987, the US Ambassador declared that a 'disaster' existed in Mozambique and that the country was eligible for aid from the Office of Disaster Assistance. The ambassador requested, on behalf of the government of Mozambique, that the US Office of Foreign Disaster Assistance send a child psychiatrist and a social worker to Mozambique with the intent of providing evaluation and consultation to approximately 50 village children. The children were 6–16 years of age, had been kidnapped by the guerrilla forces (RENAMO), forced into military training, and coerced into participating in military activities against their own villages and government forces. A number of these children were recaptured by government forces. Some of the children spent as long as four years with the guerrillas. The government was concerned about their capacity for rehabilitation and expressed fears that a whole generation of children would be lost to the guerrilla forces.

Trauma in children has been defined as 'any condition which seems definitely unfavorable, noxious, or drastically injurious to their development' (Greenacre, 1952). The exposure to war with its multiple adversities is a significant interference with the child's development. Yet the cognitive immaturity, plasticity, and adaptive capacities of the child have often veiled the effects of war in a certain obscurity. There is a conflicting and controversial literature debating the existence, frequency, and configuration of psychiatric morbidity in children exposed to war.

It is surprising how often children and adolescents are reported to adapt to the conditions of war with little evidence of manifest distress. Freud and Burlingham (1943) noted that children over two years of age who had witnessed air raids over England in World War II were able to distinguish between falling bombs and anti-aircraft weaponry, and that, after three years of war, the idea of fighting, killing and bombing had ceased to be extraordinary and was accepted as a part of everyday life. Gillespie (1942) described as a remarkable feature of the English home front the low incidence of child psychiatric casualties compared to the number anticipated. Yet Dunsdon (1941) found that children remaining under fire in Bristol, England demonstrated eight times more incidence of psychological distress when compared to those evacuated.

There are contradictory reports from Israel regarding the effects of shelling on youth. A study of the dreams and sleep habits of Israeli youth on a border town subject to terrorist activities indicated that they slept longer, and had fewer dreams, manifesting fewer horror, sexual, and aggressive themes than did their counterparts in a nonborder town. Using measurements of anxiety, Rofe and Lewin (1982) and Ziv and Israeli (1974) discovered that children from frequently shelled kibbutzim were no different from nonshelled kibbutzim. There is some evidence that communal solidarity, group cohesion, and common purpose shared by civilian and military participants of war may provide protection against anxiety (Zuckerman-Bareli, 1982). Milgram and Milgram (1976) compared preand wartime measurements of anxiety during the Yom Kippur War and demonstrated that the general level of anxiety in fifth and sixth graders doubled. There was, however, no predictable relationship between wartime stress and anxiety, but rather a correlation with being a boy and/or being an upper-middle-class child, and anxiety level.

Some of the confusion regarding the responsivity of children to the exposure of the chaotic violence and life threat of war is explained by developmental effects. The preschool child living within the security of a constantly available and supporting family often mirrors the family response to the stressor. Where there is parental injury, exaggerated parental emotional response, premorbid parental psychopathology, reversal of the dependency role, and excessive intolerance of the child's proclivity to regressive behavior, there may be an emotional derivative effect on the child.

The young child lacks the cognitive capacities available to the adult. His/her theories of causality are egocentric. Children are rarely able to talk about their frightening experiences. Unable to transform their internal conflicts and feelings into words, they are expressed in repetitive re-enactments, intrusive visual images, trauma-specific fears, aggressive and regressive activities, and other behavioral states (Terr, 1991).

Several observers studied children as the victims of war (Carlin, 1979, 1980; Lin et al., 1984; Arroya and Eth, 1985; Sack et al., 1986; Dyregrov et al., 1987; Kinzie et al., 1989). There is considerable evidence that the posttraumatic effects are serious and enduring. Sack et al. (1986) noted that 50 percent of the Cambodian-war refugee children had a diagnosis of posttraumatic stress disorder (PTSD). There was considerable comorbidity. Other prominent diagnoses were major depressive disorder, generalized anxiety disorder, and intermittent depressive disorder. In a 3-year follow-up study, 48 percent continued to exhibit PTSD and 41 percent depression. The course was variable with eight subjects having PTSD at both interviews, while eight subjects had a variable course (Sack et al., 1986). Arroya and Eth (1985) studied 30 refugees, less than 17 years of age, who had taken flight from Central America and who were referred to a mental health clinic. Many had been separated from their families. Often the parents had preceded the child to this country, leaving the child behind with relatives. The child was left with the perception of having been abandoned to the repeated violence of war. The investigators noted that approximately 33 percent of these youngsters exhibited posttraumatic stress disorders. Other diagnostic categories included adjustment disorders, separation anxiety disorder, somatoform disorders, major depressive disorder, and dysthymia.

Dyregrov *et al.* (1987) studied the effects of war in Uganda on a cohort of adolescents and noted their resiliency in the face of extreme stress. There was a proclivity for these adolescents to identify with the 'helper professions,' and to prepare in an anticipatory way for future positions in a society hopefully without war or violence. They exhibited little evidence of 'identification with the aggressor.' The children often expressed a wish to be doctors, lawyers, etc. The authors noted that adults who killed, robbed, and maltreated the villagers were regarded as strangers, 'belonging to an army hated for its cruelty and lack of discipline.' They appeared to be rejected as role models. The authors add a word of caution, however, describing themes of uncertainty, depression, and anxiety beneath the manifest coping and adaptive strivings of these youth.

Consultation

Upon entry into the country, the authors were met by representatives of the US Embassy. An Italian child psychologist with the Italian Aid Program had interviewed many of the children. She noted that they were placed in Centro de Lhanguene, a temporary shelter, a Catholic school, where they were being housed and provided some opportunities for schooling, play, and re-education. While she noted that many of the children had been beaten and tortured by RENAMO, suffered from malnutrition, experienced losses of family members, and in some instances participated in attacking and killing villagers, she felt that the children were not experienceing psychiatric problems.

We soon met with the Mozambique Vice-Minister of Health and the Deputy National Director of Health. There was a controversy in the government as to whether the children should be treated as prisoners of war or as victims of war. There was disagreement as to the treatment approach. How long should the children be kept at a 'special center' for treatment? Should they be returned to their families, placed for adoption, or assigned to group homes till they reached maturity? They expressed fears that these children would grow up to be delinquents and criminals without loyalty or fidelity to the country. They communicated their concerns that children who had participated in killing would come to enjoy their aggressivity and would prey on their fellow citizens. The Vice-Minister requested a treatment plan be provided the ministry.

Evaluation

The children were housed at Centro de Lhanguene, a Catholic school in downtown Maputo, the capital of Mozambique. The Director of the center introduced the group of refugee boys, who were marched before us, dancing to the sound of music. They were led by one of the older boys into portraying, in dramatic form, their experiences in captivity, the killing of an innocent village woman, and their eventual triumph over the guerrilla soldiers. They sang songs glorifying the revolution and the need to win victory over the 'bandidos.' There was a marked contrast between those children who were with the center 4–8 weeks and those who had just been captured by government forces and brought to the center. Approximately 10 new arrivals were sitting off by themselves separate from the group. Their heads were shaved to remove lice. Protuberant abdomens, a sign of malnutrition, were evident among 20 percent of the arrivals. They exhibited tattered clothing, bare feet, frozen emotionality, passivity, and a lack of relatedness with each other. They seemed resigned to whatever would be imposed upon them.

It was decided to evaluate 11 of the children individually and to meet with a larger group of 20 for the purpose of acquiring drawings related to several themes, i.e., the worst moment of captivity, the moment you were freed, and what you would like to be in the future.

Individual evaluations

The children were evaluated through an interpreter who spoke both Portuguese and the tribal dialect common to the southern provinces. Questions were taken from the parent's version of the Diagnostic Interview for Children and Adolescents (DICA-P) (Reich and Welner, personal communication), and the revised Frederick and Pynoos PTSD Reaction Index Scale (R. S. Pynoos, personal communication). The limitations of language and the need to translate from English to Portuguese, and frequently to a tribal dialect, made the use of instrumentation unreliable. While it was possible to make clinical judgments as to the existence of manifest psychiatric morbidity, the limits of enculturation of the instruments made it difficult to derive empirical data.

Table 4.1 depicts the presence of posttraumatic symptomatology along the three dimensions of mood, intrusive thoughts/imagery, and ego restrictions using a four-point scale. There is a suggestion of a relationship between the length of captivity and the severity of posttraumatic symptomatology.

Table 4.1 Posttraumatic symptomatology in a group of Mozambique children

	Age	Time captivity months	Time free months	Mood	Intrusive images	Ego restriction
Alfonso	12	1	6	+	+	++
Pauli	16	1	2	++	+++	++
Carlos	16	2	6	+	+	++
Angelo	14	2	5	+	++	+
Josai	14	2	6	++++	+++	+++
Israel	12	3	5	+	++	+
Fernando	15	6	14	++	+++	++
Carlos J.	10	6	3	++++	+++	++++
Firinice	6	6	1.5	++++		++++
Vasco A.	15	24	2	+++	+	+++
Ernesto	10	48	1.5	++++	+++	++++

Clinical vignettes

A few clinical vignettes are presented to illustrate the spectrum of experiences associated with these children's victimization by war.

Israel is a handsome 12-year-old boy who was originally from Gaza Province. He was captured by RENAMO in May 1987, and held a prisoner for three months (Fig. 4.1). The village where he lived was surprised and overrun by the bandidos who proceeded to loot and to take him and six others (including his mother, sister, and niece) prisoner. They were immediately forced to serve as porters, carrying food, sugar, rice, ammunition, and radios to the bandido village. They marched for approximately 14 hours and went without food or water for 24 hours. They were told that if they cried out or wept they would have their ears and/or fingers cut off with a machete. They continued to walk for two days before they reached the bandido village.

They were guarded at all times. Israel was not allowed to see or talk with his mother or other family members. They were told that they would be kept captive until 'Independence Day.' Israel was assigned as an aide to a bandido lieutenant and he was responsible for carrying and providing water. He felt that the bandits were always angry with him.

Soon after reaching the village, he was forced to participate in military training every morning from sunrise to noon. He and the other prisoners were required to train, and if they failed to do so, they would be beaten. If they performed well, they would be given water.

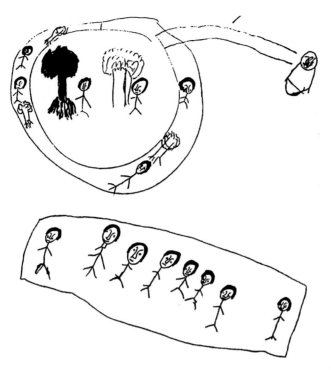

Figure 4.1   This drawing by Israel portrays the enemy camp in the circle and the captives being guarded and held prisoner away from the camp.

Israel reported a repetitive dream which he has experienced since his captivity. In the dream he is running away from the bandido camp to his home in the village. When he arrives, his brother asks him, 'How did you know how to get home?' He responds, 'How can anybody not know the way home?'

Approximately two months after his capture he learned that his mother had escaped. In the third month he escaped with a group of five boys. They pretended to be playing a game and gradually worked their way out to the periphery of the camp where they suddenly ran away. He was held prisoner and interrogated by the government forces for three months before he was sent to the center. His mother is back in her village, but he refuses to return home, preferring to stay in the safety of Maputo, away from the bandidos.

Firinice, a 6-year-old boy, was accosted by the bandidos at a river near his home. He was forced to lead them to his home where he was made to set fire to his family's hut. As his parents fled, they were killed and decapitated. His parents had been leaders in the militia. A man wrapped a Frelimo flag around the mother's head and noted that, 'This is what Frelimo buys you.' All his older siblings were killed. This account of Firinice's story occurred only months after his recapture by Frelimo. For

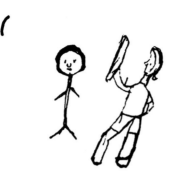

Figure 4.2   Josai's drawing shows the time when the bandido cut off the fingers of his left hand and his left ear. Notice the diminutive size of the helpless child before the threatening machete. Initially drawing in red (on the colored original), Josai quickly switched to a less emotionally loaded color.

many weeks he was virtually mute, unresponsive, emotionally frozen, and passively malleable, complying with whatever was expected of him.

Josai is an anxious and nervous 14-year-old boy who made a conspicuous effort to hide his left hand as well as to present a profile that would keep his left ear out of visual awareness. The four digits of his left hand had been chopped off with a machete and a good portion of his left ear had also been removed (Fig. 4.2). In a reticent manner he described how bandidos had entered his village, killed his father, and demanded to know which villagers were in the militia. When he responded that he did not know, they proceeded to cut off his fingers and subsequently his left ear. He has a recurring dream in which bandidos catch him while he is running away. They ask him, 'Why do you run away? We want you to kill government forces. If you don't, we're going to kill you.' He often thinks of revenge and imagines how he would cut off the hand of the man who attacked him.

Ernesto is a slightly built 10-year-old boy with signs of malnutrition who spent four years with the bandidos. The bandidos attacked his village, overran it, and set up their headquarters. His parents soon joined the bandidos. Ernesto initially served as a porter, but he was subsequently forced into military training. He learned to fire an AK-47 and participated in attacks on other villages. He denied killing anybody, noting that the recoil of the rifle would knock him down. After four years, his guerrilla band was defeated by government forces and he was taken captive. They treated him as a bandit and wanted to kill him. As a prisoner of war he was incarcerated for approximately six weeks in an army jail. He was beaten many times before he was released to the Centro de Lhanguene.

Ernesto graphically described his experiences as a bandido, and how at one point, he refused to participate in training and was threatened with death. Just before being killed, another bandit killed the one threatening him and the victim's brains flew out all over Ernesto. He described a repetitive dream of being watched by the bandidos, who kill him and he sees his own funeral.

Fernando is a 15-year-old boy with a deformity of the neck suggesting a rupture of neck muscles, resulting in his head being tilted over to the side. He related the injury to being forced to carry a 50-kg load on his head as a porter, while being held captive.

He admitted to participating in a number of attacks and killing six people. He exhibited little remorse or regret. He was preoccupied with being big and strong, expressing a wish to be a soldier and to drive a big truck. Both his parents had been killed, and at the time of his capture he was living with his grandparents. The village was surprised by child warriors with guns. As many of the villagers fled, they ran into an ambush and were killed by the adult bandidos.

After being captured, he was taught to fire an AK-47 and served as a guard for the prisoners. To prove his loyalty to the bandidos, he was forced to kill a prisoner or be killed himself. He participated in attacks on several villages, killing three villagers, and reports that in his last firefight he killed three bandidos. It was difficult to judge the veracity of this statement as he wanted to ingratiate himself with the government army. On one occasion, he indicated that he did it on purpose. On another occasion, he suggested it was an accident in which he killed them in a crossfire and subsequently fled fearing retribution. Upon his capture he was treated as a prisoner of war. He was held in an army jail for 10 months. The government forces were afraid that he would return to the bandidos. He was interrogated and tortured by Frelimo. There were scars on the inner aspects of his calves where a stick had been bored into his muscle. He was more afraid of Frelimo than he was of the bandidos. Upon his release from jail he was sent to Centro de Lhanguene where initially he carried a stick with him at all times to ensure his safety.

Vasco Albamo is a tall athletic 15-year-old boy, who wants only to play soccer. He was taking care of a herd of 13 cows when he was surprised by bandidos who took him prisoner and appropriated his herd. He lived with the bandidos for two years. He served as a porter and was trained as a guard (Fig. 4.3). He denied ever killing others, although he participated in numerous attacks on villages. He spoke of the safety he experiences in the Centro de Lhanguene and how he never wants to go back to the country. He has repetitive dream of being beaten and waking up afraid. He described the group life in the center: 'We live like brothers, we have the same problems, we love each other, we dance, sing and play football.'

Alfonso is a 12-year-old boy, who was held captive with the bandidos for one month (Fig. 4.4). He was kidnapped by the guerrillas while working in the field along with his father, mother, and brother. They fired shots into the ground warning them not to try to escape. He was forced to be a porter, carrying water, and to participate in military training. His mother's hand was cut off. One day while he

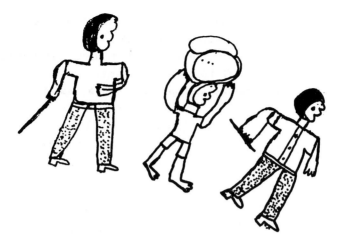

Figure 4.3   This drawing by Vasco Albamo shows him being forced to be a porter carrying food to the base camp being guarded by two bandidos.

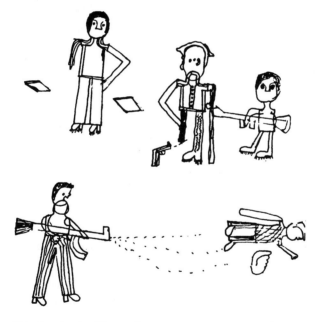

Figure 4.4   This drawing by Alfonso demonstrates two scenes. The upper scene shows a man having his leg cut off after he tried to escape. The lower scene shows the bandidos killing innocent people they meet in the forest.

was supposed to carry water to the base, he escaped. He returned to the village where he was turned over by the villagers to the government forces. He expressed feelings of sadness concerning the whereabouts of his parents. He feared going home as he would be taken once again by the bandidos.

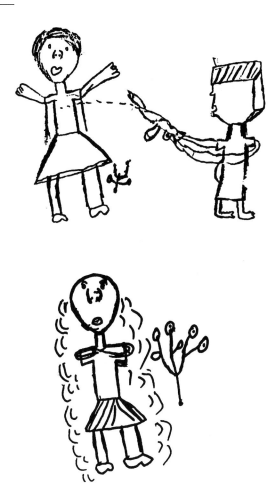

Figure 4.5   This drawing by the younger Carlos depicts the killing and burial of his aunt by the bandidos.

Carlos, a 10-year-old boy, saw the bandidos shoot his aunt dead and then bury her (Fig. 4.5).

Discussion

What are the psychological consequences of war and armed conflict on those children who were abducted by guerrilla bandits, and forced into military activities to become the 'pupils of war'? In some instances, these children not only participated in military action, but also killed others.

The child who was forced to participate in military activities and atrocities is similar to other victims of overwhelming disastrous life events. He may manifest posttraumatic stress symptomatology with its peculiar configuration of ego restrictions, disturbances in arousal, and a propensity to experience intrusive imagery and repetitive thoughts associated with the stressful experience (Terr, 1979, 1983, 1985, 1991; Pynoos and Nader, 1988).

The child's psychological response to an overwhelming stressor is determined by biological and psychosocial risk factors, the level of emotional and cognitive development, the degree of exposure to the stressor with its particular intensity and duration, the degree of injury or life threat, the losses of family members, and the disruption of the continuity of community/school/family (Pynoos and Nader, 1988). The essence of the traumatic situation is the particular meaning that the stressful experience has for the individual and the difficulty in processing that experience into his or her preconceived cognitive view of the world (Horowitz, 1974; Shaw, 1987; Ulman and Brothers, 1988).

The children in Mozambique were exposed to multiple stressors, i.e., life threats, witnessing brutal killings, physical beatings, dislocation from village life, enforced migration, separation from loved ones, exposure to marginal sustenance with food and water, coercive military training, and participation in military attacks on villages with the killings and assaulting of innocents.

The children were forced to be aggressive and violent in war when all they wanted to do was to take flight from violence. The normal child struggles to achieve control over his aggressive and destructive impulses. He controls his impulses by both conscious and unconscious self-regulation. The child who is forced to be aggressive at a time when he is learning to control aggression is traumatized in a particularly cruel manner. How much more traumatized is the child who is forced to aggressively attack members of his own family and village. The youngster who is exposed to sudden violence at a time when he is struggling to control his own aggression is in danger of having his own control over his aggressive impulses undermined and becoming more aggressive himself. We know that children who have been abused often grow up to abuse their own children (Dodge *et al.*, 1991). They identify with the 'aggressor.' Children exposed to war and conflict situations are reported to have a propensity to outbursts of hostility and aggression. Dyregrov *et al.* (1987) noted that as war and violence become an integral part of the child's life there is a risk that these children will become the 'pupils of war.' Fernando, the 15-year-old boy cited above, expressed a desire to be a soldier, yearning for a sense of powerfulness that would protect him from the captors and violent forces around him.

It is apparent that the exposure to the sudden realities of mutilation and death, the realistic limitations of the protective power of loving parents, and the sudden and unexpected impact of violence and brutality may undermine the child's illusion of safety. The child's reaction to the traumatic situation is greatly influenced by his underlying fantasy life, and his interpretation of events. When overt traumatic experiences resonate with an underlying fantasy, the experience may lead to a fixation on the trauma, in contrast to those traumatic experiences which are interpreted as incidental (Greenacre, 1952). This fixation may, in turn, lead to a compelling need to repeat the traumatic experience in a continuing effort to achieve mastery over the traumatic situation.

The peculiar brutality of the bandidos in Mozambique is evident in their kidnapping of children from local villages, coercing them into military training, and forcing them to fight against their own villagers and families. Failure to comply resulted in the cutting off of an ear, the fingers of one's hand, or even death.

An evaluation of 11 of these children, who were recaptured by government forces, indicated a high frequency of posttraumatic stress symptomatology, dysphoria, and anxiety. There was a proclivity for these children to see themselves as victims of war. There was a tendency, nevertheless, to identify with future career patterns where they would be helpers to other 'victims.' They thought of themselves as future priests, doctors, and bureaucrats. A few imagined working in the mines in South Africa where they would be able to make enough money to support themselves and their families. With one exception, the children indicated they did not want to be soldiers, but rather yearned for peace and freedom from war. Although separated from their families who lived in the country controlled by the bandidos, the majority asked to remain in Maputo, where they would be free from the risk of recapture.

It is also apparent that there is considerable variation in the child's response to the trauma contingent upon the intensity, type, and duration of the traumatic experience, the degree of participation in forced military activities, victimization by mutilation, the witnessing of the killing of parents, family members, and other villagers, the child's developmental phase, and his particular subscribed measuring to these experiences.

A prevention–intervention program

A written 'Psychosocial Treatment Plan for Children Traumatized by War at the Centro de Lhanguene' was presented to the government of Mozambique. The primary features of the program are noted in Table 4.2. The objective was to provide a transitional psychosocial program to facilitate the child's reorganization of his life, enabling him to once again meet the normal developmental expectations of childhood and be an effective participant in communal and family life.

Phase I focuses on assessment and evaluation procedures. Upon referral of a child to the Center, the first task is to assess the child's physical and nutritional needs. Next is the assessment of emotional and mental status, i.e., posttraumatic symptomatology and dysphoria, etc., followed by assessment of: level of maturity, cognitive capacities, the social and family situation; the severity, duration, and

Table 4.2 Prevention–intervention plan

Phase I	Assessment and evaluation
	Physical and nutritional status
	Emotional and mental status
	Coping and adaptive style
	Severity, duration, and type of traumatic exposure
	Inventory of losses
	Current stressors
	Child's definition of the situation
Phase II	Participation in a residential therapeutic program
	Security and protection
	Normal school experience
	Social and group activities
	Recreational opportunities
	Range of therapeutic experiences
	Ongoing assessment
Phase III	Reintegration in the community

type of traumatic experiences; current stressors; and coping and adaptive style. An inventory of the child's losses should be conducted, i.e., loss of community, home, mother/father, siblings, neighbors, and body mutilations, etc. Finally, the child's definition and understanding of the traumatic situation should be determined.

Phase II focuses on the child's active participation in a therapeutic residential treatment setting in which one can feel safe and protected. The Center will provide an organized program that encourages participation in a full schedule of events that includes practical living arrangements, normal schooling, organized play, sports, and group and social activities. The child should have an opportunity to express his feelings and to re-experience the traumatic situation through the safety of play, dance, song, drawings, and conversation.

Preferably, a mental health professional who is familiar with posttraumatic symptomatology should work with the child individually or in a group experience in an effort to facilitate abreaction, reconstruction of the traumatic situation, and 'working through'.

The Centro de Lhanguene was particularly skilful in its use of group play and dance to facilitate the child's sense of mastery over the feeling of helplessness that is the essence of the traumatic situation. In a form of psychodrama, the child participants would enact their experiences in captivity through song and dance, turning passive into active, and achieving mastery over the experience of helplessness before their captors.

The younger children are given an opportunity to draw or play out their experiences and then to talk about them. So that he won't be alone with his feelings, the child is encouraged to verbalize general feelings, questions, and concerns. It is sometimes helpful to provide emotional labels for common reactions such as 'You are feeling guilty,' 'You think you should have done more to resist,' 'You are afraid of your anger,' 'You want to have revenge,' etc. Clarification for confusion is provided. The older child is encouraged to express his fears, anxiety, anger, and sad feelings. He needs to talk about the event, to discuss his guilt, shame, grief, and sense of helplessness in being forced to do something he did not want to do.

If he has killed, he must talk about the feelings he experienced when he killed. Did he feel sadness, shame, guilt, or even a sense of power? The child needs to have the opportunity to mourn and grieve, to experience shame and guilt over his betrayal of his own standards of morality, and to be reassured, when possible, that he could not realistically have done anything else without being killed or mutilated himself. Fantasies of revenge and impulses toward aggressive, reckless behavior need to be discussed. There should be encouragement to share bad dreams and worries.

All children need to have emotional support from the group. They can do this by sharing experiences and talking about traumatic events with each other in a group setting. Realistic information is provided about what happened to him, the family and village, how it happened, and what he might expect in the future. Throughout, there is an ongoing assessment of the child's emotional response to the rehabilitation program, and his capacity to maintain progressive development.

Phase III focuses on the reintegration of the child into the community. As the child begins to reorganize his life, to 'work through' his traumatic situation, and to enhance his progressive adaptive capacities, plans are made for a more permanent setting. Emphasis must now be placed on finding an extended solution. Psychosocial evaluation will determine the choice of a social setting for the child. Primary emphasis should be placed on returning the child to his family. If this is not possible, consideration of adoption or foster home placement should be given. A program should be developed to follow these children into the future. It will rarely be necessary to refer a child to a group home or institution.

The proposed prevention and intervention program was accepted by the government of Mozambique and is currently being implemented under the leadership of Neil Boothby (Duffy, 1989).

Conclusions

Mozambique suffered the effects of an enduring civil war. The government of Mozambique requested psychiatric consultation to develop a prevention–intervention program for children who were kidnapped by bandidos and forced into military activities against their own villages and government. Following evaluation and consultation a three-phased prevention–intervention program was presented to the government of Mozambique that would reduce psychiatric morbidity and promote the child's developmental and adaptive capacities. Phase I provides the opportunity for immediate assessment of physical status, medical morbidity, coping and adapting styles, and an appraisal of the traumatic experience. An evaluation is made of the child's exposure to physical violence, the threats of injury and death, physical and psychological hardships, voluntary or forced participation in military activities upon others, and the child's definition and understanding of the traumatic experience. Phase II provides the opportunity to explore the child's psychiatric morbidity and psychosocial adaptation in a safe and organized residential milieu. Individual and group psychosocial interventions are provided, as well as realistic information as to what happened, to whom, and what will happen. The overall thrust is to extend and reinforce the child's support system, and to promote the child's adaptive capacities. Phase III is concerned with finding an extended solution and promoting the reintegration of the child into family and community.

There is evidence that many of these children can be rehabilitated when they are rightfully perceived as the victims of war and not as criminals or prisoners of war. The psychosocial program serves as a parental surrogate providing a milieu in which the child will be safe and secure, where he can normalize his daily activities in community and school life in a way that will provide him therapeutic avenues for his distress. Lastly, the program promotes the reintegration of the child back to the larger community, family, and village life, and hopefully, with restoration of his momentum, enables him to progress along his developmental and emerging psychosocial tasks.

REFERENCES

Arroyo, W. and Eth, S. (1985). Children traumatized by Central American warfare. In *Posttraumatic Stress Disorders in Children*, eds. S. Eth and R. Pynoos. Washington, DC: American Psychiatric Press.

Carlin, J. E. (1979). Southeast Asian refugee children. In *Basic Handbook of Child Psychiatry, vol. 1, Development*, ed. Noshpitz, pp. 290–300. New York: Basic Books.

Carlin, J. E. (1980). Boat and land refugees: Mental health implications, for recent arrivals compared with earlier arrivals. *Annual Meeting of the American Psychiatric Association*, San Francisco, CA.

Dodge, K., Bates, J. and Pettet, G. (1991). Mechanisms in the cycle of violence. *Science*, **00**, 00–00.

Duffy, B. (1989). An American doctor in the schools of hell. *US News and World Report*, January 16.

Dunsdon, M. I. (1941). A psychologist's contribution to air raid problems. *Mental Health*, **2**, 37–41.

Dyregrov, A., Raundalen, M., Lwanga, J. and Mugisha, C. (1987). Children and war. *Annual Meeting of the Society for Traumatic Stress Studies*, Baltimore, MD.

Freud, A. and Burlingham, D. T. (1943). *War and Children.* New York: Ernst Willard.

Gersony, R. (1988). *Mozambique Health Assessment Mission: Summary of Mozambican Refugees' Accounts of Principally Conflict-Related Experience in Mozambique.* The Indiana State Board of Health: Division of Media and Publications.

Gillespie, R. D. (1942). *Psychological Effects of War on Citizen and Soldier.* New York: WW Norton.

Greenacre, P. (1952). *Trauma, Growth, and Personality.* New York: WW Norton.

Horowitz, M. (1974). Stress response syndromes. *Archives of General Psychiatry*, **31**, 768–781.

Isaacman, A. (1987). An African war ensnarls the US ultra-right. *Los Angeles Times*, June 28.

Kinzie, J., Sack, W., Angell, R., Clarke, G. and Ben, R. (1989). A three-year follow-up of Cambodian young people traumatized as children. *American Academy of Child and Adolescent Psychiatry*, New York.

Lin, K., Masuda, M. and Tazuma, L. (1984). Problems of eastern refugees and immigrants: Adaptational problems of Vietnamese refugees Part IV. *Psychiatric Journal of the University of Ottawa*, **9**, 79–84.

Milgram, R. M. and Milgram, N. A. (1976). The effect of the Yom Kippur War on anxiety level in Israeli children. *Journal of Psychology*, **94**, 107–113.

Pynoos, R. S. and Nader, K. (1988). Psychological first aid and treatment approach to children exposed to community violence: Research implications. *Journal of Traumatic Stress*, **1**(4), 445–474.

Rofe, Y. and Lewin, I. (1982). The effects of war environment on dreams and sleep habits. In *Stress and Anxiety*, vol. 8, eds. C. D. Spielberger, I. G. Sarason and N. A. Milgram. Washington, DC: Hemisphere Publishing Co.

Rosenblatt, R. (1983). *Children of War.* Garden City, NJ: Anchor Press.

Sack, W. H., Angell, R. H. and Kinzie, J. D. (1986). The psychiatric effects of massive trauma on Cambodian children. II: The family, the home, and the school. *Title of Journal*, **25**, 377–83.

Shaw, J. (1987). Unmasking the illusion of safety: Psychiatric trauma in war. *Bulletin at the Menninger*, **51**, 49–63.

Terr, L. (1979). Children of Chowchilla: Study of psychic trauma. *Psychoanalytic Study of the Child*, **34**, 547–623.

Terr, L. (1983). Chowchilla revisited: The effects of psychic trauma four years after a school bus kidnapping. *American Journal of Psychiatry*, **140**(12), 1543–1550.

Terr, L. (1985). Children traumatized in small groups. In *Posttraumatic Stress Disorder in Children*, eds. E. Spencer and R. S. Pynoos, pp. 47–70. Washington, DC: American Psychiatric Press.

Terr, L. (1991). Childhood traumas: An outline and overview. *American Journal of Psychiatry*, **148**, 10–20.

Ulman, R. and Brothers, D. (1988). *The Shattered Self.* Hillsdale, NJ: Analytic Press.

Ziv, A. and Israeli, R. (1974). Effects of bombardment on the manifest anxiety levels of children living in the Kibbutz. *Journal of Consultations in Clinical Psychiatry*, **40**, 287–291.

Zuckerman-Bareli, C. (1982). The effects of border tension on the adjustment of Kibbutzim and Moshavim on the northern border of Israel. In *Stress and Anxiety*, vol. 8, eds. C. D. Spielberger, I. G. Sarason and N. Milgram. Washington, DC: Hemisphere Publishing Co.

5

The children of Oklahoma City

Betty Pfefferbaum

When a terrorist bomb exploded in front of the Alfred P. Murrah Federal Building on April 19, 1995, the impact extended far beyond the immediate tragedy of the 168 people who died and the hundreds more who sustained injuries. A community and nation recognized their vulnerability to terrorism. Despite earlier incidents – the first attack on the World Trade Center in 1993, for instance – most had dismissed or ignored the possibility of a major terrorist assault on US soil. The fact that the perpetrator was an American citizen, indeed one who considered himself a patriot, added to the horror.

It was widely believed that children were a target of the Oklahoma City attack. Nineteen children were among the dead. Fifteen of them were in the day care center in the Federal Building and four were visiting the building. Only five children in the day care center survived, and all were injured and hospitalized. Fifty-two children and nine staff in the neighboring downtown YMCA building were also injured. In addition, over 200 children lost one parent in the explosion and 30 were orphaned (American Psychological Association, 1997).

The death and injury of infants and children was alarming for all who contemplated it. Rescue and recovery workers found removal of their remains the most excruciating of the work they did (Tucker *et al.*, 1999; North *et al.*, in press). Families of these young victims mourned, sometimes openly, but also in their own private hell. The community wept, dealing with the trauma by displaying the children's pictures and their stories for all to see. Other children were now aware, in some unspoken way, that they too were vulnerable. This chapter is dedicated to the children and to those whose losses and suffering have provided the grim lessons that accompany terrorism.

Initial mental health response and services

In the chaos of the event on the morning of April 19, 1995, mental health professionals rushed downtown to join the intense rescue effort. Under the direction

Table 5.1 School-based services

Clinical needs assessment
Classroom coping exercise
Training for teachers and staff on:
    effects of trauma and grief on children
    holiday and anniversary reactions
    stress management
    use of projective techniques
    conflict mediation

of the State Medical Examiner's office, death notification and family support activities were established at the newly formed Compassion Center, a church three miles from downtown Oklahoma City. Multiple agencies, including the American Red Cross, Salvation Army, and various local, state, and federal government entities participated. Child mental health professionals joined death notification teams and offered their services providing crisis support therapy and assisting with a telephone bank. The center remained open for 18 days (American Psychological Association, 1997).

Using the Federal Disaster Response Plan, organized under the direction of the Center for Mental Health Services of the Substance Abuse and Mental Health Services Administration, meant that services were established expeditiously. On May 15, 1995, less than 1 month after the explosion, the Oklahoma Department of Mental Health and Substance Abuse Services opened Project Heartland (Call and Pfefferbaum, 1999).

School-based services

In May, the US Department of Education sent a team of experts to consult with the Oklahoma City Public Schools helping to initiate the development of an impressive school-based program. At the time of the bombing, approximately 40 000 students were enrolled in Oklahoma City Public Schools which employed a staff of over 5000. The bomb site was within the boundaries of the school district. Six schools were situated within five miles of the site; one school was damaged and one evacuated students and staff. To facilitate access to services, Project Heartland provided consultation, education and training, outreach, counseling, and support services at neighborhood schools (Table 5.1). Services were also provided to students and staff in surrounding public and private schools (Pfefferbaum *et al.*, 1999b).

Clinical needs assessments

While the school district had a roster of children and staff whose family members were killed or injured in the explosion, the extent of other forms of exposure and of distress were not known. Parents may underestimate distress in children (Burke *et al.*, 1982; Handford *et al.*, 1986; Sack *et al.*, 1986; Applebaum and Burns, 1991; Almqvist and Brandell-Forsberg, 1997). Therefore, in May 1995, days before the close of school for summer recess, a clinical needs assessment was conducted to determine exposure and to identify students in need of services. More than 3000 middle and high school students in 19 schools completed the assessment. Over 60 percent of the participating students reported hearing and/or feeling the explosion. Relationship to direct victims was extensive but involved mostly friends and acquaintances (Pfefferbaum *et al.*, 1999c). Similar to findings of adults in a telephone survey (Smith *et al.*, 1999), over one-third of the children surveyed reported knowing deceased or injured victims. Striking also was the level of television exposure. Approximately two-thirds of the children reported that 'most' or 'all' of their television viewing was bomb-related (Pfefferbaum *et al.*, 1999c).

Approximately 1150 elementary school children enrolled in grades three through five were assessed in the next academic year, 8 to 10 months after the incident. These children also experienced high levels of interpersonal exposure with almost one-fourth reporting that a relative had been killed or injured and almost 30 percent reporting that a friend or acquaintance had been killed or injured. Bomb-related television exposure was associated with higher levels of posttraumatic stress response (Gurwitch *et al.*, in press).

Classroom coping exercise

One novel clinical intervention used in classrooms was a group assessment and coping interview. The structured interview addressed both cognitive and emotional functioning and was designed to identify at-risk children and to facilitate sharing among children regarding coping strategies. The exercise was conducted over a 6-month period, ending just prior to the 1-year anniversary in April 1996. Approximately 6500 school children in both public and private schools participated. Almost 10 percent of the children were identified as needing further screening. Of those, approximately one-third received more intensive counseling (S. Allen *et al.*, 1999).

Training, services, and administration

In the summer of 1995, teachers and staff received training about the effects of trauma and grief on children, holiday and anniversary reactions, stress management, use of projective techniques, and conflict mediation (Pfefferbaum *et al.*, 1999b).

Federal funding to establish the full panoply of school-based services was not received until November 1995, but services were in place by the winter holidays and fully operational in early 1996. School-based services continued until the spring of 1997 (Pfefferbaum *et al.*, 1999b).

Students and trainees from local academic institutions of higher education, under the supervision of their faculty and Project Heartland staff, were enlisted to provide school-based services. This meant that a core of dedicated counselors was available at low cost. It also fostered multidisciplinary experiences and training in trauma response (Pfefferbaum *et al.*, 1999b). Concern was voiced by some, however, about the ability of these novice counselors to identify children in need of more comprehensive and sophisticated treatment.

The Oklahoma City Public Schools established a steering committee to review and coordinate bomb-related activities. The steering committee screened media inquiries, requests from various public and private groups proposing school-based clinical and educational activities, and research proposals. This required assessing the appropriateness of programs for school settings. Some administrators and teachers discouraged continued attention to the bombing, feeling that it prolonged recovery. A tension developed between those advocating school-based interventions and those focused exclusively on normalization. While the steering committee addressed these issues, many decisions regarding school-based activities rested with principals and teachers at individual schools, resulting in considerable variation in programs across the district (Pfefferbaum *et al.*, 1999b).

Preschool children

One of the neighboring buildings downtown, the YMCA, was destroyed in the explosion. The effects of the bombing on the preschool children enrolled in the day care center in the building were of particular concern. While no children or staff died or suffered serious or life-threatening injuries, most sustained minor injuries such as multiple cuts and bruises resulting from falling debris and glass in the building. These children experienced intense media attention during their evacuation and in the aftermath of the event (Gurwitch *et al.*, in press).

Gurwitch and colleagues (1996) evaluated a sample of these children approximately 6 months after the explosion. Most of the children evidenced re-experiencing and arousal symptoms. Posttraumatic play and peer discussions about the incident were extensive (Gurwitch *et al.*, in press). Avoidance was evident in many of these children who did not want to return to day care and in their hesitation to go near windows in the relocated center distant from the site (Gurwitch *et al.*, 1998). On the other hand, the children appeared to welcome opportunities to express their reactions to the event. Relatively absent were restricted range of affect and sense of a foreshortened future (Gurwitch *et al.*, in press) though these are difficult to identify in children. Arousal was evident in exaggerated startle responses, sleep disturbance, irritability, tantrums, and decreased concentration (Gurwitch *et al.*, 1998). Sleep disturbance and nightmares, not uncommon at this age, intruded even during naptime. Regression in language and toileting skills was noted with children needing increased assistance with self-care (Gurwitch *et al.*, 1998).

Clinical research findings

Exposure to trauma may occur directly through physical presence or indirectly, for example, through interpersonal relationship to victims or through the media. Research has demonstrated the relationship of physical exposure (Pynoos *et al.*, 1987; Breton *et al.*, 1993; Goenjian *et al.*, 1995; March *et al.*, 1997) and interpersonal exposure (Milgram *et al.*, 1988; Pfefferbaum *et al.*, 1999c, d; McCloskey and Walker, 2000) with symptom development. Television coverage has also been implicated (Nader *et al.*, 1993; Pfefferbaum *et al.*, 1999c; Pfefferbaum *et al.*, in press). We explored these types of exposure in our assessments of middle and high school students in Oklahoma City Public Schools in the spring of 1995 and elementary school students in the next academic year.

While many children in the middle and high school sample reported hearing and feeling the blast and/or knowing direct victims, most were in school at the time of the explosion and, therefore, not in direct physical proximity to the incident. More than one-third reported knowing someone killed and more than 40 percent reported knowing someone injured, though most of these were related through extended family, friends, and/or acquaintances rather than immediate family. Posttraumatic stress symptomatology at 7 weeks was directly correlated with female sex, relationship to direct victims, and bomb-related television viewing (Pfefferbaum *et al.*, 1999c).

Of those with interpersonal exposure, children who reported a sibling injured had the highest level of posttraumatic stress disorder (PTSD) symptoms, higher than those reporting a parent killed or injured (Pfefferbaum *et al.*, 1999c). Relatively little is known about reactions to sibling adversity (Applebaum and Burns, 1991; Hogan and Greenfield, 1991), but death or injury of an age-mate may create a sense of personal vulnerability at least as great as the loss of protection a child must feel when a parent is killed or injured. Loss or injury of a child may also be overwhelming for parents and prevent them from fulfilling their usual nurturing role with surviving children. In addition, surviving children may model their grief behavior after that of their parents.

Virtually nothing except bomb-related coverage aired on the major local television stations for days after the bombing. Television was a primary source of

Table 5.2 Predictors of posttraumatic
stress symptoms at 7 weeks in middle
and high school students

Female sex
Relationship to direct victims
Television viewing

information. Intense coverage continued for months with repeated stories about the deceased and injured. Uncertain what impact coverage of the event would have, we included an assessment of it in the needs assessment survey. In Oklahoma City middle school children, both interpersonal and television exposure were associated with posttraumatic stress at 7 weeks (Table 5.2). Among those with no physical or interpersonal exposure, television exposure was directly related to posttraumatic stress response (Pfefferbaum *et al.*, in press). The most obvious interpretation is that television viewing led to symptom development, but we cannot discount the possibility that symptomatic children were drawn to television coverage of the incident and that no clear causality exists.

We also explored, retrospectively, the children's peritraumatic reactions. The diagnostic criteria for PTSD require an initial reaction of intense fear, helplessness, or horror as part of the stressor criterion (American Psychiatric Association, 1994). A number of studies have demonstrated the importance of this initial reaction (Schwarz and Kowalski, 1991; Garrison *et al.*, 1995; Asarnow *et al.*, 1999; Pfefferbaum *et al.*, 1999d). In our middle school sample, initial emotional reaction – especially feeling nervous and afraid and being scared a friend would be hurt – was a strong predictor of PTSD symptomatology and of lingering safety concerns and worry (B. Pfefferbaum *et al.*, unpublished data).

Our findings must be discussed in light of the characteristics of the needs assessment sample, which was largely made up of indirect victims – children not physically present or closely related to direct victims. A sample of direct victims, one with a higher concentration of direct victims, or one in which relationships to direct victims were closer, would likely yield different results with respect to the relative importance of physical and interpersonal exposure.

Children geographically distant from Oklahoma City

Oklahoma is a sparsely populated state with few major metropolitan areas; therefore, we suspected that people throughout the state might have known victims. Because the identity of the perpetrators was not immediately known and the potential for continued or repeated attack was real, we were concerned that children geographically distant from Oklahoma City might have experienced a sense of personal threat associated with the bombing. We also recognized the potential impact of media exposure (Pfefferbaum *et al.*, 1999c, in press). Indeed, Terr and colleagues (1999) have proposed a 'spectrum PTSD' classification for indirect trauma. The spectrum classification includes distant trauma, reaction to a real event observed at the time but from a distant site; indirect trauma, reaction to an event not directly observable; and vicarious trauma, reaction to a highly threatening event that was not directly observable but was nationally threatening. Therefore, we studied exposure and symptoms in a sample of sixth-grade students in a community about 100 miles from Oklahoma City 2 years after the incident.

A number of students in the distant sample reported indirect interpersonal exposure, having a friend who knew someone killed or injured. Like the sample in Oklahoma City, interpersonal and media exposure predicted posttraumatic stress responses in this sample. Print coverage, as well as the more commonly examined broadcast coverage, appeared to have an impact. Broadcast and print exposures have distinct characteristics. Televised scenes, for example, tend to be fast-moving while printed portrayals are available for view for longer periods and may capture the most dramatic scenes. Television and radio coverage may be 'tuned out' by children who are accustomed to it in the background while print exposure is commonly associated with an intentional effort which may reflect the child's interest. The results of our studies suggest that children, even those whose immediate safety is not in jeopardy, may have lingering reactions to terrorist incidents and to media coverage of these incidents (Pfefferbaum *et al.*, 2000).

Clinical observations and issues

The mothers

A recounting of the impact of the Oklahoma City tragedy might well begin with the mothers – and in some cases, grandmothers – who searched frantically for their babies in the chaos and who later faced the grim realization that they would no longer be able to nurture and guide their young. The grandmothers who were raising their children's children described dual loss – loss of the grandchild and pain witnessing their own adult children grieve; yet, they felt left out at times, their grief minimized as attention focused on the mothers. Nothing in this tragedy was more poignant than their mourning. Many of the mothers were young. Some lost their first and only child. Some lost more than one child. Some lost other relatives as well. Many knew other children who shared the initial common grave of the Federal Building. Their grief lay bare for all the community to see. In some strange way they became celebrities as we tried to contemplate a loss none could imagine (J. Allen *et al.*, 1999).

Wanting to understand the elements of unimaginable grief, we longed to work with these women. We established a group for them – a chance to come together to teach us, we explained, so that maybe we could help others. Telling us that no one could possibly understand their private hell, a number came to our first sessions. No longer able to identify with those whose fate had spared them similar tragedy, these women decried that their loss was unknowable except perhaps by parents of murdered children. Few continued to attend the sessions, perhaps to avoid the traumatic reminders or perceived voyeurism associated with the activity. All maintained dignity in their insufferable grief. They taught us immeasurably through the group sessions they did attend and in individual therapy we had with some of them.

Mothers told of their guilt, the guilt of modern motherhood, for putting their children in day care in the first place. They bemoaned their belief that a day care center in a federal building would be the safest place for their children, an assumption we no doubt all held prior to April 19, 1995. Some spoke of their regrets for taking their children to day care on that particular day. Some described their child feeling sick that morning or simply not wanting to go that day. Several said they had a premonition that something ominous would occur. Their loss too deep, the guilt and grief was not to be assuaged.

When asked how the September 11, 2001 incidents had affected her, one mother, who long ago built an emotional shield around herself, said that she was dreadfully sorry for what had occurred but that nothing could really touch her again since the loss of her own child. Some mothers also minimized the effects of trauma and loss on surviving Oklahoma City siblings. These children were imbued with presumed resilience perhaps simply because they had survived by not being present at the day care or perhaps because their mothers could not tolerate the added burden of recognizing another loved one's grief.

Some were cautioned about the potential for problems associated with having 'replacement' babies. Declaring that nothing could replace their losses, a number did not heed the warning but chose instead to have additional children or start new families. Some have remarried and some have started life again quite literally by giving birth. Forever somber with their grief and hopeful with their love, they have chosen to reinvest in the future.

Children's play

Children experience posttraumatic stress responses similar to those in adults though they may have difficulty verbalizing their distress. Their play is a window to their feelings and posttraumatic play can alert us to experiences and feelings they cannot or do not verbalize. A recounting of the rescue effort through play was a favorite. In one scenario, a group of children divided themselves into rescuers and witnesses.

The rescuers gathered their equipment and donned their hats before entering the make-believe structure of the demolished building. When they emerged from the building with a survivor, the witnessing peers sent up a chorus of cheer. When the rescuers brought out an imaginary deceased, the witnesses, not knowing what to do, simply sat with a stunned look on their faces, fully capturing the shock of the community, heavy with emotion so difficult to process.

Avoidance

Avoidance was one of the clinical issues that impressed us greatly in our work with children and families. A teenager whose mother died in the explosion ran away after the incident because the thought of attending her funeral was unbearable. Children refrained from discussing loss with their peers to avoid the emotions such discussions inevitably brought. Children also experienced the consequences of the avoidance of others. For example, after removing the pictures and other remembrances of his deceased wife, one bereaved widower sent his children out of state for the summer assuming that by the time they returned for school in the fall they would 'be over' the loss of their mother.

Avoidance was also prominent in the therapeutic environment where it presented as canceled appointments, late arrivals, or termination of treatment altogether (Whittlesey et al., 1999). Whittlesey and colleagues (1999) identified avoidance stemming from a variety of sources. Parents commonly avoided treatment, for themselves and their children, because it led to painful memories. For example, almost 10 percent of the children participating in the classroom coping interviews the year after the bombing were identified as being at risk and in need of further screening. One-third of these children received no further assessment, however, because they were unavailable or because a teacher, counselor, or parent indicated that counseling was not needed (S. Allen et al., 1999). It is important to educate parents and children about the posttraumatic stress process early in treatment so they can anticipate and understand what may occur (Whittlesey et al., 1999).

Interpersonal awareness

The literature documents the tendency of parents to underestimate distress in children (Handford et al., 1986; Sack et al., 1986; Almqvist and Brandell-Forsberg, 1997). This may represent denial on the part of parents too distressed to notice the suffering of others or seeking to avoid the additional distress that acknowledgement of it would bring. Children are also commonly aware of the distress of their parents and conceal their own reactions to avoid further burdening the parent. One parent totally ignored the needs of a quiet compliant older child whose infant sibling died in the blast. Many teachers denied the effects of the incident on children in their classrooms refusing to even mention the bombing declaring that their students were obviously without problems.

Contagion, overreporting, and fabrication

There is a contagious quality to stress which can occur through both interpersonal relationships and the media (Terr, 1985; Pfefferbaum and Pfefferbaum, 1998). A number of clinical reports have described interpersonal spread of symptoms through family relationships – parent to child (Rosenheck and Nathan, 1985) and sibling to sibling (Terr, 1981, 1983) – and through peers (Terr, 1983; Milgram *et al.*, 1988). While we did not examine interpersonal contagion directly in our research in Oklahoma City, we certainly saw it in our clinical work. Overreporting of interpersonal exposure was evident in both clinical work and research (S. Allen *et al.*, 1999; Pfefferbaum *et al.*, 1999a; J. Allen *et al.*, 2000). Children participating in the classroom coping exercise fabricated interpersonal exposure (S. Allen *et al.*, 1999). A child participating in one of our research studies also fabricated loss, perhaps a manifestation of symptom contagion akin to mass hysteria, of psychological problems, of attention-seeking, or out of a desire to belong to the community in which this overwhelming trauma had occurred (Pfefferbaum *et al.*, 1999a). Another psychotic child under clinical care incorporated fabricated loss of a relative into his delusional system (J. Allen *et al.*, 2000).

Conclusions

At the time, the Oklahoma City bombing was the deadliest act of terrorism on US soil, made worse by reports that children were targeted. Children, therefore, have constituted a major focus of the clinical work and research conducted as the community recovers. Drawing from the work of others and aided by consultation with colleagues from other institutions, we established a range of services for children. School-based programs were accessible and developmentally appropriate. We learned a great deal about the reactions of children as we tried to meet their clinical needs. Recognizing the importance of documenting the effects of this deadly experience, research became a priority.

The September 11, 2001 attacks on the World Trade Center in New York City and the Pentagon in Arlington, Virginia forever changed the national perspective. Subsequent biologic attacks are grim reminders of new peril. America's children will no longer feel the unconditioned freedom of a safe and open society. Our Oklahoma City experiences provide a foundation for new clinical observations and studies about the impact of terror in the twenty-first century.

REFERENCES

Allen, J. R., Pfefferbaum, B., Hammond, D. and Speed, L. (2000). A disturbed child's use of a public event: Cotard's syndrome in a ten-year-old. *Psychiatry*, **63**, 208–213.

Allen, J. R., Whittlesey, S., Pfefferbaum, B. and Ondersma, M. L. (1999). Community and coping of mothers and grandmothers of children killed in a human-caused disaster. *Psychiatric Annals*, **29**, 85–91.

Allen, S. F., Dlugokinski, E. L., Cohen, L. A. and Walker, J. L. (1999). Assessing the impact of a traumatic community event on children and assisting with their healing. *Psychiatric Annals*, **29**, 93–98.

Almqvist, K. and Brandell-Forsberg, M. (1997). Refugee children in Sweden: Post-traumatic stress disorder in Iranian preschool children exposed to organized violence. *Child Abuse and Neglect*, **21**, 351–366.

American Psychiatric Association (1994). *Diagnostic and Statistical Manual of Mental Disorders*, 4th edn. Washington, DC: American Psychiatric Association.

American Psychological Association (1997). *Final Report: Task force on the Mental Health Response to the Oklahoma City Bombing*. Washington, DC: American Psychological Association.

Applebaum, D. R. and Burns, G. L. (1991). Unexpected childhood death: Posttraumatic stress disorder in surviving siblings and parents. *Journal of Clinical Child Psychology*, **20**, 114–120.

Asarnow, J., Glynn, S., Pynoos, R. S., *et al.* (1999). When the Earth stops shaking: Earthquake sequelae among child diagnosed for pre-earthquake psychopathology. *Journal of the American Academy of Child and Adolescent Psychiatry*, **38**, 1016–1023.

Breton, J., Valla, J. and Lambert, J. (1993). Industrial disaster and mental health of children and their parents. *Journal of the American Academy of Child and Adolescent Psychiatry*, **32**, 438–445.

Burke, J. D., Jr, Borus, J. F., Burns, B. J., Millstein, K. H. and Beasley, M. C. (1982). Changes in children's behavior after a natural disaster. *American Journal of Psychiatry*, **139**, 1010–1014.

Call, J. A. and Pfefferbaum, B. (1999). Lessons from the first two years of Project Heartland, Oklahoma's mental health response to the 1995 bombing. *Psychiatric Services*, **50**, 953–955.

Garrison, C. Z., Bryant, E. S., Addy, C. L., *et al.* (1995). Posttraumatic stress disorder in adolescents after Hurricane Andrew. *Journal of the American Academy of Child and Adolescent Psychiatry*, **34**, 1193–1201.

Goenjian, A. K., Pynoos, R. S., Steinberg, A. M., *et al.* (1995). Psychiatric comorbidity in children after the 1988 earthquake in Armenia. *Journal of the American Academy of Child and Adolescent Psychiatry*, **34**, 1174–1184.

Gurwitch, R. H., Messenbaugh, A., Leftwich, M., Corrigan, S. K. and Pfefferbaum, B. (1996). Brief intervention with children following the Oklahoma City bombing. In E. M. Vernberg (chair) *Symposium Evaluating Postdisaster Interventions*, presented at the meeting of the American Psychological Association, Toronto, Canada.

Gurwitch, R. H., Sitterle, K. S., Young, B. H. and Pfefferbaum, B. (in press). Helping children in the aftermath of terrorism. In *Helping Children Cope with Disasters: Integrating Research and Practice*, eds. A. La Greca, W. Silverman, E. Vernberg and M. Roberts. Washington, DC: American Psychological Association.

Gurwitch, R. H., Sullivan, M. A. and Long, P. J. (1998). The impact of trauma and disaster on young children. *Child and Adolescent Psychiatric Clinics of North America*, **7**, 19–32.

Handford, H. A., Mayes, S. D., Mattison, R. E., *et al.* (1986). Child and parent reaction to the Three Mile Island nuclear accident. *Journal of the American Academy of Child Psychiatry*, **25**, 346–356.

Hogan, N. S. and Greenfield, D. B. (1991). Adolescent sibling bereavement symptomatology in a large community sample. *Journal of Adolescent Research*, **6**, 97–112.

March, J. S., Amaya-Jackson, L., Terry, R. and Costanzo, P. (1997). Posttraumatic symptomatology in children and adolescents after an industrial fire. *Journal of the American Academy of Child and Adolescent Psychiatry*, **36**, 1080–1088.

McCloskey, L. A. and Walker, M. (2000). Posttraumatic stress in children exposed to family violence and single-event trauma. *Journal of the American Academy of Child and Adolescent Psychiatry*, **39**, 108–115.

Milgram, N. A., Toubiana, Y. H., Klingman, A., *et al.* (1988). Situational exposure and personal loss in children's acute and chronic stress reactions to a school bus disaster. *Journal of Traumatic Stress*, **1**, 339–352.

Nader, K. O., Pynoos, R. S., Fairbanks, L. A., Al-Ajeel, M. and Al-Asfour, A. (1993). A preliminary study of PTSD and grief among the children of Kuwait following the Gulf crisis. *British Journal of Clinical Psychology*, **32**, 407–416.

North, C. S., Tivis, L., McMillen, J. C., *et al.* (in press). Coping, functioning, and adjustment of rescue workers after the Oklahoma City bombing. *Journal of Traumatic Stress*.

Pfefferbaum, B., Allen, J. R., Lindsey, E. D. and Whittlesey, S. W. (1999a). Fabricated trauma exposure: An analysis of cognitive, behavioral, and emotional factors. *Psychiatry*, **62**, 293–302.

Pfefferbaum, B., Call, J. A. and Sconzo, G. M. (1999b). Mental health services for children in the first two years after the 1995 Oklahoma City terrorist bombing. *Psychiatric Services*, **50**, 956–958.

Pfefferbaum, B., Nixon, S. J., Krug, R. S., *et al.* (1999c). Clinical needs assessment of middle and high school students following the 1995 Oklahoma City bombing. *American Journal of Psychiatry*, **156**, 1069–1074.

Pfefferbaum, B., Nixon, S. J., Tivis, R. D., *et al.* (in press). Television exposure in children after a terrorist incident. *Psychiatry*.

Pfefferbaum, B., Nixon, S. J., Tucker, P. M., *et al.* (1999d). Posttraumatic stress responses in bereaved children after the Oklahoma City bombing. *Journal of American Academy of Child and Adolescent Psychiatry*, **36**, 1372–1379.

Pfefferbaum, B. and Pfefferbaum, R. L. (1998). Contagion in stress: An infectious disease model for posttraumatic stress in children. *Child and Adolescent Psychiatric Clinics of North America*, **7**, 183–194.

Pfefferbaum, B., Seale, T. W., McDonald, N. B., *et al.* (2000). Posttraumatic stress two years after the Oklahoma City bombing in youths geographically distant from the explosion. *Psychiatry*, **63**, 358–370.

Pynoos, R. S., Frederick, C., Nader, K., *et al.* (1987). Life threat and posttraumatic stress in school-age children. *Archives of General Psychiatry*, **44**, 1057–1063.

Rosenheck, R. and Nathan, P. (1985). Secondary traumatization in children of Vietnam veterans. *Hospital and Community Psychiatry*, **36**, 538–539.

Sack, W. H., Angell, R. H., Kinzie, J. D. and Rath, B. (1986). The psychiatric effects of massive trauma on Cambodian children. 2: The family, the home, and the school. *Journal of American Academy of Child Psychiatry*, **25**, 377–383.

Schwarz, E. D. and Kowalski, J. M. (1991). Malignant memories: PTSD in children and adults after a school shooting. *Journal of American Academy of Child and Adolescent Psychiatry*, **30**, 936–944.

Smith, D. W., Christiansen, E. H., Vincent, R. and Hann, N. E. (1999). Population effects of the bombing of Oklahoma City. *Journal of the Oklahoma State Medical Association*, **92**, 193–198.

Terr, L. C. (1981). Forbidden games: Post-traumatic child's play. *Journal of the American Academy of Child Psychiatry*, **20**, 741–760.

Terr, L. C. (1983). Chowchilla revisited: The effects of psychic trauma four years after a school-bus kidnapping. *American Journal of Psychiatry*, **140**, 1543–1550.

Terr, L. C. (1985). Psychic trauma in children and adolescents. *Psychiatric Clinics of North America*, **8**, 815–835.

Terr, L. C., Bloch, D. A., Michel, B. A., *et al.* (1999). Children's symptoms in the wake of Challenger: A field study of distant-traumatic effects and an outline of related conditions. *American Journal of Psychiatry*, **156**, 1536–1544.

Tucker, P., Pfefferbaum, B., Nixon, S. J. and Foy, D. W. (1999). Trauma and recovery among adults highly exposed to a community disaster. *Psychiatric Annals*, **29**, 78–83.

Whittlesey, S. W., Allen, J. R., Bell, B. D., *et al.* (1999). Avoidance in trauma: Conscious and unconscious defense, pathology, and health. *Psychiatry*, **62**, 303–312.

6

Individual and organizational interventions after terrorism: September 11 and the USS *Cole*

Thomas A. Grieger, Ralph E. Bally, John L. Lyszczarz, John S. Kennedy, Benjamin T. Griffeth, and James J. Reeves

The Medical Corps of the United States Navy has a longstanding history of providing psychiatric services to Navy personnel and civilians following disasters (Moore and Dembert, 1987). Support missions have deployed following collisions, fires and explosions at sea, aircraft crashes, and natural disasters. The Navy Special Psychiatric Rapid Intervention Teams (SPRINT) have been utilized for these missions during the past two decades (McCaughey, 1985, 1987; Golberg *et al.*, 1996). These teams are multidisciplinary and designed to deploy rapidly to disaster sites anywhere in the world. The teams are composed of psychiatrists, psychologists, social workers, psychiatric nurses, and enlisted psychiatric technicians. At the Navy's tertiary care hospitals these teams are preselected and receive training in postdisaster interventions. These teams can be augmented as with active duty and reservist members. At overseas hospitals, SPRINT teams are often assembled as needed with training provided at the time of deployment.

SPRINT teams have multiple objectives. They provide situational assessment of the psychological effects of traumatic events, direct support of affected individuals and units, brief psychiatric treatments, and consultation to commanders on how to mitigate negative emotional and behavioral outcomes.

The Navy also has the capacity to provide extensive medical, surgical, and psychiatry support around the world through deployment of its two hospital ships, USNS *Comfort* and USNS *Mercy* (Pentzien and Barry, 1992; Hooper, 1993; Dinneen *et al.*, 1994; Slusarcick *et al.*, 1999a, b). One ship is available on each coast of the United States. They are staffed by the medical personnel at the National Naval Medical Center in Bethesda, Maryland and the Naval Medical Center in San Diego, California.

In 2000 and 2001 the Navy experienced a new source of psychological stress, terrorist acts against Navy personnel and civilians aboard ships overseas and in the

United States. Three psychiatric deployments occurred; to Yemen and to Norfolk, Virginia following the bombing of the USS *Cole* in 2000, and to the Pentagon and New York City following the attacks on September 11, 2001. Each mission was unique, but there were elements common to all. These elements include planning and training, situational assessment, definition of the mission, logistical considerations, establishing the role as a consultant, supportive and consultative interventions, and terminating the deployment with appropriate follow-on services defined. The following sections demonstrate how each of these elements was approached in vastly different postdisaster environments.

The attack on the Pentagon

On September 11, 2001 at 8.10 a.m. American Airlines Flight 77 departed from Washington Dulles airport bound for Los Angeles with 58 passengers and 6 crew members. The plane was hijacked somewhere over West Virginia or Kentucky, reversed course, and was flown into the Pentagon at 9.43 a.m., minutes after the United States had witnessed the crashes of American Airlines Flight 11 and United Airlines Flight 175 into the North and South towers of the World Trade Center in New York. No one on the plane survived. Its impact and the resultant fire and building collapse resulted in the death of 125 military and civilians who worked in the Pentagon. Of these about one-fourth were assigned to Navy units. Survivors were exposed to death, danger, destruction, and dislocation.

Planning, preparation, and training

The National Naval Medical Center in Bethesda, Maryland is a tertiary care teaching hospital located approximately 10 miles from the Pentagon. It is also the center of one of the Navy's SPRINT teams. The team was augmented to include a total of three psychiatrists, two psychologists, two psychiatric nurses, two chaplains, and two psychiatric technicians. Eight psychiatry residents also participated on a part-time basis. Each member of the team had training in principles of postdisaster debriefing techniques. At the time of the Pentagon attack, about half of the team members had previously been deployed with a SPRINT team; one member had served as the team leader of the Sigonella team that had responded to the USS *Cole* attack. Psychiatry residents working with the team initially observed team interventions until such time as they were able to demonstrate competence in assisting with debriefing activities. They provided a large percentage of individual supportive services and evaluations for use of pharmacological treatments.

Senior hospital leadership was immediately aware of the Pentagon attack. Many were watching televised news releases from the attack on the World Trade Center when word was received that an aircraft had struck the Pentagon and that there was an ongoing threat of additional terrorist attacks. Hospital staff was placed on an alert status and ordered to remain at the hospital and prepare to accept casualties from the Pentagon and other potential sites. The SPRINT team was notified that it should be ready to deploy within 24 hours. Because of the complexity of the Pentagon command structure and high rank of officers in that structure, the SPRINT team was augmented with a senior psychiatrist who had experience with multiple prior similar missions and who had background experience with working with senior Navy leadership.

The Arlington Annex is a federal office building located approximately one half mile from the Pentagon. It also contains a small Navy clinic that provides care to Pentagon and Annex staff. Much of the building had been vacated when a major component of the Navy staff had been relocated to offices in another state during the preceding two years. On September 12, 2001 the clinic requested deployment of the SPRINT to their site. At 9.00 a.m. the final composition of the team was determined. The team arrived at the Annex at approximately 1.00 p.m. Arrival was substantially delayed because major travel routes near the Pentagon had been blocked. Security was greatly enhanced and this resulted in the closure of parking lots at the Pentagon and at the Annex. Additionally, all nonactive duty personnel who did not have federal building passes were banned from the buildings. Active duty members entering the buildings had to produce two forms of picture identification, sign in, and have all packages searched.

Situational assessment

The team arrived with minimal information concerning the nature of the attack, the number killed or wounded, or the nature of the exposures of the survivors. The team met with the clinic staff, but they too had limited information. A senior Navy physician serving as the preventive medicine officer to the US Marine Corps learned that the team had arrived and offered his assistance. He was highly familiar with the mission and assets of SPRINT as a result of working with one of the senior psychiatrists on a planning committee to establish doctrine for operational stress management. He was able to brief the team on the nature of the attack, number of deaths, injuries, and disruption that had occurred at the Pentagon. He also arranged for the team to meet with the senior Navy physician assigned to the Marine Corps. This contact greatly accelerated the team's ability to conduct its assessment and begin work.

The SPRINT mission was defined by the attack and the ongoing threat. The Navy command center in the Pentagon had been destroyed and had been relocated to the Annex. Virtually no Navy personnel remained in the Pentagon. They were being relocated to the Annex or to other federal office buildings in the area. In addition to the Annex, there were at least four other major sites that were going to house displaced navy personnel. The Navy staff was operating at a wartime tempo, with most active duty members working 12 to 14 hours per day and often working on the weekends. The Army and Air Force were establishing separate psychiatric teams to work with the Army and Air Force staff at the Pentagon.

The mission defined

The team based its operation in the Arlington Annex and provided outreach services to the other sites. Three levels of services were provided: informational/educational briefings, group debriefing, and individual supportive services. These services were provided to beneficiaries of the military health care system and to civilian employees. Beneficiaries could also be provided psychiatric and medical services. Civilian employees were referred as appropriate to providers in their health insurance programs.

Logistical considerations

In order to operate effectively the team required office spaces, telephone communications, debriefing rooms, and computers with database, word processing, and email capabilities. The team utilized cell phones initially and throughout the operation. The clinic put the team in contact with building management personnel and within 24 hours staff at the Annex had provided all other logistical support. The team established databases with contact points, appointment schedules, and running totals of services provided to each operational unit. The team obtained use of a government van for transportation to other sites. With increased security at all government office spaces, new identification cards and parking permits were required. These were obtained with the assistance of the Annex clinic staff.

Despite a well-planned approach, the dispersal of Navy offices in the capital area resulted in a challenge. Travel between sites often required up to an hour and finding the offices at other sites was often difficult. Some meetings had to be rescheduled.

Establishment of consultant role and credibility

The team began to perform informational briefings on September 13, 2001. The plan was to have one or two team members meeting with groups of between 10 and 80 individuals to provide information about the availability of services and the nature of physiological, psychological, and behavioral symptoms that might be experienced and recommendations for managing these. During the first meeting six individuals attended. No one attended the second scheduled meeting and the team recognized that the operational tempo and mass relocation activities required a different type of approach.

Senior team leadership met with senior Navy leadership to obtain their sponsorship and support. Coincidence again played a role. One of the team members had previously worked with the aide to the Director of the Navy Staff. The aide arranged for members of the team to meet with the Director. She posed two questions: What evidence did the team have that its interventions had a positive effect, and how could we justify pulling personnel from their jobs for one to two hours as the country prepared to respond to the terrorist attacks? The team could not provide scientific data, but was able to persuade her that units involved with prior SPRINT interventions routinely provided positive feedback about the nature of the interventions. The team also agreed limit the amount of time required to provide informational briefings. The Director endorsed the SPRINT mission and passed information to the leadership of all major Navy commands in the national capital area.

With command endorsement the work of the team rapidly increased. During the next two weeks the team ran between four and 10 debriefings each day. These debriefings involved one to three team members and three to 30 participants. Generally these were performed in work groups with the goals of determining the experiences of the members, lessons learned, and the nature of symptoms experienced. This provided an ongoing situational assessment. Another goal of the groups was to enhance communication within groups to foster the process of 'natural supports.' Additionally, some participants used this setting as a means of self-referral for individual supportive services. Leaders who participated were able to find out first-hand how their workers were doing.

Communication and ongoing consultation

Approximately every two days the team leadership transmitted a situation report via email to the executive assistants of the senior Navy leadership. These reports outlined the nature and location of the team's activities, number of contacts made, and a general description of findings. The reports also outlined the process for obtaining SPRINT services. Copies of the reports were forwarded to the offices of the Navy Surgeon General so that his staff was updated on the potential need for additional medical assets. Senior team members also communicated with the Army and Air Force mental health units operating at the Pentagon and at other sites.

Nature of findings

SPRINT team members estimated the following exposure information from their interactions with the survivors. Within the Navy population approximately 20 percent were in direct danger of death or serious injury, and 20 percent knew someone who was killed or seriously injured in the attack. Nearly 100 percent perceived an ongoing threat of additional attacks during the next few hours and nearly 100 percent had colleagues or friends who worked in the Pentagon. It took from several hours to days to determine the number of casualties in each operational unit. Nearly everyone faced significant disruption to his or her work routine. Approximately 20 percent had their offices destroyed and lost personal possessions, 40 percent were dislocated transiently or permanently, and 80 percent were forced to reconfigure their offices to accept those dislocated from the Pentagon. In addition, a number of survivors witnessed the plane, the crash, or the resultant fire from their sites at the Annex, Henderson Hall, or Crystal City. It took many individuals hours to contact their families to assure them that they were not harmed.

The following symptoms were reported during and after the attack: transient sleep disruption; peritraumatic dissociative symptoms (feelings of unreality or disturbance in the passage of time); a heightened degree of vigilance or autonomic arousal; intrusive thoughts about the attack that were either spontaneous or triggered by external stimuli; bereavement; anxiety about additional acts of terrorism; and fatigue lasting several days. In summary, there were multiple levels of exposure and diverse psychological and physiological responses. Nearly equal number of individuals received supportive intervention as did not, although it is not known if these groups were equally exposed or equally distressed.

Termination of team operations

By the third week of operations the team had recorded over 1800 contacts. At this time the number of new scheduled contacts began to drop to fewer than 20 per day. In addition, relocation of Navy staff to the Annex had placed office space at a premium. The majority of contacts were at sites other than the Annex. There was no longer a need to maintain a command center at the Annex and remaining group and individual services could be scheduled as needed. The team developed a plan to stand down the command center and to schedule additional services through the Behavioral Health Clinic at the National Naval Medical Center. This plan was communicated through the situational reports to the executive assistants and with their concurrence it was executed. During the following three weeks approximately 20 contacts per week were scheduled and a small number of individuals were followed individually. In total, the team had approximately 2000 contacts. The majority of contacts were in informational briefings and group debriefings. No member of the Navy staff was hospitalized for psychiatric reasons. There was minimal use of psychiatric medication. A few individuals were provided with medication to assist with sleep difficulties during the first few days following the attack.

Ongoing assessment and health surveillance

Psychiatric consequences of traumatic experiences may often be delayed for weeks to months following the experience. There was little evidence of ongoing psychiatric illness or emotional difficulty. A systematic, Pentagon-wide surveillance project was initiated, and the results of that project are under analysis. Senior Navy leadership has been reminded that ongoing care is readily available through the military hospitals and clinics in the national capital area.

Navy response to the World Trade Center attacks

In the wake of the World Trade Center attack, the United States Navy deployed USNS *Comfort* to provide medical support services to the City of New York. The urgency with which the *Comfort* deployed reflected how swiftly the tragedy struck the United States. Indeed, this was the first time an attack upon Americans was shown in 'real time.'

Predeployment

The National Naval Medical Center announced on September 12 that the USNS *Comfort* would deploy. As one of the Navy's two hospital ships, the *Comfort* is 894 feet long and displaces 70 000 tons. It has 12 operating rooms and a capacity of 1200 beds, including 80 intensive care beds. Depending on the nature of the mission, the ship deploys with various configurations of staff. During the 36-hour period prior to sailing, there were multiple negotiations as to the level of deployment as well as the mission of ship upon deployment. During this time the behavioral health team of the ship was briefed by a senior psychiatrist who had served aboard the *Comfort* during its previous deployment during the Gulf War. He was able to give specific examples of ways that behavioral health was used and supported while it served in the Gulf in 1991 (Dinneen *et al.*, 1994).

Additionally, the team received educational materials from the Center for the Study of Traumatic Stress at Uniformed Services University of the Health Sciences. These materials included articles and book chapters regarding acute stress disorder and military personnel's response to crisis and provided information that would be used by the team during deployment.

They specifically addressed the need for the internal care of the staff and crew deployed aboard ship and stressed how morale, warfare, and mental health are tied in with one another and need to be rigorously monitored during a deployment, especially an emergency deployment such as this. On Friday, September 14, the 250-bed contingency platform for the *Comfort* loaded buses to meet the ship at Earle, New Jersey. An additional psychiatrist, a psychiatric nurse specialist, and an additional psychiatric technician augmented the behavioral health team, based on the command's concern that mental health would be of utmost importance during this deployment.

Prior to departure of the ship to New York, it was determined that extensive medical and surgical assets were not needed. This prompted return of the vast majority of the contingency personnel to National Naval Medical Center. The mental health team remained aboard and deployed to New York City. This team was composed of two psychiatrists, a psychologist, a nurse clinician, and three enlisted psychiatric technicians.

Logistical considerations

The USNS *Comfort* was located at Pier 92 (51st Street and Westside Highway) approximately 2½ miles north of the World Trade Center. This distance led to fewer rescue workers traveling to the ship than was initially anticipated. Additionally, the Office of Emergency Management was located at Pier 92. It had been relocated following the collapse of its offices located at World Trade Center Building 7. Transportation between the disaster site and the *Comfort* was established within 48 hours of the arrival of the ship. The *Comfort*'s constant location facilitated the provision of care and services to rescue workers as well as support and care of the ship's personnel. No personnel were sent to isolated locations, and there was a constant base for all activities.

As part of the initial assessment of the *Comfort*'s role, an individual was assigned to provide liaison between the ship and the New York City Office of Emergency Management. The Office of Emergency Management served as the command center for the organization of the rescue and relief efforts at the World Trade Center: it also became the central coordinating organization for peripheral services such as the *Comfort* and the American Red Cross. They used Public Health Service officers assigned to New York City as their primary medical and psychiatric staff. These professionals along with the New York Police Department and Fire Department's behavioral health care systems provided the primary mental health care during this disaster. As part of the initial assessment the Public Health Service determined that it had adequate staff to handle the initial demands of the rescue workers at the site. The behavioral health contingency of the *Comfort* was asked to remain with the ship and provide care to all workers who came to the ship for relief services.

In keeping with traditional SPRINT operations, the mental health team invited participation by the two chaplains aboard. The chaplain's role has been long understood within the Navy to be dedicated to the internal care of the ship's needs, especially the morale and welfare of the ship as a whole. The team also actively encouraged the role of the enlisted psychiatric technicians. They had great insight into the below-decks atmosphere and morale of the ship.

Within four days of deployment the Public Health Service noticed the large number of rescue workers who were coming to the *Comfort*. As a result they provided two social workers from the US Public Health Service to augment the staff aboard the *Comfort*.

Upon arrival and organization of the team on September 15, one member of the team provided instruction on two models of postdisaster intervention, the Critical Incident Stress Debriefing model (CISD) and the National Organization for Violence Assistance model (NOVA). The team trained as a whole on how to organize and manage debriefing systems and discussed group and individual session's systems and back up plans. The team prepared handouts adapting educational material that had been published by the Washington DC Public Health Service and downloaded from the Internet. These handouts were available to all rescue workers as they registered aboard the ship. The handouts were also passed out on routine basis by the behavioral health team during face-to-face contact with the rescue workers, Office of Emergency Management staff, and especially with police, fire department and Emergency Medical Service supervisory personnel. These materials emphasized the needs of the individual to recognize their symptoms and the needs of the supervisor to support their personnel.

Situational assessment

On September 15 the first rescue workers and emergency personnel were brought aboard the ship for meals, support, bedding, medical care, relaxation, and debriefing. All members of the team actively engaged individuals and small groups of people while they were in the dining facility. For many workers this was their first hot meal in three or four days. What later became known as 'coffee cup therapy' started as the need to assess the overall well-being of the rescue workers. The team assessed amount of rest and sleep, amount of down time, number of meals, time away from home, and rate with which they returned to the rescue efforts at the World Trade Center. It was evident that most of the workers needed better food, more water, and more rest. Though many would admit to stress, sadness, and grief over the attacks at the World Trade Center, most acknowledged that their first and overriding concerns while aboard the *Comfort* were to supply their more primary needs. Indeed despite significant outreach by the behavioral health care team to engage in traditional debriefing groups, no individual persons or small groups of people volunteered to join any debriefing groups.

Since no one chose the group therapy approach, the best alternative that could be offered was to continue to offer the individual and small group treatments that were started during the assessment phase. Specifically, a behavioral health care worker would sit down with small groups of individuals in the dining facility. These people would be initially engaged in discussions of mundane or naturalizing subjects: weather, sports, or individual history. This allowed for not only a return to a more natural expression of emotion but also rapid rapport building between the behavioral health care personnel and the rescue workers. This also decreased the isolation of rescue workers. In an effort to decrease isolation many of these individuals were assessed or brought in with members of their natural teams. Often if the individual who was sitting alone was a policeman, firefighter or Emergency Medical Service worker they would be united with somebody else from their discipline while in the dining facility. This enhanced natural debriefing with peers as the discussions turned to the World Trade Center disaster. They discussed their individual reactions and provided normalizing reactions for one another by talking about how each had been harmed, scared, or overwhelmed by the things that they saw, heard, or felt while at the World Trade Center.

Parallel to the work in the dining facility, the behavioral health team continued with the more traditional clinician's role in the medical facility. Typically they saw people who were having greater difficulty coping. Each received individual assessment and counseling. Most often they were given the same instructions given to those in the dining facility, especially the need to avoid isolation.

Among the unusual and surprising things found during initial treatment was the number of rescue workers who had been previously diagnosed with mental illness. Some saw the *Comfort* as a place of refuge and support and sought care there despite having an already established care system. After careful assessment, these people were directed back to their traditional supports.

Challenges

Some challenges noted during the *Comfort*'s deployment to New York City were the result of the diversity of the various departments supplying the rescue and relief efforts to New York City. Specifically, as people reported aboard the *Comfort* they came in twos, threes, and fours and rarely with any supervisors. This lack of any central authority led partially to the lack of intervention groups. Conversely, for good or ill, the National Guard officers held the authority or persuasion to order personnel to attend group therapy at the Manhattan Armory. Another challenge faced by the *Comfort*'s initial intervention system was the coordination with the rescue workers' own internal systems for behavioral health support for the police and fire departments of New York City. The Police Department and Fire Department had behavioral health care workers available in their squad houses and on work shifts. They commonly used social workers and other counselors when there were particularly bad outcomes to an incident within any squad, work shift, or team. This system continued to function throughout the *Comfort*'s time in New York. The Public Health Service augmented those personnel in the firehouses and the police stations when necessary.

Another challenge that caused a shift in the focus of the *Comfort* was a change in the types of workers at the recovery site. As the work progressed from rescue into a recovery phase, the City of New York consolidated the number of workers at the site. Crews that had come from out of state or that had been moved from different parts of the city were relieved. These personnel, many of whom had stayed aboard the *Comfort*, were released to go home. Starting on September 20, 2001 many of the personnel who were seen on the *Comfort* were 'already supported.' These included personnel from the Office of Emergency Management at Pier 92, Air and Army National Guard, New York State Militia, and local construction workers.

The media was pervasive throughout the time of the *Comfort*'s deployment in New York City. The media portrayed the sailors of the *Comfort* as war heroes. Unfortunately the media also interrupted care in the ambulatory medical facility and in the dining facility when they attempted to interview rescue workers being seen by the behavioral health care or medical teams.

Collaborations

Collaboration was established between the *Comfort* and the US Public Health Service. The Public Health Service had a majority of the behavioral health care personnel assigned to disaster work. They had the infrastructure to support their behavioral health care workers and also had the organizational support of the local government. The *Comfort* team provided debriefing services for some of the Public Health Service personnel who had provided medical care at the disaster site during the early phases of the recovery operation.

The second group with whom the *Comfort* collaborated was the Disaster Psychiatric Outreach group of New York City. This group, organized by Dr Tony Ng, was a collective of psychiatrists and psychologists from the state of New York who had organized in the 1990s toward providing behavioral health care in the event of a disaster. These personnel provided mental health care directly to the rescue workers at the World Trade Center from September 12 until after the *Comfort* was ordered home. During the time that the *Comfort* was stationed in New York City, the Disaster Psychiatric Outreach group noted that they were becoming overwhelmed with the amount of work that was involved. Their health care personnel also needed to have time off and to take care of themselves. For the last three days in September, members of the *Comfort* team served with these mental health care providers at the recovery site providing behavioral health care needs to the remaining search and rescue teams and construction workers.

The *Comfort* also worked collaboratively with the Air National Guard, the Army National Guard, New York Militia, and the Army Corp of Engineers. These groups were called upon by the City of New York to provide support services, security services, and also infrastructure support to the rescue efforts at Ground Zero. These personnel were housed aboard the *Comfort* and the behavioral health care team provided debriefing for these groups. Each of these groups had good internal structure and internal behavioral care resources. They required little in the way of direct treatment from the behavioral health care team.

Internal care

The personnel aboard the *Comfort* required less care than had been initially expected. In part this was due to the brevity of the tour ($2^1/_2$ weeks) as opposed to the 8 months that the *Comfort* had deployed during the P Gulf War. Additionally there were fewer total staff aboard the ship in comparison to the P Gulf War. Lastly, the work of the Commanding Officer and Executive Officer in establishing a ship routine supported the personnel of the *Comfort*. Within a matter of two days the ship established a three-section watch. The Morale, Welfare, and Recreation personnel started functioning for relief and recreation during the times of liberty. A majority of the sailors aboard the *Comfort* maintained their usual exercise routines as well as increasing the amount of training for their duties aboard the *Comfort*. The ambulatory medical facility established daily didactics that bolstered the spirits and training of the corpsmen attached to that division. The enlisted psychiatric technicians through informal interactions in the berthing spaces did much of the care of the *Comfort* personnel. Through their contacts the behavioral health care team and ultimately the command was made aware of issues that were disquieting to the sailors aboard the *Comfort*. The command staff addressed these issues so that the sailors could return to their support roles.

The behavioral health care team established a series of group gatherings held every other day. During these meetings the chaplains and behavioral health care workers debriefed one another. Specific issues that were addressed during these debriefings included the exposure of personnel to traumatic images from the television, sharing of information and lessons learned, and realignment of personnel due to changing conditions. Senior clinicians experienced in postdisaster work at the National Naval Medical Center and Uniformed Services University of Health Sciences also provided support from a distance.

The attack on the USS *Cole*

A bomb-laden boat detonated alongside the USS *Cole* while it refueled in the port of Aden, Yemen on October 12, 2000. The destruction of the ship's galley, senior enlisted dining facility, and numerous propulsion and equipment spaces below the waterline killed 17 sailors and injured 34 more. Survivors worked around the clock for the next 96 hours, braving smoke, flooding, power loss, and the equatorial heat to stabilize the ship, stabilize the wounded, and re-establish security. In the immediate aftermath, they were unable to fight back, contact other ships, or get under way.

Planning, preparation, and training

The SPRINT at Sigonella Naval Hospital (located near Catania, Sicily) is composed of a mix of primary care providers, mental health providers, and administrative support personnel. Training includes elements of individual and group debriefing, situational assessment, and command consultation (Table 6.1). The team had responded to over one dozen small-scale incidents in the two years prior to the *Cole*

Table 6.1 Elements of Intervention

Situational assessment and triage
Education
Counseling
Debriefing
Command consultation and leader education
Group and individual support
Stress management

attack. As recently as August 2000, a Gulf Air jet crashed on approach to the Bahrain International Airport and the Sigonella SPRINT deployed to provide stress management to Bahrain-based US military personnel who assisted in the body recovery effort.

When news of the attack on the *Cole* reached the hospital, the team was placed on alert for possible deployment to Yemen. The psychiatrist was placed in charge of the team. Nine individuals were selected for the deployment. All were ready for departure within 12 hours. Immunizations were brought up to date and prophylactic treatment for Rift Valley fever was prescribed.

Situational assessment

The team flew to Aden, Yemen on October 13 and was placed under the command of the on-site senior medical officer. Team members were housed with other military and civilian personnel in the Aden Hotel. Yemeni soldiers and US Marines provided local security. The team leader met with medical personnel and chaplains who had made trips to the site and obtained the following information: (1) the recovery effort chain of command; (2) the extent of the *Cole* casualties (roughly one-sixth of the crew, with 12 dead bodies still pinned inside the wreckage); (3) the security of the remaining crew (perimeter security had been established, but it was impossible to rule out the possibility of further attack); (4) the organizational makeup and leadership structure of the *Cole* crew (21 divisions organized into five departments); (5) affected organizations (the *Cole* crew, Norfolk Naval Shipyard workers and Navy divers extracting the deceased, FBI investigators collecting evidence); and (6) the tentative timeline for the recovery effort.

The mission defined

The team decided to offer group interventions to the affected organizations, emphasizing stress management, normalization of stress symptoms, and the encouragement of social support.

Logistical considerations

The *Cole* was located 10 miles from the hotel and reachable only by armed convoys, which were difficult to arrange. Team members were ordered to wear civilian clothes to lessen their risk of becoming terrorist targets. One week after the attack, the base of operations for the relief operation was moved to the USS *Tarawa*, an amphibious assault ship located outside the harbor. This would greatly complicate access, so the team extended its local presence by remaining with the US Marines who had established a secure perimeter on the beach adjacent to the *Cole* anchorage. The team met every morning to plan its interventions for the day and met every evening to discuss the day's operations and 'debrief the debriefers.' The team leader briefed the operation's medical officer once or twice per day, the Sigonella Naval Hospital Commanding Officer by telephone every evening, and the Joint Task Force Commander once per week.

Establishment of consultant role and credibility

An 'advance party' consisting of the team leader, team administrator, and senior enlisted member traveled to the *Cole* on 15 October. The *Cole* Commanding Officer and Executive Officer met with the group upon their arrival. The team leader first verified that the Commanding Officer was amenable to the team's assistance, then briefed him on the team's mission: to minimize stress symptoms, to foster unit cohesion, and to facilitate normal grieving. The Commanding Officer expressed interest in the team's assistance and promptly requested guidance on how best to send the remaining dead bodies ashore as they were extracted, and how best to arrange collection of the personal effects of the deceased. The team leader recommended that the bodies be sent ashore in a ceremonial fashion if possible – analogous to a burial at sea – and that someone who knew the victims well conduct the handling of personal effects in a formalized, respectful way. The Commanding Officer accepted these recommendations and arranged for the SPRINT team to come aboard the following day. Team members would establish ties with middle-level leaders in preparation for the provision of support to the crew members under their supervision.

Stress management interventions

The team leader was trained in combat stress control and command consultation. The three mental health providers were trained in operational crisis intervention. The team leader prepared a set of instructions for the initial interventions (Table 6.2) and reviewed them with the team on the morning of October 16, Upon arrival later that day, team members received a tour of the ship and were paired up with members of the shipboard leadership. The crew was not operating according

Table 6.2 Guidelines for organizational consultation

Goals

1. Maintain the integrity of the chain of command.
2. Assist the command in maintaining its mission focus.
3. Contribute to organizational effectiveness and unit cohesion.

Techniques

1. Obtain direct briefings from identified organizational leaders. They should serve as a source of education and information.
2. Provide support – discuss recent events and identify effective responses to operational problems that arose.
3. Identify potential weaknesses in these individuals' communication with those above, below, or laterally in the organization.
4. Identify 'work groups' – teams of individuals with identified leaders tasked with specific missions on an ongoing basis.
5. Participate in team intervention briefing twice daily.

---

to its normal organizational structure but was instead employing hastily assembled work parties to carry out tasks. In this rapidly evolving environment, SPRINT members provided one-to-one support to identified individual crew members experiencing more pronounced stress symptoms. Team members met with scores of individuals and spontaneous assemblies of crew members. During his briefing with the Executive Officer that evening, the team leader suggested that he consider reinstituting the preattack crew organization and daily routine. In that manner unit leaders could augment the team's efforts in managing the stress of their sailors. The team decided not to attempt stress management interventions with randomly collected groups, but to wait until the crew were again operating within their normal unit structure and use this structure for group interventions (Table 6.3).

The advance party again assessed the status of the crew next morning. The Executive Officer had ordered traditional work groups to reinstitute their routine morning meetings. The work tempo remained high, but was more coordinated, along traditional organizational lines. This change permitted the team to begin more structured group interventions. The remainder of the team came aboard and that evening made contact with working groups in close group leaderships.

The team conducted another round of group stress management meetings two days later. At other times each day team members continued to work with individuals and spontaneous small groups. Many of the crew could not perform their traditional duties due to the loss of power and the destruction of workspaces. Over the ensuing days most were transferred to other duties assisting the recovery effort. Daily all-hands assemblies rendered honors as bodies of the deceased were moved ashore.

Table 6.3 Techniques for group interventions

Goals

1. Permit psychological decompression of members of ongoing work groups.
2. Assist work groups in maintaining their mission focus.
3. Contribute to organizational effectiveness and unit cohesion.

Techniques

1. Use one or two debriefers.
2. For a first intervention, meet during 'down time' and have the team leader introduce the members of the team.
3. Ask the team leader to discuss the team's work during the previous shift – what was accomplished, what is yet to be accomplished; which processes worked, which did not. Encourage problem-solving.
4. Provide the team members with the opportunity to add their comments.
5. Provide teaching on stress symptoms (use handout) and offer suggestions.

Each member of the crew was given the opportunity to spend a night aboard one of the American warships outside the harbor, where they were greeted as heroes and were able to obtain a hot shower and a good night's sleep. Crew members reported that this opportunity provided a major source of stress relief.

Team members maintained an informal liaison with two Navy chaplains from Bahrain, who visited the crew daily. The team leader established liaison with the Norfolk Naval Shipyard workers, the Navy divers, and the FBI investigators. The Navy divers were experienced in the recovery of human remains and they demonstrated no obvious signs of stress. No formal interventions were provided, but many expressed appreciation for the presence of the team. The Norfolk Naval Shipyard workers, on the other hand, were not accustomed to this work and found it very difficult. Half of the group returned to Norfolk after less than one week and the team leader notified the Portsmouth Naval Hospital SPRINT of their possible need for a stress management intervention. The remaining workers completed their tasks on October 22. They were offered a summary debriefing experience. They accepted and the intervention was provided aboard the *Cole* prior to their departure.

Ongoing consultation

The team leader met with the *Cole* Commanding Officer and Executive Officer at the start and finish of each day. As a psychiatrist, he also provided medical consultation to the *Cole*'s Independent Duty Corpsman, a senior enlisted member with some training in physician assistant skills (the ship's 'doc'), and supplemented the ship's pharmacy with benzodiazepines brought from the hospital. A brief course of medication was prescribed to sailors experiencing severe acute insomnia and was reportedly of great benefit. The team leader maintained communication with the task force medical leadership but did not establish any method of providing detailed information on the team's interventions. The team leader was able to obtain a cellular telephone, which he used to provide ongoing briefings to the Commanding Officer of Naval Hospital Sigonella and the Leader of the Portsmouth Naval Hospital SPRINT, who would assume stress management duties upon the *Cole* crew's return to nearby Norfolk.

Nature of findings

SPRINT team members estimated the following exposure information from their interactions with the survivors. Approximately 30 percent were in direct danger of death or serious injury, 100 percent knew someone who was killed or seriously injured in the attack, and nearly 100 percent perceived an ongoing threat of additional attacks throughout the course of the team's interventions. At least one-third of the crew were experiencing overt psychological responses to the attack and its aftermath. These responses included hypervigilance, startle, insomnia, irritability, numbing, and mood lability. All were deemed to be consistent with a normal response to a combat scenario.

After one week the crew's responses were becoming less overt and there were fewer requests for individual assistance. The crew turned their attention more and more to mission-oriented tasks. The ship's assigned chaplain had been serving aboard another ship at the time of the blast; he returned to the *Cole* on October 19. Upon arrival he was apprised of the team's observations and interventions and he reintegrated with the crew. He was warmly received. Once the last body was sent ashore, he planned and conducted a memorial service. The team was present but maintained a low profile.

Termination of team operations

The team determined that a summary debriefing would not be appropriate so long as the crew remained aboard the ship in the port of Aden. The team leader raised this issue with the Commanding Officer and Executive Officer who agreed that such an intervention should not take place until they had arrived at a location they perceived as safe. With a chaplain, Independent Duty Corpsman, and well-prepared leadership present to address continued stress management needs, the team sought a timely conclusion to its presence, thereby sending a strong message to the crew of their own inherent capacities. The Task Force Commander and the *Cole* Commanding Officer asked that the team leader remain aboard to provide ongoing command consultation. The remainder of the team returned to Sigonella on October 24. They conducted their own debriefing upon their return.

Completion and termination of command consultation

With the consent of the Commanding Officer, the team leader conducted an informal stress survey aboard the *Cole* 2 weeks after the attack. The results demonstrated a significant continuing level of stress. The 'show of hands' method of collecting data probably underestimated the actual prevalence. In light of the continued stress responses and particularly the prevalence of an avoidance response, the team leader proposed that the crew be given an opportunity to tour the damaged areas of the ship. The Commanding Officer agreed and assigned Division Officers to make arrangements for all crew members who wished to take part. A member of the Engineering Department led the tours. He described the mechanism of the blast damage, where the deceased had been recovered, and the methods by which the stateside shipyard would repair the damage.

The team leader worked closely with the ship's chaplain during this largely consultative period. Both he and the chaplain continued to provide support to identified crew members and to advise the ship's leadership. The majority of the *Cole* crew would travel by air to the ship's home port in Norfolk, Virginia. Once the ship was towed out of the harbor the chaplain and the SPRINT team leader accompanied the crew on its trip to Rhine Main Airbase in Germany, then on to Norfolk Naval Station. One hour before landing in Norfolk, the team leader used the plane's public address system to provide the crew with a final stress management briefing, covering education on expected stress symptoms, encouragement to make use of social support and available professional services, discouragement of alcohol use, and anticipation of follow-up monitoring.

Ongoing assessment and health surveillance

One month after their return from Yemen, the crew completed a questionnaire gauging their residual anxiety. Standardized measures included the Impact of Events Scale (IES) and the Beck Depression Inventory (BDI). One month after that, the IES and BDI were repeated and those scoring in the clinical range were referred for a psychiatric assessment. These data are in the process of analysis.

Conclusions

The US Navy and its Medical Department respond quickly to natural and human-made disasters around the world. Each disaster poses unique problems in the delivery of supportive services to survivors. Situational assessment and defining the mission are the first steps. Logistical considerations and establishing a role as a consultant are often the most challenging tasks when working with groups not familiar with the role of mental health following disasters. Without command support, survivors often tend to focus on the mission at the expense of their own well-being. Attention must be given to housing, sleep, hydration, hygiene, food, and safety. Interventions, and especially group interventions, work best among pre-established groups, routinely found in military settings. Response teams need to be flexible in adjusting their services to match the groups and individuals being served, as well as the current operational tempo. Group self-reliance and natural supports are primary tools in the mental health response.

REFERENCES

Dinneen, M. P., Pentzien, R. J. and Mateczun, J. M. (1994). Stress and coping with the trauma of war in the Persian Gulf: The hospital ship USNS *Comfort*. In *Individual and Community Responses to Trauma and Disaster: The Structure of Human Chaos*, eds. R. J. Ursano, B. G. McCaughey and C. S. Fullerton, pp. 306–329. New York: Cambridge University Press.

Goldberg, G. M., Lefever, B. E. and True, P. K. (1996). *The U.S. Navy Special Psychiatric Rapid Intervention Team: Past, Present and Future*. Portsmouth, VA: Portsmouth Naval Medical Center.

Hooper, R. R. (1993). United States hospital ships: A proposal for their use in humanitarian missions. *Journal of the American Medical Association*, **270**, 621–623.

McCaughey, B. G. (1985). US Coast Guard collision at sea. *Journal of Human Stress*, Spring, 42–46.

McCaughey, B. G. (1987). US Naval Special Psychiatric Rapid Intervention Team (SPRINT). *Military Medicine*, **152**, 133–135.

Moore, G. R. and Dembert, M. L. (1987). The military as a provider of public health services after a disaster. *Military Medicine*, **152**, 303–307.

Pentzien, R. J. and Barry, P. D. (1992). Sister services first to aid: USNS *Mercy* (T-AH 19) and USNS *Comfort* (T-AH 20) deploy to the Persian Gulf. *Journal of the US Army Medical Department*, **92**, 13–16.

Slusarcick, A. L., Ursano, R. J., Fullerton, C. S. and Dinneen, M. P. (1999a). Life events in health care providers before and during Persian Gulf War deployment: The USNS *Comfort*. *Military Medicine*, **164**, 75–82.

Slusarcick, A. L., Ursano, R. J., Fullerton, C. S. and Dinneen, M. P. (1999b). Stress and coping in male and female health care providers during the Persian Gulf War: The USNS *Comfort* hospital ship. *Military Medicine*, **164**, 166–73.

Part III

Interventions in disaster and terrorism

7

Applications from previous disaster research to guide mental health interventions after the September 11 attacks

Carol S. North and Elizabeth Terry Westerhaus

Introduction

Tragically, there will probably always be another disaster. To be prepared, we must learn from past events and apply what we have learned to the next time.

Never has there been a disaster like the September 11, 2001 terrorist attacks. Separating this event from other disasters are its unprecedented scope and magnitude, as well as other unique characteristics. The September 11 home strike into the nerve center of the United States and the very symbols of our country constituted new external threats to American security nation-wide. Media coverage brought the immediacy of the evolving attacks directly into our homes in living Technicolor with repeated images of planes crashing into World Trade Center towers.

The September 11 incidents may be expected to generate unparalleled mental health consequences among the victims who escaped with their lives. Widespread mental health effects may also ripple through the population, distributed far more widely than in any disaster in American history. The existing mental health system does not have the necessary resources in place to meet the volume of psychiatric disorders anticipated.

We look to disaster research literature to guide the development of mental health interventions after these profoundly tragic events. We can only extrapolate from previous experience and the existing literature to anticipate mental health effects and direct programs to help the affected populations.

Posttraumatic stress disorder (PTSD) is the classic diagnostic consideration in populations afflicted by disasters. Most of what we know about PTSD, however, derives from studies of other populations affected by other kinds of traumatic events. Studies of combat veteran populations are a large source of existing data on

PTSD (Brewin *et al.*, 2000). Community victims of episodic accidents and violent crime, typically studied in treatment settings or among volunteers solicited from advertisements, provided another important source of information about PTSD. The field of research on disasters has advanced in recent years, but its contribution remains relatively small compared to the larger existing literature on PTSD studied in other settings.

It is likely that PTSD following disasters represents a different phenomenon than the presentations of PTSD we have observed in populations of combat veterans (Brewin *et al.*, 2000) and victims of sporadic violence in the community. Characteristics of the population that put them at risk for PTSD are many of the same ones that generate risk for adverse outcomes, including PTSD (Breslau *et al.*, 1995, 1998; Breslau, 1998). For the most part, disasters represent equal-opportunity events that select people randomly. Floods are an important exception striking low-income populations who choose to live on flood plains because the land is affordable. Therefore, disasters provide opportunities to study the effects of trauma in its purest representation. Data on mental health effects from studies of disasters are needed to guide the field in the wake of the tragedies of the September 11 terrorist attacks.

This chapter will synthesize available data from existing research to anticipate the mental health effects of the September 11 disasters and suggest directions for intervention based on the existing knowledge base, relying especially on experience in the Oklahoma City bombing. The chapter will delineate different effects on various populations, describe the expected course of PTSD over time based on findings from other studies, and provide data-guided principles for intervention.

Identifying affected populations

Intensity of disaster exposure can be conceptualized as a series of concentric circles spreading out from the epicenter of the point of direct impact. After disasters, psychiatric disorders cluster most densely at the disaster epicenter and diminish outward, generating ever smaller waves as ripple effects reach the periphery. Those injured and others who fled for their lives from the burning World Trade Center towers and the Pentagon can be anticipated to suffer the most prevalent and severe mental health consequences including PTSD and comorbid disorders, most commonly major depression. The thousands of bereaved who lost loved ones in the World Trade Center, the Pentagon, and in the planes that crashed will also be at risk to develop PTSD and, in a proportion of cases, major depression complicating the bereavement process.

Others deeply affected will be the rescue and recovery workers who risked their lives and also lost valued colleagues from among their ranks, especially the approximately 15 000 firefighters of the New York Fire Department who were personally endangered in the collapse of the Twin Towers and who lost more than 300 of their members in the disaster. Other worker groups potentially at risk with significant exposure to the disaster include police, hospital personnel, and Red Cross and mental health volunteers, insurance adjusters, and media personnel. Yet other affected segments of the population may include family and close friends of those who survived the perilous escape from the World Trade Center, people who evacuated from nearby buildings, and schoolchildren located so near the World Trade Center that they had to evacuate.

As the concentric circles spread ever outward toward the periphery in space and time following a disaster, other related psychological effects may emerge. These effects may be evident among businesses in lower Manhattan, especially those closest to the disaster site that were devastated by loss of the physical location of the business or inconvenienced by suspension of business. New York City as a whole may be negatively affected by loss of commerce such as the tourism trade. The ripple effects may further extend to those who witnessed the disaster unfolding from a distance, including people watching the towers collapse from the New Jersey shoreline.

The first requirement of *DSM-IV* criteria for PTSD, known as the 'Stressor A criterion,' dictates that only (1) direct exposure or (2) eyewitness to a traumatic event or (3) secondary exposure through experience of a loved one in the event can result in PTSD. Exposure to a traumatic event through seeing it in a movie or on the television news does not qualify. Therefore, the millions of people across the country who viewed repeated images of the airplane flying into the second World Trade Center tower and the dramatic collapses of the Twin Towers and graphic images of people leaping from the upper levels of the flaming towers will not be diagnosed with PTSD based on this media exposure alone. This is not to say that these images were not distressing, however, or that they could not arouse strong emotional responses and considerable psychological upset. A study of school children 100 miles away from the Oklahoma City bombing two years after the bombing found significant posttraumatic symptoms related to the bombing in 16 percent, reflecting distant effects of disasters on the psychological status of the population (Pfefferbaum *et al.*, 2000).

A Pew poll (Associated Press, 2001) shortly after the terrorist attacks found that seven out of 10 people acknowledged feeling depressed, nearly one in two reported trouble concentrating, and one in three had trouble sleeping. Longstanding assumptions of national safety have apparently been supplanted by a new sense of widespread personal vulnerability. How this may translate into nation-wide psychiatric casualties that could potentially overwhelm the mental health treatment system is unknown.

An overlooked group is the established psychiatric population, especially people being treated in the state mental health systems. Heightened needs for psychiatric care among established patients in the wake of the tragedies may further stress the mental health system.

Subsequent events have further traumatized the population, first in the form of anthrax delivered through the US postal system and then the untimely crash of an American Airlines airplane in Queens, a neighborhood that had experienced significant losses in the World Trade Center attacks. The original catastrophe of September 11 may have primed the population for increased vulnerability to effects of the second and third waves of traumatic events (Ford, 1997). The occurrence of this repetitive traumatization can be expected to complicate assessment of mental health effects as well as application of interventions. The associated economic downturn following the September 11 tragedies can be expected to be followed by the increase in psychiatric problems in the population typically seen in times of economic distress (Bland, 1998).

Risk factors

As discussed above, proximity and intensity of the individual's exposure to a disaster event is a risk factor for PTSD. Following the Oklahoma City bombing, PTSD was statistically associated with the number of injuries sustained in the disaster (North *et al.*, 1999). Although it is intuitive that degree of exposure would predict likelihood of developing PTSD, exposure variables are not routinely predictive of PTSD (Sungur and Kaya, 2001) and may be more predictive of either short-term (McFarlane, 1989) or long-term morbidity (Sungur and Kaya, 2001).

The most robust predictors of PTSD after disasters consistently emerging from disaster studies are female gender and pre-existing psychiatric illness (North *et al.*, 1999) (Table 7.1). Higher rates of PTSD among women compared to men after disasters are not surprising, given the higher rates of anxiety and depressive disorders well documented among general-population women (Blazer *et al.*, 1991; Eaton *et al.*, 1991; Weissman *et al.*, 1991). Researchers have suggested that pre-existing psychiatric illness is most significant among more distantly exposed populations and moving closer to the direct source of the disaster impact finds that relationship diminishes in importance as more and more people with no history of psychiatric illness succumb to psychiatric disorders (Hocking, 1970; Shore *et al.*, 1986; Feinstein and Dolan, 1991; Breslau and Davis, 1992; Smith *et al.*, 1993).

Taking this information into account, it has previously been suggested that disaster mental health efforts to identify psychiatric casualties might improve their efficiency by focusing on the most highly exposed, women, and individuals with prior psychopathology (McFarlane, 1989; Smith *et al.*, 1993). Previous studies have

Table 7.1 Those at higher-risk for PTSD

Persons highly exposed to trauma
Women
Individuals with prior psychopathology

found this strategy successful: in a study of a jet plane crash into a hotel, two-thirds of acute postdisaster psychiatric disorders were identified among survivors with previous psychiatric histories (Smith *et al.*, 1990).

Other studies have identified additional personal predictors of risk for postdisaster psychiatric problems that may include advanced age, lack of education, lower socioeconomic status, and litigation, but these variables do not uniformly provide the predictive impact of gender and pre-existing psychopathology (North, 1995). Some of these other factors may be associated with risk for PTSD only through other variables, such as through confounding of lower educational achievement with female gender found in the study of the Oklahoma City bombing (North *et al.*, 1999).

Assessment of the disaster-affected population

Studies of disasters have reported widely varying rates of PTSD, as low as 2 percent following a volcano eruption (Shore *et al.*, 1986), 4 percent after torrential rain and mudslides (Canino *et al.*, 1990), and 4 to 8 percent following flooding and exposure to dioxin contamination (Smith *et al.*, 1986). Other researchers have reported much higher rates of PTSD: 44 percent after a dam break and flood (Green *et al.*, 1990), 53 percent following bushfires (McFarlane, 1986), and 54 percent following an airplane crash landing (Sloan, 1988).

It is thought that disasters perpetrated by terrorists may produce the most severe mental health consequences of all types of traumatic events (North, 1995). Experience with mental health issues following the bombing in Oklahoma City and other disasters can help disaster workers anticipate the magnitude of mental health problems and the need for treatment. Following the Oklahoma City bombing – the most severe act of terrorism in history at the time – one out of three people in the path of the bomb blast developed full-blown PTSD, and another 10 percent had some other psychiatric disorder, most often major depression (North *et al.*, 1999). The exponentially greater magnitude and consequences of the New York and Pentagon attacks compared to that at Oklahoma City can be expected to deposit significantly more psychiatric casualties in its wake, as well as persistent symptoms in the community.

A useful principle that emerged from research on the Oklahoma City bombing involves recognition that two distinct populations may emerge with different intervention needs (North *et al.*, 1999). An applicable dichotomization of disaster-affected populations is by presence or absence of postdisaster psychiatric disorders that can be used to direct individuals to the most appropriate form of treatment for their needs.

Based on the Oklahoma City bombing findings, those without psychiatric illness after a disaster can be reassured that their disturbing reactions and emotions afterward do not necessarily indicate that the individual is becoming psychologically unraveled or psychiatrically ill, and that their symptoms can be expected to diminish with the healing effects of time. Because the vast majority of individuals directly exposed to disasters report responses such as intrusive memories, difficulties concentrating, and sleep difficulties, these normative experiences can hardly be called symptoms because no disease is present. This experience can be conceptualized as reactions involving normal responses to abnormal events. This kind of psychological upset may be best characterized as *subdiagnostic distress* in recognition of the suffering it generates yet not escalating the reaction to a pathological level.

In contrast, the needs of individuals with PTSD and other psychiatric disorders are best served when they can be identified and triaged for psychiatric treatment. Although some clinicians may wish to resist burdening individuals with a psychiatric diagnosis just because they have problems coping with a catastrophic event they have been unfortunate enough to experience, the potential benefit of recognizing psychiatric disorders and directing people to appropriate treatment that may greatly reduce suffering far exceeds concern over stigma attached to psychiatric labeling.

Research has suggested that people developing psychiatric problems after disasters can be identified early on by certain characteristics and symptom patterns. Findings from the Oklahoma City bombing and the Northridge earthquake (North *et al.*, 1999; McMillen *et al.*, 2000) found that Group C PTSD symptoms of avoidance and numbing were highly predictive of PTSD. In Oklahoma City, 94 percent of those meeting the avoidance and numbing criteria developed the full panoply of symptoms qualifying them for a diagnosis of PTSD. These symptoms also predicted functional disabilities, psychiatric comorbidity, pre-existing psychopathology, treatment seeking, and use of medications and alcohol for coping. Thus, people so traumatized by the disaster that they are emotionally numbed and can cope only by avoiding all reminders of it appear to be at particularly high risk. These findings suggest that individuals with prominent avoidance and numbing symptoms might be effectively targeted for psychiatric interventions. On the other hand, intrusive re-experience (Group B) and hyperarousal (Group D) symptoms in the absence of avoidance and numbing did not predict any of the above associations. Intrusion and hyperarousal symptoms alone, experienced by the vast majority of the survivors, were like noise in the system – creating a roar initially but not amounting to much in the long run.

The Oklahoma City bombing study further found that psychiatric comorbidity identified the most severe PTSD and cases with the greatest functional disability. Comorbidity thus served as a marker of severity and impairment complicating cases of PTSD. Therefore, it is important to perform a full diagnostic assessment, not stopping once the diagnosis of PTSD is elicited.

In the Oklahoma City study, the majority of PTSD cases occurred in the presence of an additional psychiatric disorder, most often major depression. Major depression is the signature diagnosis for treatment efficacy in psychiatric practice, and overlooking it will necessarily miss significant opportunities to reduce morbidity of this eminently treatable disorder.

Researchers have also described personality disorders as important predictors of PTSD (Southwick *et al.*, 1993). It is intuitive that predispositional personality characteristics would greatly affect people's ability to assimilate the experience and heal. Psychiatric assessment should not stop with Axis I disorders. Clinicians are cautioned, however, that in the short term, behaviors in the context of extreme situations and other psychopathology should be considered as potentially transient responses rather than features of personality traits. Observation over time and gathering additional information about the individual's predisaster social history can help tease out the origins of the behaviors.

Although self-medication with drugs and alcohol is a potential concern after traumatic events, the Oklahoma City bombing study demonstrated no new cases of drug and alcohol abuse materializing after disasters, and no studies have documented increased postdisaster substance use disorders. However, disasters represent opportunities to screen populations for substance abuse problems along with other psychiatric issues and bring people to treatment who otherwise might not be identified and therefore not interface with opportunities for treatment.

Expected course

In Oklahoma City, three-fourths of people in the direct path of the bomb blast who developed PTSD reported its onset as occurring the same day as the bombing (North *et al.*, 1999). By 1 week, 94 percent of those destined to have PTSD were already symptomatic, and the rate increased to 98 percent in 1 month. There were no delayed PTSD cases as defined by *DSM-IV*'s requirement of 6 months' delay in onset (North *et al.*, 1999). Other disaster research has also failed to identify delayed PTSD (North *et al.*, 1997). An exception was the Buffalo Creek dam break and mudslides in which 11 percent of PTSD cases found were identified as having a delayed onset. This sample was nonrepresentative, however, in being a large group of litigants (Grace *et al.*, 1993). The concept of delayed PTSD may have originated in studies of Vietnam veterans in which 16 percent of post-Vietnam PTSD cases had delayed onset (Helzer *et al.*, 1987). This finding is another indicator that PTSD in other populations such as veterans may be quite different from the PTSD seen following disasters. Although PTSD is not delayed after disasters, seeking treatment is often quite delayed, if it occurs at all (Weisaeth, 2001).

In the general population, studies have shown that PTSD tends toward chronicity (Kessler *et al.*, 1995). The average duration of PTSD in community settings was found to be 3 years, with women having four times the duration of men. In a significant proportion, approximately one-third, chronicity extends to 10 years or more. Among Oklahoma City bombing survivors, all PTSD identified was chronic (lasting at least 3 months per *DSM-IV* definition) (North *et al.*, 1999). In a study of a mass murder episode in Killeen, Texas about one-half of the PTSD cases had remitted by the year following the disaster (North *et al.*, 1997). Few predictors of recovery were identified. In other studies, chronicity has been predicted by the presence of pre-existing psychiatric disorders, neuroticism, a history of early separation from parents in childhood, and family history of anxiety or antisocial behavior (Breslau *et al.*, 1991), as well as litigation (Binder *et al.*, 1991). Among people not developing PTSD, however, healing appears to be much faster, so that despite the wide prevalence of symptoms initially, the majority does not sustain sufficient symptoms over a month's time to meet full PTSD criteria.

The diagnosis of acute stress disorder added to *DSM-IV* has an earlier onset (within 4 weeks of the event) and a shorter duration (only 2 days' to 4 weeks' duration). The utility of this diagnosis has not been convincingly demonstrated and its ability to predict PTSD and other psychopathology is unknown (Ursano *et al.*, 1995). An argument for its utility is that a psychiatric diagnosis is needed before the elapsed month required by *DSM-IV* for meeting criteria for PTSD. The key to the utility of the acute stress disorder diagnosis will lie with the ability of future research to demonstrate associated disability and significant suffering as well as response to treatment. The diagnosis of acute stress disorder shares with PTSD a need for diagnostic validation. This diagnosis based on symptoms that by definition must resolve in 4 weeks or less after a disaster suggests that it may tap normative distress responses of traumatized populations. Diagnostic validation of these disorders will require more effort to demonstrate delineation from other disorders, family transmission, and follow-up studies demonstrating fidelity of the diagnoses over time.

Designing therapeutic interventions

Probably the most helpful principle in planning postdisaster mental health interventions is to start by dichotomizing the population based on identification of psychiatric disorders (especially PTSD). The controversy over treatment may lie in part with failure to consider this dichotomy. The pitfall of approaches that fail to differentiate normal responses from psychiatric illness is application of inappropriate treatment to the needs of the affected. In amorphous nondiagnostic approaches to disaster populations, proponents of treatments based on talking such as psychotherapy and debriefing therapies may advocate for universal application of these interventions without consideration of individual needs. The prominent association of avoidance and numbing symptoms among individuals with PTSD would suggest that therapeutic interventions that require them to relive or think about the event may be traumatizing to the individual not ready to face such material. In this case, debriefing might even be harmful.

Alternatively, provision of psychiatric diagnoses to facilitate psychiatric treatment for all people who seem to be upset by the disaster may inappropriately pathologize the majority with strong emotional responses that are part of normative responses to the most extreme traumatic events and expose them to potentially harmful treatments such as medications that are not indicated.

The vast majority of disaster survivors indicate that the most commonly used method of coping is talking with trusted others about the experience (North *et al.*, 1999). Cognitive processing, making meaning of traumatic life events, and obtaining a perspective of the events in the fabric of the individual's life are part of the healing process. People can be encouraged to reach out for the support of loved ones, the most relied-upon and effective coping tool. Those around them can be encouraged to provide support by offering their presence and engaging in active listening. Even good emotional support, however, does not necessarily preclude or prevent the onset of PTSD in those who may be predisposed (McFarlane, 1989), again emphasizing the importance of assessing the individual's needs in order to apply the right treatment.

The rapidity of onset of PTSD suggests that evaluation of disaster-affected populations can begin soon after the event. Women and people with pre-existing psychiatric disorders should receive especially careful surveillance for PTSD. When prominent avoidance and numbing profiles are identified, individuals should be referred for skilled psychiatric evaluation and treatment. The advent of effective medications for PTSD, combined with psychotherapy, has made this an eminently treatable disorder. Although only sertraline has received FDA approval for a PTSD indication, studies have also provided promising data for other selective serotonin reuptake inhibitor antidepressant agents as well (van der Kolk *et al.*, 1993; Tucker *et al.*, 2001).

Individuals experiencing disturbing intrusive re-experience and hyperarousal responses in the absence of prominent avoidance and numbing may benefit from education and reassurance about their responses. Providing crisis counseling and forums for people to gather and share their experiences, mourn their losses, and begin to process and make meaning of events can facilitate healing. Resumption of normal routines as soon as possible can be encouraged along with maintaining good self-care such as regular nutritional meals, exercise, and avoidance of excesses in alcohol and other habits. Those with established faith and ties to religious communities can be encouraged to tap these resources, which can be especially helpful.

Because posttraumatic disorders often become chronic, mental health resources will need to remain in place to manage the long-term consequences and serve the many who do not seek treatment right away. Applying emergency emotional first aid in the short run only to abandon people in their long-term need will be shortsighted.

Needed resources and other considerations

Research has provided many insights into the psychiatric consequences of disasters. Among the important points learned are that the majority of people do not go on to develop psychiatric disorders after disasters, and most symptoms and strong emotions tend to dissipate with time, reassurance, and support from loved ones. Psychiatric illnesses that develop after disasters are eminently treatable with medications and psychotherapy, and those at risk can be identified early and encouraged to seek treatment.

Just as emergency rooms are quickly overrun with the wounded and dying in the first hours after disasters, existing mental health infrastructures may be overwhelmed in the months ahead. The mental health system will need an infusion of resources to manage the influx of individuals needing services to avoid compromising the already strained resources reserved for those with severe and persistent mental illness.

Tasks ahead include finding people with psychiatric illness, getting them into the treatment system, and directing resources into the mental health system. In order to do this effectively and quickly, it is necessary to identify those at a level of high risk as described above. Public education to overcome the stigma of mental illness will be needed so that people are willing to seek services. Reducing the stigma of mental illness through community education will hopefully encourage those troubled with symptoms to come forward and seek treatment sooner, thus reducing the likelihood of chronicity of illness. Psychiatrists and other mental health professionals specializing in the treatment of disaster victims may make use of the media to educate the public and facilitate community outreach. To identify needs, workers may need to knock on doors and visit employers to locate and encourage those who are reluctant to talk and seek treatment.

Assurance of the availability of appropriate care is needed for people with no insurance coverage and for those whose mental health plans do not provide sufficient coverage for mental health treatment in the wake of this tragedy. This effort should insure that all people affected by this and future disasters receive quality mental health services in a timely fashion. Mental health programs will be needed as soon as possible and should continue into the unforeseen future.

A high level of government commitment and involvement at federal, state, and local levels is critical for accomplishing these tasks. This also includes a collaborative effort between the government and private mental health communities. Employers, particularly in fire and police departments involved in the rescue and recovery operation, can help by providing access to mental health services and time off work to obtain treatment and by ensuring that confidentiality is not violated in procedures for filing medical insurance claims.

Preliminary work suggests that enlistment of the aid of community leaders can help extend the tightly stretched resources of postdisaster periods. Clergy, teachers, employers, and family members can be trained to provide support to those who are distressed, identify individuals needing treatment, and direct them to the appropriate mental health professionals providing services. Treatment is best provided in communities where people live and work. Specialized instruction on identification and management of cases may improve the effectiveness of health care professionals in primary practice with this population (North and Hong, 2000). Psychiatric intervention in the wake of disasters should be implemented through community outreach and focus on identifying high-risk groups, fostering recovery as a community and not just on individual basis, and minimizing perturbance of established social supports and settings (Ursano *et al.*, 1995).

Psychological effects of disasters do not have to be all negative. Despite the numerous negative consequences incurred in disasters, some people are able to see benefit (McMillen *et al.*, 1997; McMillen, 1999). Research shows that victims of traumatic experiences are sometimes led to reorganize their lives, placing new emphasis on the priority of values of family and country and goals perhaps lost before the incident (Ursano *et al.*, 1995). If we do not think to consider positive outcomes, we may miss them altogether.

Conclusions

Amidst all of the suffering and destruction of the September 11 attack, not to be overlooked is people's resilience people after disasters (North, 1995). In spite of the overwhelming prevalence of PTSD symptoms after extreme traumas, the majority of survivors do not become psychiatrically ill. Reassuring these individuals that their symptoms represent normal responses to extreme events, supporting them, and helping them re-establish their balance can go a long way toward helping them cope with such extreme situations. This must be balanced, however, with ability to recognize psychiatric illness and direct it to appropriate sources of intervention.

Unfortunately, the September 11 attacks may be a harbinger of things yet to come. Following a disaster of this scope and magnitude, it will be prudent to invest in organized research conducted with the most careful scientific methodology to help us learn from this experience to ensure a better future. In the midst of our tragedy and suffering, let us not overlook the need to learn more about mental health issues so that next time we will be even more prepared.

REFERENCES

Associated Press (2001). *Poll: Americans Depressed, Sleepless.* September 19, 2001. Retrieved from http://www.msnbc.com/news/631188.asp.

Binder, R. L., Trimble, M. R. and McNiel, D. E. (1991). The course of psychological symptoms after resolution of lawsuits. *American Journal of Psychiatry,* **148**, 1073–1075.

Bland, R. C. (1998). Psychiatry and the burden of mental illness. *Canadian Journal of Psychiatry,* **43**, 801–810.

Blazer, D. G., Hughes, D., George, L. K., Swartz, M. and Boyer, R. (1991). Generalized anxiety disorder. In *Psychiatric Disorders in America: The Epidemiologic Catchment Area Study,* eds. L. N. Robins and D. A. Regier, pp. 180–203. New York: Free Press.

Breslau, N. (1998). Epidemiology of trauma and posttraumatic stress disorder. In *Psychological Trauma,* ed. R. Yehuda, pp. 1–29. Washington, DC: American Psychiatric Press.

Breslau, N. and Davis, G. C. (1992). Posttraumatic stress disorder in an urban population of young adults: Risk factors for chronicity. *American Journal of Psychiatry,* **149**, 671–675.

Breslau, N., Davis, G. C. and Andreski, A. (1995). Risk factors for PTSD-related traumatic events: A prospective analysis. *American Journal of Psychiatry,* **152**, 529–535.

Breslau, N., Davis, G. C., Andreski, P. and Peterson, E. (1991). Traumatic events and posttraumatic stress disorder in an urban population of young adults. *Archives of General Psychiatry,* **48**, 216–222.

Breslau, N., Kessler, R. C., Chilcoat, H. D., *et al.* (1998). Trauma and posttraumatic stress disorder in the community. *Archives of General Psychiatry,* **55**, 626–632.

Brewin, C. R., Andrews, B. and Valentine, J. D. (2000). Meta-analysis of risk factors for posttraumatic stress disorder in trauma-exposed adults. *Journal of Consulting and Clinical Psychiatry,* **68**, 748–766.

Canino, G., Bravo, M., Rubio-Stipec, M. and Woodbury, M. (1990). The impact of disaster on mental health: Prospective and retrospective analyses. *International Journal of Mental Health,* **19**, 51–69.

Eaton, W. W., Dryman, A. and Weissman, M. M. (1991). Panic and phobia. In *Psychiatric Disorders in America: The Epidemiologic Catchment Area Study,* eds. L. N. Robins and D. A. Regier, pp. 115–179. New York: Free Press.

Feinstein, A. and Dolan, R. (1991). Predictors of posttraumatic stress disorder following physical trauma: An examination of the stressor criterion. *Psychological Medicine,* **21**, 85–91.

Ford, C. V. (1997). Somatic symptoms, somatization, and traumatic stress: An overview. *Nordic Journal of Psychiatry*, **51**, 5–13.

Grace, M. C., Green, B. L., Lindy, J. L. and Leonard, A. C. (1993). The Buffalo Creek disaster: A 14-year follow-up. In *International Handbook of Traumatic Stress Syndromes*, eds. J. P. Wilson and B. Raphael, pp. 441–449. New York: Plenum Press.

Green, B. L., Lindy, J. D., Grace, M. C., *et al.* (1990). Buffalo Creek survivors in the second decade: Stability of stress symptoms. *American Journal of Orthopsychiatry*, **60**, 43–54.

Helzer, J. E., Robins, L. N. and McEvoy, L. (1987). Posttraumatic stress disorder in the general population. *New England Journal of Medicine*, **317**, 1630–1634.

Hocking, F. (1970). Psychiatric aspects of extreme environmental stress. *Diseases of the Nervous System*, **31**, 542–545.

Kessler, R. C., Sonnega, A., Bromet, E., Hughes, M. and Nelson, C. B. (1995). Posttraumatic stress disorder in the National Comorbidity Survey. *Archives of General Psychiatry*, **52**, 1048–1060.

McFarlane, A. C. (1986). Posttraumatic morbidity of a disaster: A study of cases presenting for psychiatric treatment. *Journal of Nervous and Mental Disease*, **147**, 4–13.

McFarlane, A. C. (1989). The aetiology of posttraumatic morbidity: Predisposing, precipitating and perpetuating factors. *British Journal of Psychiatry*, **154**, 221–228.

McMillen, J. C. (1999). Better for it: How people benefit from adversity. *Social Work*, **44**, 455–468.

McMillen, J. C., North, C. S. and Smith, E. M. (2000). What parts of PTSD are normal: Intrusion, avoidance, or arousal? Data from the Northridge, California, earthquake. *Journal of Traumatic Stress*, **13**, 57–75.

McMillen, J. C., Smith, E. M. and Fisher, R. H. (1997). Perceived benefit and mental health after three types of disaster. *Journal of Consulting and Clinical Psychiatry*, **6**, 733–739.

North, C. S. (1995). Human response to violent trauma. *Ballière's Clinical Psychiatry*, **1**, 225–245.

North, C. S. and Hong, B. A. (2000). Project C.R.E.S.T.: A new model for mental health intervention after a community disaster. *American Journal of Public Health*, **90**, 1–2.

North, C. S., Nixon, S. J., Shariat, S., *et al.* (1999). Psychiatric disorders among survivors of the Oklahoma City bombing. *Journal of the American Medical Association*, **282**, 755–762.

North, C. S., Smith, E. M. and Spitznagel, E. L. (1997). One-year follow-up of survivors of a mass shooting. *American Journal of Psychiatry*, **154**, 1696–1702.

Pfefferbaum, B., Seale, T. W., McDonald, N. B., *et al.* (2000). Posttraumatic stress two years after the Oklahoma City bombing in youths geographically distant from the explosion. *Psychiatry*, **63**, 358–370.

Shore, J. H., Tatum, E. L. and Vollmer, W. M. (1986). The Mount St. Helens stress response syndrome. In *Disaster Stress Studies: New Methods and Findings*, ed. J. H. Shore, pp. 77–79. Washington, DC: American Psychiatric Press.

Sloan, P. (1988). Posttraumatic stress in survivors of an airplane crash-landing: A clinical and exploratory research intervention. *Journal of Traumatic Stress*, **1**, 211–229.

Smith, E. M., North, C. S., McCool, R. E. and Shea, J. M. (1990). Acute postdisaster psychiatric disorders: Identification of persons at risk. *American Journal of Psychiatry*, **147**, 202–206.

Smith, E. M., North, C. S. and Spitznagel, E. L. (1993). Posttraumatic stress in survivors of three disasters. *Journal of Social Behavior and Personality*, **8**, 353–368.

Smith, E. M., Robins, L. N., Przybeck, T. R., Goldring, E. and Solomon, S. D. (1986). Psychosocial consequences of a disaster. In *Disaster Stress Studies: New Methods and Findings*, ed. J. H. Shore, pp. 49–76. Washington, DC: American Psychiatric Association.

Southwick, S. M., Yehuda, R. and Giller, E. L. (1993). Personality disorders in treatment-seeking combat veterans with posttraumatic stress disorder. *American Journal of Psychiatry*, **150**, 1020–1023.

Sungur, M. and Kaya, B. (2001). The onset and longitudinal course of a man-made post traumatic morbidity: Survivors of the Sivas disaster. *International Journal of Psychiatry in Clinical Practice*, **5**, 195–202.

Tucker P., Zaninelli, R., Yehuda, R., *et al.* (2001). Paroxetine in the treatment of chronic posttraumatic stress disorder: Results of a placebo controlled, flexible-dosage trial. *Journal of Clinical Psychiatry*, **62**, 860–868.

Ursano, R., Fullerton, C. S. and Norwood, A. E. (1995). Psychiatric dimensions of disaster: Patient care, community consultation, and preventive medicine. *Harvard Review of Psychiatry*, **3**, 196–209.

van der Kolk, B. A., Dreyfuss, D., Michaels, M., *et al.* (1993). Fluoxetine in posttraumatic stress disorder. *Journal of Clinical Psychiatry*, **55**, 517–522.

Weisaeth, L. (2001). Acute posttraumatic stress: Nonacceptance of early intervention. *Journal of Clinical Psychiatry*, **62**, 35–40.

Weissman, M. M., Bruce, M. L., Leaf, P. J., Florio, L. P. and Holzer, I. C. (1991). Affective disorders. In *Psychiatric Disorders in America: The Epidemiologic Catchment Area Study*, eds. L. N. Robins and D. A. Regier, pp. 53–80. New York: Free Press.

8

A consultation–liaison psychiatry approach to disaster/terrorism victim assessment and management

James R. Rundell

Introduction

Physicians and mental health professionals involved in disaster/terrorism response planning should understand the importance of considering behavioral symptoms among trauma victims within the context of concurrent medical–surgical assessment and treatment. In addition, having medical or surgical injuries or conditions following a disaster or terrorist attack increases the likelihood a psychiatric condition is also present. This chapter will identify how postdisaster patient triage can incorporate behavioral/psychiatric assessment, merging behavioral and medical approaches in considering the differential diagnosis of common psychiatric syndromes among medical–surgical disaster or terrorism casualties.

Integrating psychiatric and other behavioral considerations into disaster victim medical–surgical triage

Types of terrorism and disaster threats

Disasters include natural disasters as well as human-made disasters such as terrorist attacks with explosives, chemicals, and biological agents. In cases of disaster or terrorism, particularly when the scope of potential casualties could overwhelm local response capabilities, the ability to separate medical–surgical casualties, psychiatric casualties, mixed casualties, and the worried well becomes crucial to targeting aid to the correct patients. The principles of differential diagnosis discussed in this chapter are aimed to be clinically useful across the range of disaster etiologies.

The ATLS® primary and secondary surveys

Since 1980, the American College of Surgeons has taught Advanced Trauma Life Support®, an approach for providing care to people suffering major, life-threatening physical injury. ATLS® is accepted world-wide as a standard for immediate posttrauma care. The underlying concept of ATLS® is simple; the greatest threats to life are treated first – loss of airway, loss of breathing ability, loss of circulating blood volume, and effects of an expanding intracerebral mass (American College of Surgeons, 1997a). The rapid, targeted examination of the patient necessary to identify these life-threatening injuries is called the 'primary survey.' The primary survey is a structured approach to assuring that rescuers and triagers focus on these critical elements first. The victim's airway is checked for obstruction, while taking care to protect the spine and spinal cord. Next, adequate air flow to the lungs is ensured, and provided to the patient by artificial means if needed. Next, blood circulation is assessed, points of hemorrhage addressed, fluids replaced, and cardiac compressions administered if indicated. A brief alertness assessment is made; the patient is described as alert, responsive to verbal stimuli, responsive to painful stimuli, or unresponsive. The more alert the patient, the more reassured the triager is that the individual is stable for the moment. The final step of the primary survey is to completely undress a patient and observe for obvious injury, taking care to prevent hypothermia.

Once the primary survey of a trauma victim is completed, resuscitative efforts are well established, and the patient has stable vital signs, the 'secondary survey' is initiated. The secondary survey (American College of Surgeons, 1997a) is a 'head to toe' evaluation of the trauma patient – each region of the body is systematically examined. Available and relevant aspects of medical history are reviewed at this juncture as well: especially allergies, current medications, significant past illnesses, and events related to the injury.

The 'tertiary' psychiatric survey: early identification of psychiatric casualties

Military psychiatrists stationed in Europe are highly encouraged to have ATLS® training, and are required to maintain current certification in Advanced Cardiac Life Support (ACLS) (American Heart Association, 1997). There is a good case to be made that all psychiatrists likely to participate in disaster or terrorism response should have this training. The history and examination findings collected during the primary and secondary surveys are the very data needed for the differential diagnosis of psychiatric symptoms in the medical–surgical and trauma settings. Psychiatrists who are skilled in or at least understand ATLS® and ACLS concepts can be highly effective in the disaster or emergency room setting when the time comes to evaluate potential victims. First, they have credibility with medical–surgical colleagues because they speak the language inherent in ACLS and ATLS® algorithms and understand the concepts of those two approaches. Credibility with disaster leaders is key to influencing their leadership behaviors (Bartone *et al.*, 1994). Second, they can apply the triage philosophies behind ATLS® and ACLS to the differential diagnosis of neuropsychiatric symptoms and to early identification of psychiatric disaster casualties.

A postdisaster or postterrorism psychiatric screening examination to triage and identify early psychiatric casualties can be thought of as a 'tertiary survey' that focuses on the most common psychiatric sequelae (Ursano and Rundell, 1994; Rundell and Ursano, 1996; Holloway *et al.*, 1997) and those most likely adversely affect medical–surgical outcome. There will be time for a more comprehensive mental health evaluation later, along with debriefings, psychotherapy, and medication evaluations. The screening psychiatric examination of the disaster, terrorism, or trauma victim is easy if the primary and secondary surveys are unremarkable. Psychiatric examination findings in that instance are likely to represent the warning signs of primary psychiatric disorders. However, when there are behavioral signs as well as significant primary and secondary survey findings, differential diagnosis can be difficult, and multiple disorders may be present. Table 8.1 summarizes key principles of psychiatric screening of medical–surgical disaster victims following primary and secondary surveys and medical stabilization.

The mental status examination in critically injured patients

Conducting a good mental status examination in a critically injured patient is a challenge, but it is indispensable for differential diagnosis. First, note the patient's level of consciousness. Next, establish a method of communication. If the patient cannot communicate verbally, have him or her write answers on a tablet. Writing may show spatial disorientation, misspellings, inappropriate repetition of letters (perseveration), and linguistic errors. If a patient is unable to speak or write, use either an eye blink method of communication (one blink for yes, two blinks for no), or have the patient squeeze your finger with his or her hand (one squeeze for yes, two squeezes for no). Phrase questions to allow for a yes or no response (e.g., 'Are you feeling frightened?'). To determine whether a patient is confused, insert nonsense questions, such as 'Do catfish fly?' 'Do beagles yodel?' (Rundell and Wise, 2000). If the patient looks surprised or amused and properly answers the question, a secondary psychiatric disorder (medical or toxic etiology) is not as likely.

Differential diagnosis of psychiatric signs in medical–surgical disaster casualties

Table 8.2 identifies key psychiatric conditions that data obtained from a psychiatric screening survey can help establish a risk level for.

Delirium

In the disaster or terrorism victim with major injuries, volume depletion and metabolic derangements can cause delirium, also known as acute confusional state: clouded consciousness, agitation or diminished responsiveness, and disorientation.

Table 8.1 Screening psychiatric examination of medical–surgical disaster casualties: The 'tertiary survey'

Examination parameter	Finding increases likelihood of:
History	
Physical injuries during traumatic event	Secondary psychiatric disorder,[a] ASD,[b] PTSD,[c] dissociation
Past history of psychiatric illness	That psychiatric illness or condition
Patient is on routine medications	Substance intoxication, substance withdrawal, secondary psychiatric disorder[a]
Received ATLS® or ACLS medications	Secondary psychiatric disorder[a]
Physical findings	
Elevated heart rate, blood pressure	Substance withdrawal, generalized anxiety disorder, panic disorder, PTSD,[c] ASD,[b] secondary psychiatric disorders[a]
Easy startle	PTSD,[c] ASD,[b] generalized anxiety disorder
Lateralizing neurological signs	Head or vertebral column injury, secondary psychiatric disorder[a]
Physical complaints out of proportion to objective findings	Conversion disorder, hypochondriasis, factitious disorder, malingering,[d] undiagnosed physical condition
Mental status examination	
Disoriented	Delirium, secondary psychiatric disorder[a]
Clouded Consciousness	Delirium, secondary psychiatric disorder,[a] substance intoxication, dissociation
Decreased response to verbal or painful stimuli	Delirium, secondary psychiatric disorder,[a] dissociation
Dysarthria	Substance intoxication, head injury
Dysgraphia, dyscalculia	Head injury, delirium
Impaired short-term memory	Head injury, substance intoxication, delirium, generalized anxiety disorder, panic attack
Hallucinations or delusions	Substance intoxication, secondary psychiatric disorder,[a] substance withdrawal, primary psychotic disorder

[a] Psychiatric disorders due to general medical conditions or due to toxins/psychoactive substances.
[b] Acute stress disorder.
[c] Posttraumatic stress disorder.
[d] Malingering is not a psychiatric disorder; it is a legal accusation.

Table 8.2 Differential diagnosis of
psychiatric signs in medical–surgical
disaster casualties

Delirium
Acute stress disorder
Posttraumatic stress disorder
Dissociation
Effects of disaster medications

While medication treatment of the delirious patient can help decrease agitation and
mitigate a safety problem, this is not the ideal management. The medications used
to manage agitation can further complicate medical assessment and can further
complicate an already difficult clinical course. Symptomatic management of the
patient's behavioral problems with sedating medication should be initially reserved
to protect the life or safety of the patient and other patients or staff. Resolution of
the delirium itself should be the primary goal, and requires resolving the metabolic
sequelae of the injury. Common causes of delirium in the trauma victim include hy-
povolemia, hypoxemia, central nervous system mass effect, infection, and adverse
effects of ATLS® and ACLS medications.

Acute stress disorder and posttraumatic stress disorder

Acute stress disorder (ASD) and posttraumatic stress disorder (PTSD) do not occur
in a vacuum. When one of these disorders exists, it is highly probable that other
psychiatric conditions exist as well, especially major depressive disorder, panic
disorder, substance use disorder, and generalized anxiety disorder (Ursano *et al.*,
1995). In the aftermath of terrorism or disaster, patients do not divide easily into
those who have physical injuries and those who have psychiatric sequelae. Having
a physical injury makes one at higher risk of, not immune from, ASD or PTSD.

Dissociation

Dissociation is generally underrecognized in the immediate aftermath of a traumatic event or disaster. Among the USS *Cole* casualties evacuated to Landstuhl
Regional Medical Center in October 2000, dissociation was the most common behavioral response observed (J. R. Rundell, unpublished data). Following a fatal
Amtrak train crash in Silver Spring, Maryland in February 1996, the author lived
nearby and was a first responder. At least four of the first 12 initial casualties brought
to a hastily arranged medical triage area initially labeled as 'urgent' casualties because of apparent unresponsiveness were later found to simply be dissociating.

Their misidentification as potential head injury patients resulted in misdirected rescue resources early in a mass casualty situation with heavy demands on local rescue resources.

Dissociation may adaptive in the immediate aftermath of a trauma – dissociating may prevent the eruption of intolerable affects or the unleashing of potentially dangerous impulses or behaviors (e.g., to flee the scene). It is easy to confuse dissociation and diminished neurological responsiveness. A key role of a psychiatrist in the immediate aftermath of a disaster, while primary and secondary surveys are occurring, can be to help identify dissociation. Gently tap the patient on the shoulder and ask if there is anything they need and do they know where they are/what day it is. Watch for a muted but appropriate response in a dissociating person; this indicates his or her level of consciousness and orientation is grossly intact. Identifying otherwise uninjured disaster victims who are simply dissociating frees up scarce evaluation and treatment resources for other emergency patients. If dissociation subsequently becomes frequent, ongoing, and disabling, it may then be formally diagnosed as a psychiatric disorder – dissociative disorder. Serial examinations of the patient can help differentiate adaptive dissociation from dissociative disorder.

Effects of disaster medications

A mainstay of managing patients under ATLS® and ACLS paradigms are medications, many of which can cause neuropsychiatric or autonomic symptoms. It is important to find out what medications an injured patient has received, in what amounts, over what time period. Agents such as intravenous fluids (water), epinephrine, lidocaine, atropine, sedatives, nitroglycerin, and morphine are commonly used and have significant psychiatric or autonomic effects. These can resemble primary psychiatric disorders. For example atropine causes significant anxiety and anticholinergic effects. Epinephrine causes blood pressure and heart rate elevations, and causes patients to feel anxious or panicky. Morphine causes sedation and impairs orientation and responsiveness.

It is also important to know what substances a patient has *not* been exposed to. Following a faked chemical or biological agent threat, there may be a large number of individuals who fear they have been exposed and will present with realistic symptoms based on their knowledge of the alleged agent and vital sign abnormalities produced by anxiety/fear (Fullerton *et al.*, 1996). To minimize the effects of mass hysteria, disaster leaders need accurate information from investigating authorities, as soon as it can be provided, along with a preplanned public information campaign.

Clinical issues in medical–surgical casualties

The main clinical issues in medical–surgical casualties are shown in Table 8.3.

Table 8.3 Clinical issues in medical–surgical casualties

Burn patients
Loss of body parts and functions
Disfigurement and body image
Guilt
Grief
Dead and dying
Heroes in hospitals

Burn patients

During the first 24–72 hours after a severe burn, there is typically a brief period of initial lucidity, during which patients usually are told their prognosis. After that, between 30 percent and 70 percent of hospitalized severe burn patients develop delirium, presumably caused by biologic stress and burn-induced metabolic disturbances (Rundell and Wise, 2000). Watch closely for substance withdrawal syndromes; unfortunately, the time courses for most withdrawal syndromes coincide with the critical periods of burn patients' medical courses. Substance withdrawal can greatly complicate medical care if not managed early and aggressively.

Strongly consider the possibility of a medically induced secondary mood syndrome when burn patients appear depressed (Pasnau *et al.*, 1999). Burn patients lose water at a rate several times faster than normal; hypovolemic shock is common. Following the shock phase is a period of intense catabolism and negative nitrogen balance. The usual anorexia, weight loss, exhaustion, and lassitude of this period may lead unsuspecting clinicians to diagnose primary depression.

Pain is a continuing and critical issue for the burn patient; it becomes especially important during dressing changes and debridement. Narcotics are the drugs of choice for treating acute burn pains – this is not the time to worry about addiction. Dressing changes often require preemptive analgesia.

Losses of body parts and functions

The larger the disaster or terrorist event, the higher the probability that medical–surgical needs will outstrip available resources, particularly in the crucial 'golden hour' following an event. This means that there will be a number of victims who have lost body parts and functions that might have been salvaged if the disaster had been on a smaller scale. For example, victims who might have received early comprehensive intervention at a trauma center following a car accident might be triaged into a less emergent category and attended to much later following a large train accident. This can become an important psychotherapy issue after the initial survival crisis, when inevitable 'what if' and 'if only' thoughts emerge. When there is acute vision loss, there is a high risk for delirium, psychosis, and dissociation.

Disfigurement and body image

Facial disfigurement and facial burns usually cause more psychological difficulty than injuries and burns to other body areas. Give patients honest explanations and prognoses, but do not force a patient to view a deformity until ready; he or she may choose to wait several days or even weeks before looking in a mirror. Longer-term individual or group psychotherapy is sometimes required to help severely injured or burned patients adjust to permanent disfigurement and changes in body image. In one study, 35.3 percent of burn patients met criteria for PTSD at 2 months, 40 percent met the criteria at 6 months, and 45.2 percent met the criteria at 12 months postinjury (Perry *et al.*, 1992).

Guilt and grief

It is a rare disaster or terrorist event where bereaved families are not offered a great deal of grief counseling or therapy. However, survivors and their families will also have to face important grief and guilt issues – particularly over losses of body parts and body functions. Having a serious injury doesn't make one immune from the survivor guilt experienced by those disaster victims who walk away uninjured. Unassuaged survivor guilt may complicate and slow psychotherapy aimed at body image and disfigurement issues. There also may be secondary effects among surviving children of victims of terrorist events or other disasters.

The dead and the dying

It is often easy in a busy postdisaster setting to ignore those individuals who are 'expectant.' It is a fact that people die in disasters, and sometimes not instantly – avoid avoiding them. The dead deserve a respectful transition from disaster scene to family funeral director. When resources are available, a great deal can be done to ease the suffering of disaster victims who are dying (Shuster *et al.*, 1999; Wiener *et al.*, 1999). The dying patient is generally comfortable talking about death. It is usually the family, and sometimes the disaster management team, who are reluctant to engage in such conversations. Don't underestimate the importance of religious faith and the belief in an afterlife in dying patients. Discuss 'Do not resuscitate' orders, wills, and comfort measures early.

In a postdisaster hospital or hospice setting, depression is common. The usefulness of antidepressant medications is limited by the several weeks needed for the agents to be effective. The threat of impending death can also obviously cause a great deal of anxiety. If an individual does not mention fears of dying, inquire either indirectly (e.g., 'You look scared. How are you doing?') or inquire directly (e.g., 'Are you worried that you may die?'). If death is imminent, ask the patient 'What frightens you the most about dying?' Three common fears are abandonment, uncontrollable pain, and shortness of breath (Cassem, 1991). Therapists should not be afraid to speak the unspeakable or confirm reality (Blacher, 1987). Anti-anxiety medications are very effective for dying patients if symptomatic or disabling anxiety persists after psychological support and the opportunity for abreaction is provided (Rundell and Wise, 2000). Benzodiazepines, however, can also result in lethargy and/or confusion.

Heroes in hospitals

Being a hero presents unique psychological challenges. Released prisoners of war, disaster victims who saved others' lives, and rescue personnel who went beyond the efforts of their peers frequently become public heroes. A recent example is the attention given to injured firefighters and policemen who responded to the World Trade Center terrorism event. The hero must meet expectations of adoring audiences and communities. They must grin when they might want to cry. They must avoid or be extremely cautious in how they publicly discuss their own survivor guilt and grief. Heroes' families may insist on special treatment for themselves and their hero relatives. Medical personnel may, with the best of intentions, set up scenarios which make heroes' own postdisaster psychological recoveries more problematic.

Case example

This author, in many years of consultation–liaison psychiatry experience, has only witnessed one case of iatrogenically induced drug addiction, where the medical team itself was primarily responsible for a drug dependence disorder. The nursing staff on a 'VIP' ward continued to offer round-the-clock narcotic analgesics to a hospitalized war hero with minor injuries who actually no longer complained of nociceptive pain. The hero continued to accept the opiate analgesic because it helped relieve his psychological pain, guilt, and suffering. After an attending physician realized the patient now had opiate withdrawal signs, he sought psychiatric consultation. The VIP ward team had to be re-educated in the art of managing heroes, who are at least as vulnerable to psychological regression as any other type of hospitalized patient.

Hospitalized heroes become the centers of politician, press, and busybody attention. Then when the public's short attention span wanders to other topics, they must become regular people again. This dizzying rise and steep fall need to be addressed in psychotherapy. Preventing posttraumatic psychiatric syndromes in these unique individuals requires that they be protected from overstimulation during the immediate postdisaster period. Dedicated and jealously protected individual 'quiet time' is one way to achieve this. Hospitalized heroes' real achievements should be acknowledged and rewarded, but pampering and overinflating achievements increases the likelihood of psychological 'crash and burn.' Beware the overuse of analgesic or sedative–hypnotic medications.

Medico-legal considerations

Informed consent

In general, informed consent requires an informed patient (i.e., an informed patient can understand the information provided, and is capable of making a reasoned judgment about the treatment or procedure). However, in a medical emergency or in a mass disaster or terrorism setting, when a physician administers appropriate treatment in a medically emergent situation where the patient or other people are endangered, and it has proven impossible to obtain either the patient's consent or that of someone authorized to provide consent for the patient, the law typically 'presumes' that consent is granted (Simon, 1999). When a nonemergency patient does not have the capacity to provide consent, it is obtained from a substitute decision-maker, normally the next of kin when available (Howe, 1988).

Rejection of resuscitative treatment

A competent patient has the right to reject or insist upon resuscitative treatment (Miles *et al.*, 1982). That right is rarely overruled (Simon, 1999). One exception is when the rights of a spouse or child are considered more important than the patient's decision (Miles *et al.*, 1982). If a patient has a major psychiatric disorder such as major depressive disorder and rejects resuscitation because death is sought as an 'appropriate deserved' outcome, the patient is generally considered incompetent (Simon, 1999).

Scope of practice, standards of care, and negligence

Any psychiatrist, but particularly those active in disaster management and response teams, may find himself or herself at a disaster or terrorism scene. Though a physician happening upon a disaster or terrorism scene is not legally required to undertake rescue (American College of Surgeons, 1997b), ethical and moral obligations cause most physicians to do so. Once engaged in a rescue or disaster management operation, a physician *is* under a legal duty to act in accordance with recognized standards of care. For a disaster victim, these considerations can be complex, and are determined by the nature of the medical injuries and the resources available to the clinician. A psychiatrist who engages, for example, in rescue practices of ATLS® is held to the standard as to 'what a reasonably competent ATLS® doctor would do under the circumstances of a particular case' (American College of Surgeons,

1997b). Because psychiatrists in the disaster management planning or operations communities are physicians and face the likelihood of being part of a disaster or emergency response, they should strongly consider completing ATLS$^®$ and ACLS training.

Fortunately, 'Good Samaritan' laws exist in every state. The potential for a successful malpractice suit against a physician responding to a disaster or accident is almost zero, unless the physician performs in a 'grossly or shockingly negligent manner' (American College of Surgeons, 1997b). An example of gross negligence would be moving the neck and head of a trauma victim around who has obvious head or neck injuries, a key consideration emphasized in virtually every portion of ATLS$^®$ training. There are four legal elements needed by a court to demonstrate negligence: a standard of care exists, the standard has been breached, the breach results in physical injury, and the breach of standard directly caused the injury (American College of Surgeons, 1997b).

Special issues of chemical and biological terrorism threats

Recognition of chemical and biological attacks

Biological warfare is not new. Since antiquity, biological and chemical agents have been used to contaminate sources of water and food, or to cause uncontrollable diseases among populations (Christopher *et al.*, 1997). In recent decades, technical capabilities of those who would use chemical or biological agents of terror have surged. While there is ample recent evidence that explosive devices can cause considerable death and destruction, an incident of chemical or biological terrorism could potentially generate tens of thousands of casualties requiring prompt medical attention. The news or rumor of a chemical or biological attack could also generate tens of thousands of people who fear they have been exposed who could rapidly overwhelm local medical resources. Local and national level response effectiveness depends as much or more on effective public education and public health efforts as on individual medical treatments. Because the signs and symptoms of chemical and biological attacks can be nonspecific and mimic neuropsychiatric syndromes, differential diagnosis by skilled clinicians may be crucial to effective triage of large populations.

Chemical and biological attacks could unfold in similar ways, known to authorities as they unfold, requiring well-defined emergency responses by local, state, or national authorities. However, it is also possible that a biological attack could unfold as the secret release of a biological agent into food, water, or air. A successful covert attack would go unnoticed until the clinical syndrome presents and it is too late for effective prevention or intervention. This contingency requires that public health officials have the ability to rapidly detect unusual disease outbreaks and begin prompt treatment of large numbers of exposed individuals (Tucker, 1997).

Agents of biological terrorism

Bacteria, viruses, or toxins of animal origin may be used as biological warfare or terrorism agents (Franz *et al.*, 1997). Examples include *Bacillus anthracis* (anthrax), botulism toxin, *Yersinia pestis* (plague), staphylococcal enterotoxin B (SEB), Venezuelan equine encephalitis (VEE) virus, and smallpox. These agents can be dispersed in aerosols, as food or water contaminants, or via the skin or mucous membranes. Given low wind speed and turbulence, aerosol administration is the most effective employment mechanism.

Anthrax has received a great deal of publicity and attention as a realistic threat for terrorists interested in biological agents. A biological attack with anthrax spores would most likely occur by aerosol delivery. Initially after inhalation there may be a preliminary (prodromal) syndrome characterized by fever, malaise, and fatigue. This prodrome may be followed by temporary improvement for two or three days or may progress directly to severe respiratory distress with shortness of breath and hypoxia. Death usually follows in 24 to 36 hours (Franz *et al.*, 1997). Once symptoms of anthrax appear, treatment is almost variably ineffective. Unfortunately, except for high fever, the symptoms of the prodrome of anthrax infection are nonspecific. The physical effects of *fear* of exposure may be the same as early physical effects of actual exposure (malaise, fatigue, anxiety). Presence or absence of fever becomes an early differentiator of those exposed and those not exposed but fearful they may have been. Obviously, public information and a calm, reasoned approach by health and political authorities in the context of threatened or potential anthrax attack is important to prevent the health care system from being overwhelmed early after rumors of a potential attack.

Community responses to terrorist attacks

There are a number of reasons and motivations for biological and chemical terrorism (Stern, 1999). They include attracting attention to the terrorists' cause, aiming to disrupt economic infrastructures, belief in the need for a cleansing apocalypse, exacting revenge, creating chaos, creating an aura of divine retribution, and copycat phenomena. The most likely perpetrators include religiously motivated groups, antigovernment forces within nations, and insurgency groups without access to conventional military technology.

Preparing effective public health, individual health, and population management strategies is crucial to managing a potential biological or chemical terrorist attack. Medical planners should assure that skilled psychiatrists or other trained clinicians are available at triage and treatment areas to rapidly assist in identifying individuals who lack specific evidence of exposure, but exhibit clear signs of anxiety and dissociative conditions, so that precious specific medical treatments can be focused on individuals with higher likelihood of toxic exposure.

Tucker (1997) recommends a number of proactive actions that planners can make to enhance response to chemical and biological terrorism. First, federal agencies should elaborate detailed coordination plans. Second, public information campaigns should be prepared in advance of a terrorist incident, not in the midst of crisis. Third, governments should distribute detection equipment for first responders such as firefighters and policemen. Fourth, early warning detection systems should be established, including close monitoring for suspicious outbreaks of disease. Finally, governmental agencies should stockpile necessary medical equipment, nerve agent antidotes, and antibiotic/antiviral medications in high-threat areas.

Conclusion

When psychiatric signs and symptoms confuse or coexist with medical–surgical injuries and conditions, psychiatric consultation early in the triage and management process can ensure more timely, accurate, efficacious, and cost-effective management of disaster or terrorism victims. Psychiatrists can increase their potential effectiveness in the disaster arena by taking ACLS and ATLS® courses, and using the programs' algorithm-based concepts to guide their own assessment and management of disaster victims.

REFERENCES

American College of Surgeons (1997a). Initial assessment and management. In *Advanced Trauma Life Support*® *for Doctors: Student Course Manual*, pp. 23–58. Chicago, IL: American College of Surgeons.

American College of Surgeons (1997b). ATLS® and the law. In *Advanced Trauma Life Support*® *for Doctors: Student Course Manual*, pp. 419–432. Chicago, IL: American College of Surgeons.

American Heart Association (1997). *Advanced Cardiac Life Support*. Dallas, TX: American Heart Association.

Bartone, P. T., Wright, K. M. and Radke, A. (1994). Psychiatric effects of disaster in the military community. In *Military Psychiatry: Preparing in Peace for War*, eds. F. D. Jones, L. R. Sparacino, V. L. Wilcox and J. M. Rothberg, pp. 279–291. Washington, DC: TMM Publications.

Blacher, R. (1987). Brief psychotherapeutic intervention for the surgical patient. In *The Psychological Experience of Surgery*, ed. R. S. Blacher, pp. 207–220. New York: John Wiley and Sons.

Cassem, N. H. (1991). The dying patient. In *Massachusetts General Hospital Handbook of General Hospital Psychiatry*, 3rd edn, ed. N. H. Cassem, pp. 343–371. St Louis, MO: Mosby Year Book.

Christopher, G. W., Cieslak, T. J., Pavlin, J. A. and Eitzen, E. M., Jr (1997). Biological warfare: A historical perspective. *Journal of the American Medical Association*, **278**, 412–417.

Franz, D. R., Jahrling, P. B. and Friedlander, A. M. (1997). Clinical recognition and management of patients exposed to biological warfare agents. *Journal of the American Medical Association*, **278**, 399–411.

Fullerton, C. S., Brandt, G. T. and Ursano, R. J. (1996). Chemical and biological weapons: Silent agents of terror. In *Emotional Aftermath of the Persian Gulf War*, eds. R. J. Ursano and A. E. Norwood, pp. 111–142. Washington, DC: American Psychiatric Press.

Holloway, H. C., Norwood, A. E., Fullerton, C. S., Engel, C. C. and Ursano, R. J. (1997). The threat of biological weapons: Prophylaxis and mitigation of psychological and social consequences. *Journal of the American Medical Association*, **278**, 425–427.

Howe, E. G. (1988). Forensic issues in critical care medicine. In *Problems in Critical Care*, ed. M. G. Wise, pp. 171–187. Philadelphia, PA: JB Lippincott.

Miles, S. H., Cranford, R. and Schultz, A. L. (1982). The do-not-resuscitate order in a teaching hospital: Considerations and a suggested policy. *Annals of Internal Medicine*, **96**, 660–664.

Pasnau, R. O., Fawzy, F. I., Skotzko, C. E., *et al.* (1999). Surgery and surgical subspecialties. In *Essentials of Consultation–Liaison Psychiatry*, eds. J. R. Rundell and M. G. Wise, pp. 307–324. Washington, DC: American Psychiatric Press.

Perry, S. W., Difede, J., Musngi, G., Frances, A. J. and Jacobsberg, L. (1992). Predictors of post-traumatic stress disorder after burn injury. *American Journal of Psychiatry*, **149**, 931–935.

Rundell, J. R. and Wise, M. G. (2000). Special consultation–liaison settings and situations. In *Concise Guide to Consultation–Liaison Psychiatry*, 3rd edn, eds. J. R. Rundell and M. G. Wise, pp. 269–302. Washington, DC: American Psychiatric Press.

Rundell, J. R. and Ursano, R. J. (1996). Psychiatric responses to war trauma. In *Emotional Aftermath of the Persian Gulf War*, eds. R. J. Ursano and A. E. Norwood, pp. 43–82. Washington, DC: American Psychiatric Press.

Shuster, J. L., Breitbart, W. and Chochinov, H. M. (1999). Psychiatric aspects of excellent end-of-life care. *Psychosomatic*, **40**, 1–4.

Simon, R. I. (1999). Legal and ethical issues. In *Essentials of Consultation–Liaison Psychiatry*, eds. J. R. Rundell and M. G. Wise, pp. 63–80. Washington, DC: American Psychiatric Press.

Stern, J. (1999). The prospect of domestic bioterrorism. *Emerging Infectious Diseases*, **5**, 517–522.

Tucker, J. B. (1997). National health and medical services response to incidents of chemical and biological terrorism. *Journal of the American Medical Association*, **278**, 362–368.

Ursano, R. J. and Rundell, J. R. (1994) The prisoner of war. In *Military Psychiatry: Preparing in Peace for War*, eds. F. D. Jones, L. R. Sparacino, V. L. Wilcox and J. M. Rothberg, pp. 431–455. Washington, DC: TMM Publications.

Ursano, R. J., Fullerton, C. S. and Norwood, A. E. (1995). Psychiatric dimensions of disaster: Patient care, community consultation, and preventive medicine. *Harvard Review of Psychiatry*, **3**, 196–200.

Wiener, I., Breitbart, W. and Holland, J. (1999). Psychiatric issues in the care of dying patients. In *Essentials of Consultation–Liaison Psychiatry*, eds. J. R. Rundell and M. G. Wise, pp. 435–450. Washington, DC: American Psychiatric Press.

9

The role of screening in the prevention of psychological disorders arising after major trauma: Pros and cons

Simon Wessely

Introduction

In this contribution I will seek to address the question of the role of screening in the prevention of psychological disorders arising after major trauma: pros and cons. I will approach this in two ways – is the role for screening, either before exposure to a potentially traumatic event or events, or soon after the event has taken place? I will use examples from the military for two reasons. First, because whilst it is very difficult indeed in civilian populations ever to be in a position to screen people before exposure to a disaster or seriously adverse event, in the military the un-equivocal association between war and trauma means this is theoretically possible. Second, because much of the literature, such as it is, on screening, comes from the military.

It has long been argued that identifying in advance those who will suffer psychiatric injury as a result of future exposure to traumatic events is a worthwhile objective, for many reasons – military, economic, and humanitarian. Over the last century this has been attempted by the military and medical authorities in many countries. I will therefore begin by discussing the history of such attempts, and then their scientific and epidemiological context.

Screening

Seeking to identify those at risk of developing an adverse outcome, but who have yet to show manifest signs of the particular outcome, involves screening. Over the years a vast research and clinical literature has grown to highlight the basic princi-ples and practices involved. Before discussing the specific case of the military and the prevention of psychiatric injury, it is essential to review these principles. These are straightforward, well understood, and crucial to understanding the general record of failure in screening for psychological vulnerability, and then psychological disorders. They are described in any textbook of screening, public health, or epidemiology (Table 9.1) (Hennekens and Buring, 1987; Muir Gray, 1997; National Screening Committee, 1998).

The first principle concerns the method used to detect those one wishes to identify, which in this situation is most likely to be a questionnaire. This must have certain properties. Technically these are known as sensitivity, specificity, positive predictive value, and negative predictive value. The instrument must detect a substantial proportion of those we wish to detect (those who either have, or will get, the disorder in question) – this is sensitivity. Likewise, it must not detect very many of those who do not have, or will not get, the disorder – this is specificity. Finally, when we are talking about detecting those who have not yet developed the disorder in question, the key statistic here is the positive predictive value – of those who are detected by our program, how many will go on to develop the disorder itself (Rose, 1992).

The second principle is that screening is worthwhile. There must be a benefit to the individual, and to society, from detecting people by this method. Several requirements must therefore be satisfied. First, one only screens for disorders for which proven effective interventions exist and are available. There is no point in screening for disorders that cannot be treated effectively. Likewise, there is little point in screening for disorders that will improve spontaneously. A knowledge of the natural history of the disorder is thus a prerequisite. Screening for conditions in which the natural history is towards recovery is hard to justify on ethical, clinical, and economic grounds. Second, screening must be cost-effective. There is little point in mounting a complex and costly screening program if there is evidence that most people with the disorder are going to be detected by existing methods or services anyway.

All screening carries a risk of harm. As Muir Gray (1997) puts it: 'all screening programmes do harm, some can do good as well.' Those detected as potentially at risk may be exposed to investigations or treatments with side effects. Screening itself has hazards – side effects of the instrument, or increased anxiety about the condition. Those who are identified by the program may not realize, and indeed probably don't realize, they are 'at risk.' Once they learn that they are now at increased risk of an adverse outcome, their behavior may change in many unforeseen ways. They may become more careful or soliticious about their health, or conversely adopt a wide range of risky behaviors – 'because it is going to happen to me anyway.' Their view of themselves as a healthy person has been altered, and their mood and psychological well-being may be adversely effected. There is a wide, extensive, and compelling literature on the adverse psychological consequences of screening (Shaw et al., 1999). For those who are identified as at risk, but actually are not going to develop

Table 9.1 National Screening Committee's criteria for appraising the viability, effectiveness, and appropriateness of a screening programme

---

The condition

The condition should be an important health problem

The epidemiology and natural history of the condition, including development from latent to declared disease, should be adequately understood and there should be a detectable risk factor, disease marker, latent period, or early symptomatic stage

All the cost-effective primary prevention interventions should have been implemented as far as practicable

The test

There should be a simple, safe, precise, and validated screening test

The distribution of test values in the target population should be known and a suitable cutoff level defined and agreed

The test should be acceptable to the population

There should be an agreed policy on the further diagnostic investigation of individuals with a positive test result and on the choices available to those individuals

The treatment

There should be an effective treatment or intervention for patients identified through early detection, with evidence of early treatment leading to better outcomes than late treatment

There should be agreed evidence-based policies covering which individuals should be offered treatment and the appropriate treatment to be offered

Clinical management of the condition and patient outcomes should be optimized by all health care providers prior to participation in a screening program

The screening program

There should be evidence from high-quality randomized controlled trials that the screening program is effective in reducing mortality or morbidity

There should be evidence that the complete screening program (test, diagnostic procedures, treatment/intervention) is clinically, socially, and ethically acceptable to health professionals and the public

The benefit from the screening program should outweigh the physical and psychological harm caused by the test, diagnostic procedures, and treatment

The opportunity cost of the screening program (including testing, diagnosis, and treatment) should be economically balanced in relation to expenditure on medical care as a whole

There should be a plan for managing and monitoring the screening program and an agreed set of quality assurance standards

Adequate staffing and facilities for testing, diagnosis, treatment, and program management should be available prior to the commencement of the screening program

All other options for managing the condition should have been considered (e.g., improving treatment, providing other services)

Source: National Screening Committee (1998).

the disorder (false positives) it will be clear that screening can only a source of harm – the question is how much.

Screening for psychological vulnerability

Background

I will use the example of the military to demonstrate the practical, theoretical, and ethical problems that exist with the otherwise tempting belief that one can use screening to reduce psychological disorder in those who are likely to be exposed to subsequent adversity.

The virtues of a successful screening have been obvious to the military for many years, and are now being advocated as well by many public services organizations such as the police or fire services. Fighting armies usually wish to exclude those who would make poor soldiers. The military, social, and economic costs of attempting to train people who would later prove unequal to the task are clear. Hence starting with the aftermath of World War I and the experiences of the American Army, there is a long history of screening programs.

Some aspects of screening programs have proven successful, so much so that their utility is taken for granted today. At its simplest, all assessment procedures used by all modern military establishments will reject those with physical disabilities that preclude effective military service. Likewise, certain characteristics that are stable, easy to measure, and associated with a high probability of unsuitability for service, such as very low intelligence or psychosis, are also the targets of screening, even if the word 'screening' is rarely used to describe such activities.

However, when it comes to screening for those vulnerable to psychiatric disorder in the event of being exposed to adversity, we encounter major difficulties (Table 9.2), which are summarized as follows:

1. There is considerable uncertainty as to what factors predict vulnerability.
2. These factors are difficult to measure.
3. It is unclear if screening is worthwhile – are psychologically vulnerable people really unsuited for military service?
4. It is unclear if the test is acceptable to the population.
5. There remains uncertainty surrounding the natural history.
6. No consensus exists as to what, if any, is the appropriate treatment for the person, or administrative response for the organization.
7. There may be adverse consequences to the individual of being labeled as psychologically vulnerable or unfit.

Screening in the military: An historical analysis

The high-water mark of screening by the military for psychological disorders and vulnerability to such disorders came in World War II. The impetus however had

Table 9.2 Challenges associated with screening for posttraumatic stress disorder

Uncertainty on what factors predict PTSD vulnerability
Factors are difficult to measure
Unclear if screening is worthwhile
Unclear if test is acceptable to public
Uncertainty surrounding the natural history of psychiatric disorders following trauma
Lack of consensus on appropriate treatment or organizational response
Adverse consequences for individual being labeled as psychologically vulnerable

come from experiences during World War I, or more accurately its aftermath. At the start of World War II the literature was full of warnings about the past, and the need to do things better this time. Reference after reference was made to the immense cost imposed by the large numbers of psychiatrically damaged servicemen after the previous conflict (Baganz, 1940; Davidson, 1940; Porter, 1941; Kiene *et al.*, 1942).

Such warnings were usually linked with a general sense of optimism that the mistakes of the past would not be repeated, and in particular that part of the answer lay in screening programs. Belief in the effectiveness of, and need for, screening had grown during the inter-war period into a firm conviction (Sutton, 1939; Hilman, 1940; Anderson, 1966). A typical quote from a large literature reads: 'If we set up filters against the defective, unstable and potentially neurotic.... We'll go far towards drying up our post war neurotics at source and so lighten the load of the Veteran's Bureau' (Davidon, 1940).

Thus the Americans, in the *Medical Circular Number 1* issued by the Selective Service System (i.e., Draft Board) of November 1940, and the *Circular Number 19* from the Surgeon General's Office in March 1941 made psychiatric screening an essential part of their mass mobilization (Deutsch, 1944).

What happened in practice? The answer was it made little difference. In the United States, despite the fact that approximately 1 600 000 of those registered for the draft were classified as unfit for military service because of mental disease, indicating a disqualification rate between six and seven times higher than in World War I (Strecker, 1945; Glass, 1966), discharges for psychiatric disorder in World War II were 2.4 times as high as in World War I (Glass, 1966). 'The evidence clearly indicates that the actual incidence of neuropsychiatric conditions is significantly higher in World War II than it was in World War I' (Appel *et al.*, 1946). There are many reasons for this surprising finding, but what seems clear is that the widespread use of psychiatric screening had not fulfilled its expectations. 'Despite high rejection rates for psychiatric disorders, large numbers of men with emotional difficulties of all severities kept turning up' (Brill and Beebe, 1952a).

A similar picture emerged in the United Kingdom. On the assumption that new screening and treatment programs either prevented psychological breakdown or effectively resolved cases, it has been widely reported that few pensions were granted for psychoneurosis in the aftermath of World War II (Ahrenfeldt, 1958; Shephard, 2000). However, this appears optimistic. Official statistics published by the Ministry of Pensions in 1953 showed that 10 percent (50 060) of all war pensions awarded to World War II veterans were for psychoneurosis and neurological disorders, excluding epilepsy. This rate was significantly higher than that for World War I when 84 681 (6.3 percent) pensions had been granted for equivalent disorders (Anonymous, 1953). These figures appear relate solely to ex-servicemen with a single diagnosis.

This came as no surprise to the more thoughtful observers. From an early stage of the war there were many voices starting to be heard warning against over-optimistic estimates about the utility of psychiatric screening. This is an American view from the same year, 1941: 'There may be enthusiasts who would carry psychiatric scrutiny of recruits to extremes, or who would sell to the Government infeasible mental hygiene schemes. Such promotions sometimes emanate from nonmedical sources. They tend to discredit the real service which the psychiatrist can render' (Anderson, 1966).

Aita (1941), also writing in 1941, sounded similar warnings, suggesting that it might be sensible to follow up those rejected on psychiatric grounds to assess the predictive value of the decision (he later did just that and showed it was extremely poor (Aita, 1949)). Kardiner himself (1941) sounded a note of caution based on his World War I experiences: 'though I have seen many hundreds of the chronic forms of these neuroses and have studied the psychopathologic picture, course, treatment, and previous personality, I should hesitate to offer any criteria that can be used to predict that a given candidate will have a traumatic neurosis.'

As the war progressed, it became obvious from the numbers of psychiatric casualties that the screening program was failing to prevent psychiatric disorder, but that was not its only failing. It was also starting to impact on the war effort itself. Time and time again it became clear, both during the war and afterwards, that screening programs rejected too many people. As the war progressed, so did the need for manpower, and so did the criticisms of the screening programs.

Policies had to be changed, and they were. In Britain there was greater reliance placed on intelligence testing, linked with personnel selection which functioned as a form of aptitude testing – avoiding the 'square pegs into round holes' problem (Crang, 1999). Now the intention was not to prevent psychiatric breakdown, but to try and ensure that recruits were placed in suitable trades or occupations.

In America, where the most optimistic claims for the screening program had been made, changes also were made. Harry Stack Sullivan, the charismatic psychiatrist and advisor to the Draft Board, was sidelined and resigned in 1943 (Deutsch, 1944). Official directives document the growing disillusionment, culminating in the War

Department Technical Bulletin issued on April 21, 1944 in the build up to the invasion of Europe, which established as a point of principle that 'individuals with minor personality defects and neurotic trends could be of service, (US Army War Department, 1944).

One could argue 'They would say that, wouldn't they?' and that the change in policy was simply the result of the manpower situation, but whilst it cannot be denied that the manpower crisis was a major catalyst for change, there was also ample evidence before and since to support the need for a change in policy. It was not just a matter of military expediency – the policy itself was flawed. As one later commentator expressed it 'as a means of avoiding psychological casualties, screening failed abysmally' (Marlowe, 2000).

Why did screening fail?

The main problems encountered during World War II and in the following, optimistic, years, can be summed up in the words 'false positives' and 'false negatives.' As already described, no screening procedure prevented later psychiatric disorder – people were being passed as fit who still broke down (false negatives). Studies also started to show the converse – no matter what instrument was tried, it rejected people who actually would have made good soldiers (false positives).

In an American study Egan and colleagues followed up 2054 men rejected by the military on psychiatric grounds during World War II, but later inducted into the Army anyway, an elegant natural experiment. Of those initially rejected, only 18 percent had later been discharged on psychiatric ground. Of the rest, nearly all had given 'satisfactory duty' – 78 percent of the total sample (Egan *et al.*, 1951). In other words three quarters of those who had been screened out on psychiatric grounds could have made adequate soldiers.

Aita (1949) carried out another natural experiment. He compared the subsequent military careers of 250 men whom he had personally interviewed in 1941 and predicted successful military careers, and another 250 about whom definite doubts were expressed. Five percent of the 'good' group had subsequently failed in one form or another, compared to 21 percent of those who had indeed been predicted to do badly. But 79 percent of those he predicted would perform poorly had in fact performed either averagely, or indeed successfully. As he put it 'for every two who proved to be failures, there were three who became successful soldiers.' Likewise, psychiatric casualties were indeed more common in those predicted to do badly, but nevertheless, 80 percent of that group had not broken down. He concluded that many recruits often enter camp with a myriad of somatic complaints or other symptoms, but with good leadership and improved motivation become entirely asymptomatic and performed well, views echoed elsewhere (Voth, 1954). Said Aita (1949), ' we were attempting to predict on the basis of what these men had been' – and yet they were about to embark on what would for many be the most challenging and testing period of their life, one which may indeed have changed them, both for better and worse. Small wonder that predicting how these very young men would perform in conditions different from anything they could have experienced in the past was a hazardous process.

One problem was that the variables used to select out those thought to be vulnerable to later breakdown did indeed, as some had suggested, have low predictive power. Brill and Beebe looked at the rates of psychiatric admission in those who did, and who did not, have a predisposition (Brill and Beebe, 1952b). In those without such a history 2 percent had been admitted to a psychiatric facility, compared to 29 percent of those who did. These confirm that the risk of admission was substantially higher in those with such a history – but the figures also show the impracticalities of screening for such predispositions. Seventy percent of those with such a history did not break down.

A different look at the same question came from American studies that evaluated how those who did have psychiatric disorders and yet still made it to combat roles performed – these studies showed that those with psychiatric disorders did perform slightly worse, but nevertheless most were very satisfactory – and although most studies do not mention the subsequent after histories one study found that of 395 men with psychological disorders who endured 50 days of combat, only 12 were lost for psychiatric reasons (Sharp, 1950). Another (Plesset, 1946) followed 138 soldiers who had shown 'sufficient adjustment difficulty during training to necessitate psychiatric attention' and from whom the author, the Divisional Psychiatrist, expected very little – 'I had anticipated seeing most of the group of 138 in the first few days of combat or perhaps even earlier, for these were the "known" problems.' The psychiatrist admitted he was wrong. After 30 days of combat (the 'Battle of the Bulge') only one had become a psychiatric casualty. The other 137 remained on active duty, and one had already received a medal for gallantry (Plesset, 1946).

Disillusion

By the time of the Korean War, and as a direct result of the experiences of World War II, the proportion of those rejected as unsuitable for American military service on psychiatric grounds had fallen dramatically, from 7.2 percent to 3.2 percent (Glass *et al.*, 1956). However, there had been a rise in those rejected on grounds of mental deficiency, as a consequence of the recognition that measures of intelligence were both more robust, and better predictors, than those of psychological vulnerability.

Nevertheless, such is the seductive power of the belief that screening must be effective that efforts did not stop after World War II. Over the next 30 years the Americans witnessed a frequent pattern of local resurgence of interest in the possibilities of screening, often inspired by the belief that newer and better instruments had finally been developed, only to be followed by yet more disillusion, as studies continued to demonstrate how screening programs for psychological vulnerability continued to fail to satisfy the requirements for such programs. As an example, the US Navy, having reintroduced recruit screening some time during the 1980s, finally abandoned it in 1998.

An important study was carried out during the Korean conflict by Albert Glass and colleagues, looking at the usefulness of psychiatric screening in routine inductees in the US Army (Glass *et al.*, 1956). This differed slightly from its predecessors, since it took those who had already been accepted for military service, and hence had already excluded those obviously unfit on medical or psychiatric grounds. Once again, psychiatric prediction failed dismally – looking at combat performance 'it is evident that none of the forecasts for below-average or poor performance was correct.' The same was true for combat support personnel as well. What psychiatrists were able to predict with rather more accuracy was those who would break down when assigned to noncombat roles in the United States. The reasons were that these people failed very early in their military careers – and that 'overt signs of psychiatric or mental abnormality can forecast later adjustment over a relatively brief period of time' – another basic rule that the accuracy of prediction of anything decreases rapidly with time. Glass goes on to make the point that 'it is the rule rather than the exception for psychiatrists and others to under estimate the capacity of individuals to perform satisfactory combat duty' – much the same could be said about questionnaires as well – the problem of excess false positives.

Psychiatric injury and the rediscovery of trauma

The concept that selection would solve the problem of psychiatric injury failed for one further reason, which now seems obvious but seemingly was not apparent at the time. As is now well known, by 1942 and 1943, the American Army was having the same experiences as the British Army had experienced on the Somme – the rate of psychiatric casualties from the Pacific and North Africa was rising inexorably, sufficient to cause widespread concern. And this was despite all the investment in screening. The reason was simple – the main cause of combat neurosis, battle fatigue, or call it what you will, in soldiers actually exposed to prolonged periods of intense fighting, was combat itself, amplified by armies such as the Americans or the Germans who kept soldiers in the front line for prolonged periods. 'One thing alone seems to be certain: Practically all infantry soldiers suffer from a neurotic reaction eventually if they are subjected to the stress modern combat continuously and long enough' (Swank and Marchand, 1946).

From this period came what are still the definitive statistical studies of the relationship between combat intensity and acute psychiatric disorder (Shephard, 2000; Jones and Wessely, 2001). As exposure to combat increased, so did both physical and psychiatric casualties, a sad lesson confirmed once more in the Arab–Israeli Wars (Levav *et al.*, 1979; Belenky, 1987). In the balance between the 'weakness of the personality,' to use their terminology, and the stress of the situation, as the stress increased, the contribution made by the personality decreased. It was indeed a 'paradigm shift' (Marlowe, 2000), from a doctrine of vulnerability due to inherited factors to one based on war-related environmental stressors.

People came to realize that screening was measuring the wrong thing at the wrong time. What mattered as regards the chances of breakdown was not scores on tests given at induction, or indeed prior to deployment. Attempts to predetermine behavior under stress were doomed to failure, because the critical variables – the circumstances of 'mission, assignment, associates, leadership, moral, hardships, hazards and other environmental variables' (Anderson, 1966, p. 742) – were unknown and unknowable at the time of screening. Indeed, some would argue are not even knowable during combat itself.

Recent research on predictors of posttraumatic stress disorder and their relevance to the screening debate

As is well known to all the readers of this book, 1980 represents a watershed in the literature on posttraumatic stress disorder (PTSD), representing the year in which the diagnosis became enshrined in *DSM-III*. One notable and welcome consequence of this change was a rapid increase in the scientific literature on all aspects of the subject. Relevant to this chapter is the new work on prediction of PTSD.

In an important study, Brewin and colleagues (Brewin *et al.*, 1998, 2000) have recently conducted a meta-analysis of risk factors for PTSD in which all the references are after 1980. The task was a familiar one, albeit expressed in modern terms – to identify reliable predictors for the development of PTSD.

Overall the results showed that no single variable was a particularly good or powerful predictor of developing PTSD. The best predictor, although by no means exceptionally strong, was the intensity of the trauma itself. This of course is not a new finding, and has already been alluded to in the World War II literature. It will also be clear that by definition such a factor cannot be used in pretrauma screening.

Associations were noted for other factors which could be reliably measured pre exposure. These included gender, age, social class, intelligence, education, family and personal histories of psychiatric disorder, and more controversially childhood abuse. All of these variables, with the possible exception of childhood abuse, can be measured relatively reliably. And all contributed very little to the overall risk.

As Brewin pointed out, the associations were statistically significant (because by using meta-analytic techniques he had increased the sample size), but actually were very small. Whilst it is true that many researchers have used combinations of pre- and postexposure variables to construct statistical models to identify those who subsequently developed illness, it remains my opinion that none has the positive predictive power to allow it to be used to identify *individuals* at risk.

Brewin concludes that 'attempts to identify a common set of pre trauma predictors of PTSD that will be equally valid across different traumatized are premature' (Brewin *et al.*, 2000). Hence there remains no reason to alter the post-Korea conclusion that 'exception is taken to the premise that brief psychiatric screening is of value in predicting possible psychiatric casualties, except in certain obvious cases' (Voth, 1954).

What happens to those identified as 'at risk'?

But there is to my mind an even greater obstacle to the use of screening as part of a strategy of preventing posttraumatic psychiatric disorder. It is the 'What happens next?' question.

If someone were to be found on the basis of screening to be indeed 'vulnerable' or at risk of developing psychiatric disorder under stress, what action follows? Clearly, some action must follow, or there is no purpose to the exercise. Continuing the military analogy, because the issues are most clear cut, one possible consequence is that the person identified as at risk would either not be deployed on active service as previously intended, or perhaps not inducted into the military in the first place.

But the consequences of such a decision are immense, both for the individual and the military, resulting in many tangible practical and ethical dilemmas (Nicholson *et al.*, 1974). The individual is now labeled as 'psychologically vulnerable,' whatever that may mean. The implications for the rest of their service are considerable, as indeed they would be in civilian employment as well. What are their chances of getting insurance? They may, and probably will, feel acutely the stigma of being labeled as psychologically vulnerable or unstable.

Almost certainly the person's view of themselves will now change, assuming they are told the results of such screening, as seems ethically imperative. They may never have considered themselves as psychologically vulnerable – but now they may do so. Their behavior may be altered in many unforeseen and adverse ways. They may actually now become anxious or depressed, simply as a result of been told that this may happen to them in the future! One can predict a large number of different psychological responses to the information, few of them helpful. An analogous situation comes from the hypertension literature. Hypertension itself is not associated with any increased risk of depression or psychological symptoms – it is itself asymptomatic – but workers informed they have high blood pressure following workplace screening responded with increased time off work, significant loss of income, and further increases in blood pressure (Birkinlager, 1993).

What if the person does not accept the result of the screening? Are they able to challenge the judgment? Presumably so. Once again, one suspects that the inevitable result will be litigation in some shape or form. We should not forget that the record of World War II shows that those who were denied the chance to enlist because of a presumed vulnerability to psychiatric breakdown under stress were not grateful for being spared military service – rather the reverse (Shephard, 2000). 'Many rejected men will find themselves in a very unpleasant position in the community and their instability will be further increased' (Bowman, 1941).

What does the employer, military or civilian, do instead with this individual identified as at risk? Presumably to deploy them in a low-stress environment – but what exactly would such an environment exist? Certainly the person could avoid combat duties, and perhaps be assigned to rear echelon roles. But all of us will have come across cases of people 'breaking down' in jobs whose 'stress levels' fall far short of combat, in both civilian and military sectors. Administration and management is hardly a stress-free environment these days. Stress seems to be a ubiquitous accompaniment of modern society. None of us is immune from 'stress,' whatever that may be.

Perhaps the person needs treatment to reduce that vulnerability – but there is no consensus at all as to what such treatment might consist of – and many of the risk factors that will have contributed statistically to rating this person as 'at risk' (such as gender, ethnicity, past history, and so on) are immutable and unchangeable. What if they refuse treatment? And what if treatment, what ever it may be, and I have little idea, makes them worse?

The consequence is that once someone has been labeled as 'at risk' of psychiatric breakdown under stress, the problems do not end, they merely begin. All of these issues need to be addressed before routine psychological screening could be commenced, and one suspects that the practical, social, public relations, and legal outcomes that would result would rapidly bring the program into disrepute.

Screening for vulnerability: Conclusion

Screening therefore is a very blunt weapon indeed. It will pick up some who will break down later, but at a cost of rejecting lots of good soldiers, policemen, or what ever occupational group we are considering, and missing many, if not most, of those who will still break down after encountering adversity. Most of the factors associated with psychiatric breakdown are not factors that can be measured at baseline, if they can be measured at all – leadership, training, and morale, for example. Once one has eliminated the grossly unsuitable, further screening for vulnerability for subsequent psychiatric disorder has never been shown to be effective in preventing subsequent breakdown in the face of adversity. Finally, in the modern era, the adverse consequences to those who are identified wrongly as being at risk, and perhaps even those who are correctly identified, would almost certainly alone prevent such a system being implemented.

'Efficient psychiatric screening requires an unusually high degree of accuracy' (Glass *et al.*, 1956). That is as true now as it was during World War II. It was not obtained then, and has not been obtained now.

Screening after exposure to trauma

So far I have considered the question of screening before exposure to trauma, and concluded that there are probably insuperable objections to such a strategy, certainly given current knowledge. But what about after exposure? Now the question is should screening be used to detect those who actually have, as opposed to might develop, disorders? I shall conclude that a better case can be made for such screening, but the evidence remains far from compelling.

Principles

I have already discussed in detail the requirements that must be satisfied before an acceptable screening program to prevent any disorder can be introduced. The requirements that need to be fulfilled before implementing a program whose purpose is to detect existing disorder, while not identical, are not radically different. The key additional factors to be considered, as well as the usual problems of reliability, and the risks of side effects, are as follows:

1. That the natural history of the disorder is well known, and that spontaneous recovery is unlikely.
2. That those who are the target of screening would not have presented anyway.
3. There is a proven intervention for those detected.
4. Evidence exists to show that the benefits of screening outweigh the risks and side effects.
5. That both the screening and treatment programs are acceptable to those targeted.

Is there any need for screening at all?

This may seen obvious, but is not. It is not disputed that psychiatric disorders such as PTSD can be associated with considerable morbidity. But psychiatric disorders are not 'all or nothing' – conditions one either has or does not have – but lie on a dimension from the normal, via distress, to frank disorder. No cutoffs or points of rarity exist, and the decision as to when the normal and understandable becomes a discrete disorder is a complex and arbitrary one. The prevalence of disorder also varies in time and place. Symptoms may be not uncommon after deployment, as we have shown after the Gulf War, but discrete disorders that affect functioning and may require treatment are considerably less so (Unwin *et al.*, 1999; Ismail *et al.*, in press). No absolute argument exists for routine screening of any group exposed to adversity – each instance must be taken on a case-by-case basis. It is my opinion that simply being exposed to a stressor is not sufficient reason for instituting a screening program, unless there is reason to believe that the expected rates of psychiatric disorder are going to be substantially elevated (see below).

The next fundamental requirement for screening is that services exist to deal with the disorder that is going to be detected, and those people who require treatment are not already accessing it. If those who are the target of that screening would have presented to medical services anyway then there is clearly no case for launching an expensive and elaborate screening system.

Again, this will differ from country and country, depending on the characteristics of different health care systems. There is less of a case for screening in countries such as the United Kingdom, in which there is a comprehensive primary health care system, which is very permeable indeed (most people see their family doctor between three and four times a year), than in the United States. Likewise, many military health systems are exceptionally easy to access. If people are accessing the care system, but are not being recognized, the solution is not screening, but better education and training of the physician.

However, even if an efficient and effective system for managing psychological disorder existed (and regrettably, despite the above, examples of efficient and effective systems for managing psychological disorder are conspicuous by their absence in all the health care systems I have knowledge of), the case for screening can still be made if those who should access the system do not do so, for whatever reason.

There are various reasons why people might not access services when they should do so, and hence are potential beneficiaries of screening. One reason may be that they have not yet actually developed the disorder in question – in this context the question of delayed PTSD. But such people will not gain from screening for obvious reasons.

What about people who have the disorder, but have not sought help? There are numerous studies describing the characteristics of those who seek treatment, since such studies are easy to perform, but what is required is studies in which those who do not seek treatment but are also suffering from psychological distress are compared to those with similar conditions who have sought assistance. This kind of data is much harder to find. Solomon, the Israeli psychologist, has carried out one of the few empirical studies on this question. Those with combat-related psychiatric disorder who failed to seek treatment after the 1982 Lebanon War had less severe symptoms and a greater sense of self-efficacy than those who had sought treatment – in other words were less ill. Given that postcombat psychological reactions lie on a dimension from the normal to the pathological, this group were far closer to, and overlapped with, the normals (Solomon *et al.*, 1989). In that study, those most in need of treatment were receiving it. Such evidence of course only applies to the specific circumstances of the Israeli military psychiatric services (which are generous) and society. Population based studies of Vietnam veterans (Kulka *et al.*, 1990) and Dutch survivors of World War II confirm that help-seeking is related to level of traumatic symptoms (Bramsen and Ploeg, 1999), but at the same time also show, as do community studies, that even so large numbers of people exist who fulfil criteria for PTSD but have not sought help (Kessler *et al.*, 1995). The question of unmet need probably does differ from country to country, and across periods.

But why do people not present? Some do not wish to, as indeed is their basic human right. Some are deeply aware of the stigma of psychiatric disorder, and either feel ashamed of their symptoms, or are concerned that others might see them as morally weak. Like the author, the readership of this book almost certainly does not share this attitude, but there can be no doubting that many others do. For some avoiding such labeling or stigma is a powerful motive. As no one is advocating compulsory treatment for posttraumatic stress and its variants, these wishes must be respected. Mental health professionals all too easily forget the low esteem in which we and our patients are held by the general public. My experiences with the military have shown that many may also feel that admitting to psychiatric disorder will have an adverse effect on their career – I do not know if this view is accurate, but it is certainly common within and without the military.

Others do not present because of the nature of traumatic psychiatric disorder. For some avoidance of reminders of the source of their distress is a powerful force. The disorder itself plays a role in preventing them for seeking help. These people may be persuaded to access services if correctly identified and sensitively managed, and are perhaps the group that stand most to benefit from screening.

A further important point to mention is that if people who could be accessing the system do not wish to do so, for whatever reason, then identifying them by a screening program is less likely to lead to any demonstrable changes since these people will still be reluctant to access the services, whether identified by screening or not. Even if they enter treatment, the results are likely to be less successful than for those who have come forward of their own volition.

Next, the issue of prognosis. One screens for cervical or breast cancer because neither spontaneously improves or results in recovery. This is not the case for the disorders we are concerned. As Solomon's study has shown, even combat stress improves over time (Solomon, 1989). Taking a wider perspective, Shalev concludes that 'a significant proportion of patients show recovery within a relatively short time after trauma, with up to two thirds of patients recovering within five months in some studies' (Shalev, 2001). This does not eliminate the case for screening, but does weaken it.

Who should be screened?

Screening is always more appropriate and also cost-effective, with a lower risk of false positives, when carried out on those who are at higher risk of disorder. In the context of this book, I will take it as accepted that those who have been exposed to major trauma are indeed at higher risk of psychiatric disorder, but we still need to address the question of exactly how high.

Crucially, the case for screening for psychiatric injury depends on the expected prevalence of such injury. The risk factors for developing these conditions will likewise vary according to the intensity of the stressor. Thus the case for instituting posttrauma screening can never be a general one, but always must depend on the nature of the trauma itself, and identifying which is the appropriate subgroup to be screened, which is no simple task.

In the military context we can make some observations, which can also inform the discussion about which groups of civilians could be candidates for screening. It is now clear that certain subgroups within the military do have an increased risk of psychiatric disorder. Examples include those exposed to prolonged, intense combat (as exemplified by classic campaigns such as the Western Front, the Italian or Pacific campaigns of World War II, or the operations of Bomber Command and the USAAF over Germany). Others are those assigned to specific duties – grave registration being one, or those who have endured gross hardship – prisoners of war being another. Finally those involved in so-called 'friendly fire' incidents seem to be another subgroup. Screening of many of these groups is now carried out in several armed forces. Turning to the civilian sector, it is beyond dispute that rates of psychiatric disorder after rape are extremely high, providing another high-risk group that might well form a suitable target for routine screening.

All of these are groups of people who satisfy the first requirement before considering a screening program, that the rates of psychiatric disorder are sufficiently high to justify some form of screening, but that in itself is not sufficient indication to commence such a program – several more requirements need to be fulfilled.

How long after exposure should screening be performed?

The next question is when should screening be carried out? Again no clear-cut answer emerges. Screening early after exposure to adversity will miss delayed-onset PTSD cases. Early screening will also be more likely to pick up people with transient disorders that will resolve spontaneously. Both scenarios decrease the efficiency and effectiveness of screening. Another possible drawback is that screen too early and people may not be ready to accept intervention. Screening late gives a higher likelihood of detecting persisting symptomatology, but will have missed the possibility of early intervention before disorders become chronic, which was one of the main points of the exercise. There remain remarkably few data on which to base this crucial question. If pressed, I would say that the best window of opportunity comes at around 3 months, but this is far from established beyond doubt.

Choice of measure

The next question is that if screening is desirable, is there an effective instrument? As already stated, the key statistics in assessing the performance of any screening instrument are its sensitivity, specificity, and positive predictive value.

There are now many instruments around that have been used to detect PTSD. Several of the newer ones have shown acceptable psychometric properties in specific populations. For example, the scale devised by Davidson, reported in 1997, has at its best cutoff a sensitivity of 0.69, a specificity of 0.95, and a positive predictive value of 92 percent, which is very respectable (Davidson *et al.*, 1997). However, those data come from the validation study in which the prevalence of PTSD was very high – 67 out of 129 subjects had the disorder. In a sample with far lower prevalences of PTSD the scale will perform far worse.

A more relevant comparison was provided by Shalev and colleagues (Shalev *et al.*, 1997). They compared the ability of four different questionnaires to predict PTSD in those attending an Accident and Emergency Department. This is more relevant to the current discussion, because the overall prevalence of PTSD was lower than in previous studies (30 percent at 1 month and 17 percent at 4 months), albeit still higher than the population.

The results showed that whereas all the questionnaires did predict PTSD better than chance alone, none had the properties required for a screening program – in particular the positive predictive values were all low, and would be unacceptable as a basis for any screening programme (Shalev *et al.*, 1997). Likewise, although I note that the US military does have a program of psychological screening in place for personnel who have served in the former Yugoslavia, a report I have read shows that 19 percent of those screened were positive on the screening instrument, but only 5 percent 'exhibited psychological distress' and were referred to a mental health professional. It is not stated how many of that group in turn continued to have significant disorder, nor what, if any, were the results of intervention, but with those statistics one wonders if the program will prove cost-effective when formally evaluated (Bienvenu, 1998).

Could it be done?

There remain doubts as to whether or not the natural history of PTSD is suitable for screening, and whether or not an effective instrument existed. But that is still not the end of the story. As a classic textbook (Hennekens and Buring, 1987) states:

> Even after a disease is determined to be appropriate for screening and a valid test becomes available, it remains unclear whether a widespread screening program for that disease should be implemented. Evaluation of a potential screening program involves consideration of two issues: first, whether the proposed program is feasible, and second, whether it is effective.

In the next sections I will examine the practical obstacles to developing such a system, and finally the empirical evidence as to whether or not any similar system has ever been shown to bring benefit in analogous situations.

Feasibility

As someone who has spent a good part of the last five years attempting to get military personnel to answer questionnaires on their health, I do not underestimate the enormous practical difficulties of any such routine program. I am sure that many other contributors to this book will have had similar experiences in many other populations. The practical obstacles to any posttrauma screening program will be considerable, and may prove insuperable in some situations.

Treatment

It is a requirement of all screening programs that there is a benefit to the person who is identified as a result of the screening – in other words that treatments of proven efficacy exist and are available. Questions of treatment will be addressed elsewhere, but at present the long-term effects of treating trauma-related psychiatric disorder are not outstanding, particularly for military samples (Foa *et al.*, 2000).

In certain conditions such as cervical cancer, where early intervention is virtually curative of what would otherwise be a fatal condition, treatment clearly passes the risk–benefit equation with flying colors, and hence the case for screening is strengthened. However, the only modest, at best, success of treatment for PTSD means that the case for screening for PTSD in this population is more problematic.

The more recent optimistic reports of the use of new treatment modalities in some populations of patients with acute stress disorders is an important step forward (Andre *et al.*, 1997; Bryant *et al.*, 1998, 1999), but may not necessarily relate to screened populations. Randomized controlled trials of treatment are almost invariably based on those who come forward spontaneously for assistance. In contrast, it seems likely that those identified by a screening program are less motivated to change, and hence less likely to gain benefits from treatment than those who form the subject of the cited statistics on treatment success and failure.

Adverse effects of a screening program

I have already noted that all screening programs carry a risk of adverse effects – the question is the balance between these and the benefits. As the UK National Screening Committee, the body charged with deciding whether or not the National Health Service will adopt a new screening program, makes clear: 'The benefit from the screening programme should outweigh the physical and psychological harm caused by the test, diagnostic procedures, and treatment'. What might the potential adverse effects of screening for PTSD be? The following is a list of some potential adverse effects. Of course, whether or not all these effects will occur would be a matter for research, but it is essential that an awareness of the possibility of harm is part of the discussion of the case for and against screening.

False positives

The pursuit of false positives consumes both patient and doctor time, leads to frustrations in both parties, and can only expose the person falsely identified, who is not in need of treatment, to unnecessary inconvenience, risk of iatrogenic harm, and possible stigma. Disenchantment with the screening program may follow. Overdiagnosis and overtreatment is a definite risk.

Stigma

I have already drawn attention to the problems of stigma of psychological disorders in society in general. Exposing individuals to this stigma, no matter how much we may not share these general views, is an adverse effect of screening, even if difficult to quantify.

Labeling

People may not come forward for treatment because they perceive their distress as, for example in the military context, an 'appropriate response to the stressors of war, and not as a psychiatric disorder that could be ameliorated' (Solomon, 1989). The important issue is that former view, a normalizing attribution, may be converted by the screening process into the latter. The benefits could be that the soldier may now accept treatment, which in turn may, or may not, help. On the other hand, it may also reduce the person's sense of control or responsibility for their symptoms, engender a feeling of helplessness, and begin the process of converting someone from being an individual with a problem into a victim of forces beyond his or her control. What was previously seen as a normal reaction has now become a psychiatric or medical problem, to be treated by a professional. I myself believe that this professionalization of distress is an important reason for the probably adverse effects of psychological debriefing (Wessely *et al.*, 2000). The subject of what is called 'labeling' has acquired a vast literature over the years, with numerous documented examples of how being labeled as having a particular disorder, especially a psychiatric disorder, has numerous adverse social, psychological, and behavioral effects.

Side effects

This is straightforward. All treatments have side effects, and hence one unwanted effect of screening is to exposing people to risk of side effects of treatment, or even to receiving ineffective treatments. That this will happen is certain – the question remains the balance between benefit and harm.

Inefficient use of resources

Screening programs are expensive. One needs to consider if it is money well spent – could the same amounts of money achieve more if, for example, used to provide better treatment services?

Is screening effective?

We now reach the final requirement, that there be evidence that the screening program is effective – that at the end of the day, there has been a demonstrable difference in health outcomes to the population that has been screened, taking into account both the positive and negative aspects of the program.

The only way in which one can assess the success or failure of such a strategy is via the randomized controlled trial, since there is no other safe way of knowing what would have happened without the screening, and no way of assessing the size and scale of any adverse effects. I have been unable to locate any such studies relevant to PTSD, but there is evidence concerning general psychiatric disorders that is relevant.

A recent high-quality systematic review, published in the *British Medical Journal* and later extended and shortly to be published on the Cochrane Database of Systematic Reviews, found nine randomized controlled trials of the results of screening for mental health problems linked with some method of feeding back the results of the tests to doctors – which would be one simple way in which post-trauma screening would be carried out in countries with reasonable primary care services (Gilbody *et al.*, 2001).

First, routine administration and feedback did not increase the overall recognition of mental disorders. Second, if only those with high scores were fed back to the doctors (removing the noise and concentrating on the signal, as it were) then there was evidence that the recognition of disorders did increase. However, even if recognition increased, it did not lead to any differences in intervention, and nor could any effect on patient outcome, which is the point of the exercise, be demonstrated. The conclusions do not support the policy of routine screening for psychiatric disorders (Gilbody *et al.*, 2001).

Likewise, another recent review detected seven studies which examined the actual results of screening for mental health problems in routine practice – 'none of these studies found an advantage for detecting patients' (Coyne *et al.*, 2000). Whilst the authors still do not discount the possibility that there may still be as yet undemonstrated benefits to such systems, 'the lack of contrary evidence is disconcerting' (Coyne *et al.*, 2000).

The answer seems to be that with the best intentions in the world, mental health programs based on screening for existing disorders have not been a success.

Conclusion

The potential benefits of a successful screening program are self-evident. Screening could call attention to unrecognized psychological distress and morbidity, and foster the resolution of suffering. It could trigger treatment for established disorder or prevent more chronic and persistent morbidity. Those who are the targets of screening may be reassured that something is being done, and that someone, be it their employers, the state, or the Health Service, takes an interest in them.

It is precisely because the benefits of successful screening seem so intuitively correct, indeed 'beguiling' (Mant and Fowler, 1990), that screening is so often advocated, and occasionally instituted, in the mental health setting, and hence why there is so much evidence of the many pitfalls, side effects, and practical obstacles to its routine use.

Some of these obstacles can be predicted from the basic principles of screening. The more common the disorder, the better the properties of the screening instrument, and the more successful the program. Thus there is a case to consider for implementing special measures in groups that can be anticipated to have very high rates of psychiatric disorder indeed. I have mentioned some military scenarios; the victims of rape are another.

Other obstacles come from the specific circumstances of psychological disorders. These include the absence of accurate case-finding instruments, disorders that have high rates of spontaneous improvement or alternatively have delayed onsets, the difficulties in separating out normal distress from clinical disorder, and the equivocal results of treatment.

I conclude that no intrinsic objection exists to routine screening for psychiatric disorders in those exposed to serious trauma, but only if and when a sound case can be demonstrated for its effectiveness. This is therefore a research question. The questions that must be asked and answered are many, and include:

Who should be screened? Which subgroups?

At what time should screening be carried out?

What instrument(s) should be used?

Has that instrument been validated in the target population?

What are the positive and negative predictive values of that instrument when used in this situation?

What would be the likely participant rates?

How can those to be screened be identified and traced?

How can confidentiality be guaranteed?

What response rates can be expected?

What happens to those who 'screened positive' anyway? How many will still improve without action?

What action is indicated following a positive score?

How many of those who will later develop disorder would be missed by the program?

What side effects are there from screening?

What do those who are the target of the screening think about this? Would they consent?

What treatments would be available to those who were identified?

How effective are these treatments?

What are the risks of these treatments?

Is there any evidence from randomized controlled trials to show that the benefits of screening outweigh the risks?

How much would the program cost?

At the time of writing we do not have sufficient answers for most of these questions. My own views are as follows. I am sceptical that routine screening for psychological disorders after trauma is justified, and am inclined to think that the resources could be better spent on better treatment facilities for those who do come forward. Likewise, I am also inclined to think that in our present knowledge we are better advised to make efforts to ensure that the population at risk is aware of the availability of services and what they can offer, and then allow those affected to make up their own minds.

Finally, one would like to think that somewhere, someone is planning a randomized controlled trial of screening for trauma-induced psychiatric injury that can prove me wrong.

REFERENCES

Ahrenfeldt, R. H. (1958). *Psychiatry in the British Army in the Second World War*. London: Routledge and Kegan Paul.

Aita, J. (1941). Neurologic and psychiatric examination during military mobilization. *War Medicine*, **1**, 769–780.

Aita, J. (1949). Efficacy of brief clinical interview method in predicting adjustment: 5-year follow-up study of 304 Army inductees. *Archives of Neurology and Psychiatry*, **61**, 170–178.

Anderson, R. (ed.) (1966). *Neuropsychiatry in World War II*. Washington, DC: Department of the Army.

Andre, C., Lelord, F., Legeron, P., Reignier, A. and Delattre, A. (1997). Etude contrôlée sur l'efficacité a 6 mois d'une prise en charge précoce de 132 conducteurs d'autobus victims d'agression. *L'Encéphale*, **23**, 65–71.

Anonymous (1953). *Ministry of Pensions, 28th Report for the Period to 31 March 1953*. London: HMSO.

Appel, J., Beebe, G. and Hilger, D. (1946). Comparative incidence of neuropsychiatric casualties in World War I and World War II. *American Journal of Psychiatry*, **103**, 196–199.

Baganz, C. (1940). The importance of a proper psychiatric survey in the enrollment of personnel of military forces. *Military Surgeon*, **86**, 471–477.

Belenky, G. L. (1987). Varieties of reaction and adaptation to combat experience. *Bulletin of the Menninger Clinic*, **51**, 64–79.

Bienvenu, R. (1998). *On-Site Psychological Screening in Bosnia*. Springfield, VA: National Technical Information Service.

Birkinlager, W. (1993). Hypertensive labeling: Does it have therapeutic implications? *Cardiovascular Drugs and Therapy*, **7**, 207–209.

Bowman, C. (1941). Psychiatric examination in the Armed Forces. *War Medicine*, **1**, 213–218.

Bramsen, I. and Ploeg, H. (1999). Use of medical and mental health care by World War II survivors in the Netherlands. *Journal of Traumatic Stress*, **12**, 243–261.

Brewin, C., Andrews, B., Valentine, J. and Rose, S. (1998). *Selection to Reduce Casualties from Post Traumatic Stress Disorder*. London: Defence Evaluation and Research Agency.

Brewin, C., Andrews, B. and Valentine, J. (2000). Meta-analysis of risk factors for posttraumatic stress disorder in trauma exposed adults. *Journal of Consulting and Clinical Psychology*, **68**, 748–766.

Brill, N. and Beebe, G. (1952a). Psychoneuroses: Military applications of a follow-up study. *US Armed Forces Medical Journal*, **3**, 15–33.

Brill, N. and Beebe, G. (1952b). Some applications of a follow-up study to psychiatric standards for mobilization. *American Journal of Psychiatry*, **109**, 401–410.

Bryant, R., Harvey, A., Dang, S. and Sackville, T. (1998). Treatment of acute stress disorder: A comparison of cognitive–behavioral therapy and supportive counseling. *Journal of Consulting and Clinical Psychology*, **66**, 862–866.

Bryant, R., Sackville, T., Dang, S., Moulds, M. and Guthrie, R. (1999). Treating acute stress disorder: An evaluation of cognitive behavior therapy and supportive counseling techniques. *American Journal of Psychiatry*, **156**, 1780–1786.

Crang, J. (1999). Square pegs and round holes: Other rank selection in the British Army 1939–45. *Journal of the Society for Army Historical Research*, **77**, 293–298.

Coyne, J. C., Thompson, R., Palmer, S. C., Kagee, A. and Maunsell, E. (2000). Should we screen for depression? Caveats and potential pitfalls. *Applied and Preventive Psychology*, **9**, 101–121.

Davidson, H. (1940). Mental hygiene in our Armed Forces. *Military Surgeon*, **86**, 477–481.

Davidson, J. R. T., Book, S. W., Colket, J. T., *et al.* (1997). Assessment of a new self-rating scale for post-traumatic stress disorder. *Psychological Medicine*, **27**, 153–160.

Deutsch, A. (1944). Military psychiatry: World War II 1941–1943. In *One Hundred Years of American Psychiatry*, eds. J. Hall, G. Zilboorg and H. Bunker, pp. 418–441. New York: Columbia University Press.

Egan, J., Jackson, L. and Eanes, R. (1951). A study of neuropsychiatric rejectees. *Journal of the American Medical Association*, **145**, 466–469.

Foa, E., Keane, T. and Friedman, M. (2000). Guidelines for treatment of PTSD. *Journal of Traumatic Stress*, **13**, 539–588.

Gilbody, S., House, A. and Sheldon, T. (2001). Routinely administered questionnaires for depression and anxiety: Systematic review. *British Medical Journal*, **322**, 406–409.

Glass, A. (1966). Lessons learned. In *Neuropsychiatry in World War II*, ed. R. Anderson, pp. 735–746. Washington, DC: Department of the Army.

Glass, A., Ryan, F., Lubin, A., Ramana, C. and Tucker, A. (1956). Psychiatric prediction and military effectiveness. Part I. *US Armed Forces Medical Journal*, **7**, 1427–1443.

Hennekens, C. and Buring, J. (1987). *Epidemiology in Medicine*. Boston, MA: Little, Brown.

Hilman, C. (1940). Medical problems encountered in military service. *Annals of Internal Medicine*, **13**, 2205–2221.

Ismail, K., Davies, K., Brugha, T., *et al.* (in press). Psychological disorders in UK Gulf War veterans: A controlled study. *British Medical Journal*.

Jones, E. and Wessely, S. (2001). Psychiatric casualties of War: An inter and intra War comparison. *British Journal of Psychiatry*, **178**, 242–247.

Kardiner, A. (1941). The neuroses of war. *War Medicine*, **1**, 219–226.

Kessler, R., Somnnega, A., Bromet, E., *et al.* (1995). Post-traumatic stress disorder in the National Comorbidity Survey. *Archives of General Psychiatry*, **52**, 1048–1060.

Kiene, H., Hassell, A. and Miller, H. (1942). Neuro-psychiatric examination at the R. I. Army Induction Station. *American Journal of Psychiatry*, **98**, 509–514.

Kulka, R. A., Fairbank, J. A., Jordan, B. A., Weiss, D. and Cranston, A. (1990). *Trauma and the Vietnam War Generation: Report of Findings from the National Vietnam Veterans Readjustment Study*. New York: Brunner/Mazel.

Levav, I., Greenfield, H. and Baruch E. (1979). Psychiatric combat reactions during the Yom Kippur War. *American Journal of Psychiatry*, **136**, 637–641.

Mant, D. and Fowler, G. (1990). Mass screening: Theory and ethics. *British Medical Journal*, **300**, 916–918.

Marlowe, D. (2000). *Psychological and Psychosocial Consequences of Combat and Deployment*. Santa Monica, CA: Rand Corporation.

Muir Gray, J. (1997). *Evidence-Based Healthcare: How to Make Health Policy and Management Decisions*. London: Churchill Livingstone.

National Screening Committee (1998). *First Report of the National Screening Committee.* London: Health Departments of the United Kingdom.

Nicholson, P., Mirin, S. and Schatzberg, A. (1974). Ineffective military personnel. 2: An ethical dilemma for psychiatry. *Archives of General Psychiatry*, **30**, 406–410.

Plesset, M. (1946). Psychoneurotics in combat. *American Journal of Psychiatry*, **103**, 87–90.

Porter, W. (1941). Military psychiatry and the selective service. *War Medicine*, **1**, 364–371.

Rose, G. (1992). *The Strategy of Preventive Medicine.* New York: Oxford University Press.

Shalev, A. (2001). What is Posttraumatic stress disorder? *Journal of Clinical Psychiatry*, **62** (Suppl. 17), 4–10.

Shalev, A., Freedman, S., Peri, T., Brandes, D. and Sahar, T. (1997). Predicting PTSD in trauma survivors: Prospective evaluation of self-report and clinician-administered instruments. *British Journal of Psychiatry*, **170**, 558–564.

Sharp, W. (1950). Fate of 395 mild neuropsychiatric cases salvaged from training period and taken into combat. *American Journal of Psychiatry*, **106**, 801–807.

Shaw, C., Abrams, K. and Marteau, T. (1999). Psychological impact of predicting individuals' risks of illness: A systematic review. *Social Science and Medicine*, **49**, 1571–1598.

Shephard, B. (2000). *A War of Nerves.* London: Jonathan Cape.

Solomon, Z. (1989). A three-year prospective study of PTSD in Israeli combat veterans. *Journal of Traumatic Stress*, **2**, 59–73.

Solomon, Z., Kotler, M., Shalev, A. and Lin, R. (1989). Delayed onset of PTSD among Israeli veterans of the 1982 Lebanon War. *Psychiatry Interpersonal and Biological Processes*, **52**, 428–437.

Strecker, E. K. A. (1945). *Psychiatry in Modern Warfare.* New York: Macmillan.

Sutton, D. (1939). The utilization of psychiatry in the armed forces. *Psychiatry*, **2**, 133–135.

Swank, R. and Marchand, W. (1946). Combat neuroses: Development of combat exhaustion. *Archives of Neurology and Psychiatry*, **55**, 236–247.

Unwin, C., Blatchley, N., Coker, W., *et al.* (1999). The health of the United Kingdom serviceman who served in the Persian Gulf War. *Lancet*, **353**, 169–178.

US Army Department (1944). *Technical Bulletin (TB MEDD 33) #33 April, 1944.* Carlisle, PA: US Army Military History Institute.

Voth, H. (1954). Psychiatric screening in the armed forces. *American Journal of Psychiatry*, **110**, 748–753.

Wessely, S., Bisson, J. and Rose, S. (2000). A systematic review of brief psychological interventions ('debriefing') for the treatment of immediate trauma related symptoms and the prevention of posttraumatic stress disorder. In *Depression, Anxiety and Neurosis Module of the Cochrane Database of Systematic Reviews*, 2nd edn, ed. M. Oakly-Browne, R. Churchill, D. Gill, M. Trivedi and S. Wessely. Oxford: Update Software.

10

Early intervention and the debriefing debate

Beverley Raphael

The concept of debriefing has been popularized as a mental health intervention in the early phases of response to disaster. Indeed, debriefing is now a powerful social movement and critical appraisal of its utility and appropriateness has been strongly resisted. Despite an increasing number of studies showing that psychological debriefing or critical incident stress debriefing (CISD) does not prevent posttraumatic stress disorder (PTSD), it is still seen by many as the most appropriate first-line response to those who have been exposed to stressors that may be psychologically traumatic. Several issues need to be addressed about psychological debriefing techniques and their place or otherwise as mental health interventions in the immediate postdisaster or posttrauma phase.

Clarifying the meaning of 'debriefing'

The term 'debriefing' as a word in the English language is widely used to suggest helping someone or assisting him or her to describe their response to a particular situation: to, as it were, 'unload' their experience. This broad meaning has psychological significance in terms of the perceived or actual psychological effect of sharing one's experience with others. A range of terms and usages are linked to this.

'Operational debriefing' is usually a thorough review of the operation or activity that has been carried out, usually by a team. Its aim is to review what happened, to learn, and to use this learning to improve effectiveness for future response. Such formats, i.e., operational review, have been in place for a long time and are seen as part of good practice, and in current terms as contributing to quality improvement.

The definitions of operational debriefing and debriefing provided by Stokes (2001) in the recent consensus meeting are of value:

> The term 'debriefing' should be restricted to its original context of 'operational debriefings' – factual reviews of the details of mission events by the participants, for the parent organization's purpose of learning what actually happened for the historical record or planning process, to improve future results in similar missions, and to increase the readiness of those being debriefed

for further action. Operational debriefings are conducted by leaders or specialized debriefers according to the organization's standing operating procedure. The debriefers and the organization should, of course, consider the potential long-term behavioral and mental health effects of their debriefing techniques, and should conduct long-term program evaluation using scientific methods.

The overuse of the term 'debriefing' to refer to a wide variety of individual and group interventions intended primarily to improve long-term mental health is misleading. Use of 'psychological debriefing' should not be sanctioned. 'Critical incident stress debriefing' should only be used in the organizational context of pre-existing teams that have experienced traumatic mission events, debriefed according to protocol with the intent of sustaining capability to continue operations.

Marshall (1947), a military historian, used a process of group review with soldiers after combat to gain detail of the nature of combat. His work with soldiers was noninterventionist in that he facilitated narrative about the experience, but made no interpretation of its meaning. These group sessions could be quite prolonged, going on until the issues had been thoroughly described. Although it has been suggested these processes may have been helpful to the soldiers, there is no information as to whether or not these sessions improved psychological adaptation or prevented adverse outcomes. Nevertheless, some recent work, which will be described below, utilizes this framework for a current form of 'debriefing' with military and other teams of responders.

Recognition of the psychiatric casualties associated with combat also focused on the need for early intervention and the search for brief, effective programs to lessen risk of psychiatric casualties. There was also the aim of sustaining the soldiers functioning in his combat role. The military psychiatry program based on principles of Proximity, Immediacy, and Expectancy (P.I.E.) has been widely utilized and is seen as effective in the aim of sustaining soldiers' functioning. However, there is little to suggest that it has prevented the development of posttraumatic stress disorder (PTSD), as repeated combat stress reactions, for which it has been applied, have been found to be associated with the development of chronic PTSD (Solomon *et al.*, 2000). Debriefing in the psychological sense is frequently related to this military model of early intervention.

The stressors faced by emergency workers were seen as contributing to job turnover and stress-related conditions, even before PTSD had been identified as a possible consequence of their exposure to death, life threat, and horrors, as well as other major stressors. These workers are familiar with operational review of team functioning after an incident. The model of psychological debriefing to assist their psychological function followed on this. For instance, after a major rail disaster 'psychological debriefing' was provided to a volunteer rescue team and other groups (Raphael, 1977). In a way this reflected the sort of talking through of what happened that many team leaders encouraged, often in a social context.

This was also a relatively noninterventionist process, and usually took place one or more weeks later. Its impact on functioning was not evaluated. Nevertheless a brief survey of emergency and other responders following this incident showed that workers were stressed, often by the frustration of not being able to fulfill their roles, or the tasks they felt they were trained for. However, many considered that they had come through the experience with outcomes such as positive re-evaluation of their lives and valuing their family relationships (Raphael *et al.*, 1984).

The 'Mitchell model' evolved as a structured format for emergency workers. It has been presented as a mental health intervention with defined stages of review and is seen as lessening the likelihood of stress related outcomes and staff turnover in emergency workers (Mitchell, 1983). While models also developed with stronger educational and other focus (Dunning, 1988), the model of CISD has been the most widely taken up and applied, both in the United States where it evolved, and internationally. Debriefing or psychological debriefing has become equated to CISD, even though as Mitchell and his colleagues suggest, it may not be applied with fidelity and integrity of the specific model.

A number of other frameworks have evolved such as 'multiple stressor debriefing' (Armstrong, 2000) which aims to deal with the multiple needs of diverse stresses experienced by disaster responders, and programs such as the Assaulted Staff Action Program (Flannery, 2000) for health workplaces. Mitchell's CISD has also been recontextualized in the broader context of critical incident stress management (CISM) (Mitchell and Everly, 2000), and more recently as 'crisis intervention' after the model of Caplan (1964).

There has been a range of critical appraisals of the effectiveness and appropriateness of debriefing as an early intervention. These will be discussed below. This has led not only to an expanding research base, but also a re-examination of the application of earlier models and their benefits or otherwise, for instance historical group debriefing (Shalev, 2000), and group stress debriefing (Weisaeth, 2000).

A number of factors have made it difficult not only to clarify what debriefing means to different people, but also to examining its role and potential effects. First, debriefing has become a powerful social movement, one that is difficult to challenge. Second, it is applied in times of distress and potentially chaos, which make its effects difficult both to standardize and to evaluate. Furthermore there is not a systematic understanding of the phenomenology of the immediate posttrauma response, except from generally retrospective data. The severity of the exposure, reactions such as dissociative states or hyper-responsiveness, natural attrition of reaction and adaptation, the potential processes of pathogenesis of disorder are all relevant and need to be better understood. Thus, there are currently poor conceptual and empirical grounds for action.

Does debriefing work?

This leads to questions of for whom, when, and for what purposes, as well as many other queries. There is now a growing body of work which must lead to concern as to the application of debriefing to postdisaster populations. This is the more so as the model most widely used, CISD, does not account for the multiple stressors that may have impact, for instance bereavement, dislocation, continuing or new threat, and the responses they may require. There is also the issue of 'to whom.' Debriefing started as a stress management program for emergency workers, and indeed that is what its originators claim for it. Yet it has been taken up and applied widely to all disaster-affected populations, after mass violence, to the bereaved, to many different workers and workplaces, to children, to culturally diverse populations, without a research base or studies to justify this, as compared to its role in 'stress management.'

The difficulties of research design and implementation in the immediate post-trauma or postdisaster circumstance have meant that there have been no 'gold standard' randomized controlled trials of CISD in the postdisaster phase for broader affected populations. The studies that contribute to knowledge about debriefing broadly come from naturalistic or systematic postdisaster studies, trials of debriefing with individuals as opposed to groups, and reports from those who have experienced it. These findings have been described in a number of reports, but will be summarized below.

Kennardy and Carr (2000) evaluated a population cohort who experienced an earthquake in Newcastle on the Australian East Coast. They sought, in this repeat-measures study, to find out if people from different sectors had been 'debriefed' or not, and how this correlated with mental health outcomes. They found that debriefing was not associated with benefit for this broadly affected population, and indicated that those debriefed had the potential for higher levels of morbidity at follow-up than others who had not been debriefed.

Watts, in a series of studies of populations exposed in major transport (bus) disasters with substantial mortality and traumatic exposure, found no correlation between the debriefing provided and positive outcomes. Although debriefing was perceived as helpful by many, others did not identify benefits. Perceived helpfulness did not correlate with outcomes (Watts, 2000).

In a series of studies of individuals exposed to motor vehicle accident trauma, Hobbs *et al.* (1996) showed no benefit of debriefing for those individuals either in the shorter or longer term.

The Cochrane Review (Rose *et al.*, 1998) concluded there was no evidence to support the effectiveness of psychological debriefing as an early intervention. It was suggested that its continued use was questionable. More recently an excellent analysis by Litz *et al.* (2002) examined the controlled trials of such applications. They reviewed studies of burn victims (Bisson *et al.*, 1997), peacekeepers in Bosnia (Deahl *et al.*, 2000), motor vehicle accident survivors (Hobbs *et al.*, 1996; Conlon *et al.*, 1999; Mayou *et al.*, 2000), and physical and sexual assault victims (Rose *et al.*, 1999). They found no benefits for CISD, and worse outcomes in some instances. Although these studies like others had methodological limitations, they nevertheless reflected the state of findings to date and are consistent in the directions of effect they report.

Studies addressing debriefing and specific aspects of the hypothesized pathogenesis of posttrauma morbidity are of interest. Shalev (2000) addresses historical group debriefing. He reports that for a group of 39 Israeli soldiers postdebriefing scores as compared to predebriefing scores decreased in terms of impact-of-event (IES) scale scores and anxiety state, and that there were increases postdebriefing in self-efficacy and group cohesion. This was not a controlled study and longer-term outcomes are not available. Shalev believes the decreased arousal reflected in these findings may be a positive factor that may lessen the risk of PTSD. However, this is not established. Homogeneity of group may mean, of course, that some are better and some are worse, and this may reflect matters of concern. This study is based on concepts from studies about the significance of arousal/anxiety in the pathway to PTSD morbidity and will be of interest in further development of this field. Of note in this context is a study by Pitman *et al.* (in press), where propranolol was given as an anti-anxiety measure for a 10-day course commencing within 6 hours of the index trauma. This is reported to have decreased physiological responsiveness by 3 months post trauma, but both groups showed equal levels of PTSD.

Another area of interest is the potential for benefit or otherwise of the 'talking' about what has happened. Much therapy is based on the belief of the value of being able to 'talk through' one's distress and/or experience. Ursano *et al.* (2000) examined medical care workers after an air disaster and evaluated the perceived benefits or otherwise of talking, and the talking of debriefing. These workers found that those with higher IES scores, intrusive scores as well as PTSD were more likely to talk about the disaster with another person. But those with higher talk scores were likely to have increased PTSD symptoms at 2 months: the talking did not appear to have prevented PTSD. Other studies have suggested that people may not wish to talk in this early phase, or if they do, it is to colleagues immediately after the experience, but the majority wanted to wait and monitor their reactions over time (Orner and Schnyder, 2003). For the most part, they did not want the intrusion of outside professionals and preferred to use their own coping strategies including humor, physical activity, keeping busy, working hard, and exercise. This is supported by other reports (e.g., Stuhlmiller and Dunning, 2000) where police and other emergency workers reported not needing debriefing and feeling it implied that they could not cope.

A further concept is that debriefing is for those that have been 'briefed.' Weisaeth (2000) suggests that it is the professional team that works together and who are briefed to respond who may benefit from debriefing, whereas informal, random, and reserve groups are less structured and are less likely to do so. He also suggests the value of the leaders of the groups being trained and supported to carry out this process, rather than the intrusion of a professional. In a small study testing this model, group psychological debriefing was found to be associated with fewer arousal symptoms 2 weeks later (Eid *et al.*, 2001). Those experiencing this debriefing also reported more lessons learned, and showed a tendency to discover new aspects of themselves after the incident. These military personnel were compared to a civilian group with the same task – firefighting. They also found that for their group as a whole, a lower number of symptoms was associated with learning from the accident, and a higher number with not being finished working through the experience. This was a small study of formal teams. It suggested some early benefits of this group approach through decreasing arousal and increasing learning. Larger studies and longer-term outcome evaluation will be important in taking these findings further, the more so as a number of studies have found more negative outcomes for those debriefed at later stages (e.g., Bisson *et al.*, 1997; Carlier *et al.*, 1998; Kennardy and Carr, 2000; Mayou *et al.*, 2000). Early benefits of decreased arousal for those with very early debriefing (10 hours compared to 42 hours after a bank robbery) have also been found by Campfield and Hills (2001) at follow-up 2 weeks post incident. These studies suggest one potential pathway of benefit for debriefing after single incident disasters/trauma, i.e., through diminishing arousal as one of the potential components of future PTSD.

Another debriefing model is that of integration of debriefing with occupational health and safety programs, as reported by Alexander (2000). Here police dealing with body recovery after an oil-rig disaster were paired in a 'buddy' system of more junior and senior officers, and provided with informal support and informal debriefing by a psychiatrist closely involved with their service. This appeared beneficial, but as with the studies outlined above, this was not a controlled trial.

As can be seen from the above and numerous other studies, there is significant evidence that individual debriefing is not helpful in preventing PTSD. Mitchell and Everly (2000) highlight other benefits including perceived helpfulness, which is found in many reports (although it has not been found to correlate with improved outcomes). Robinson (2000) also emphasizes these benefits and reports symptom reductions, improved work functioning, and reduced sick leave/job turnover. All of these features still need clarification through randomized controlled trials of appropriate power, methodological rigor, and timelines. The potential for positive outcomes, the potential for negative and the potential to do harm must all be taken into account.

At this stage, consensus would not recommend individual debriefing and would be cautious about the effectiveness of group debriefing in terms of potential for preventing PTSD. Whether for lesser stressors and formal teams it provides a component of stress management is a relevant question. Recent studies suggest outcomes that should be systematically measured include drug and alcohol intake, relationships, work performance, and so forth (Deahl *et al.*, 2000). These may be appropriate but in the face of very severe exposure, as for instance in mass violence, group debriefing may be seen as supporting the group, and individuals, to 'keep going,' to function in relevant roles, but may not protect them from post-trauma morbidity such as PTSD, depression, and other disorders. This dichotomy of ongoing functioning to continue to deal with the traumatic incident is important. However, PTSD and other morbidity may be a later cost (Solomon *et al.*, 2000).

Further questions about early intervention and debriefing

Psychological needs after exposure to 'trauma,' mass violence, and the human chaos after disaster are to date generally understood from descriptions, anecdote and narrative, observation, and retrospective surveys and studies. As noted above, the early phenomenology and course of response after exposure to psychologically traumatic experiences also needs further empirical prospective research. In addition the aura and power of the 'traumatic stress' model frequently overshadows other conceptualization so that analyses are only in terms of 'trauma' and PTSD, and infrequently in terms of other exposures, reactions, and outcomes (Table 10.1).

Physical needs in relation to survival, safety, and shelter may be primary and while threats to these are psychologically distressing, providing the appropriate safety, security, shelter, nutrition, protection, and opportunity for sleep, and addressing physical health needs are far more critical than a specific psychological intervention such as debriefing. And such intervention (i.e., addressing physical needs) is far more likely to decrease arousal and lessen vulnerability to future mental ill health effects.

For those who do not know of the fate of loved ones, or who are separated from them, particularly children, partners, or for children parents, there may be intense distress and searching behaviors. Sometimes this can place people at further risk physically. Information about the possible place of loved ones, and what has happened to them, and support to assist reunion with them will be effective in as far as these endeavors are possible, and support if there is uncertainty. Again debriefing cannot be an appropriate early intervention for such stressors.

Table 10.1 Special issues in early intervention and debriefing

Physical needs
Separation
Loss of loved ones
Dislocation, loss of home, destruction of community
Human malevolence
Making meaning
Personality and individual coping styles
Timing
Culture

Other things happen at such times and one of the most profound of these is loss of loved ones who may die in unexpected, untimely, and possibly horrific ways. While such bereavements are frequently 'traumatic,' their phenomenology is not that of 'traumatic grief' as described by Prigerson and Jacobs (2001). Rather it is a complex interplay of the phenomena of traumatic stress reactive processes and bereavement reactive processes (Lindy *et al.*, 1983; Raphael and Martinek, 1997). For instance, in the acute phase the arousal in trauma leads to scanning for cues of potential further threat. The arousal in the bereaved drives scanning for the dead person's return – for images or reminders. Anxiety for those traumatized is about threat, life threat, threat of death. For the bereaved it is intense separation anxiety/distress. The preoccupations are different for those traumatized who focus on the event; for the bereaved it is on the lost person. The reality and finality of the death and loss of a loved one are only gradually incorporated psychologically and this is more difficult if no body has been found. Adaptation is then even more complex (Singh and Raphael, 1981). While early models of traumatic stress reaction (e.g., Horowitz *et al.*, 1979) incorporated bereavement as a stressor, it has subsequently been recognized as different: Criterion A for PTSD, for instance, although the two may co-occur when the circumstances of the death are horrendous. Debriefing as an early intervention is inappropriate in that it does not recognize and provide a framework for the processes of bereavement. The only study of acute brief intervention for high-risk bereaved in the earliest days showed no beneficial effect, in contradistinction to studies of intervention in the following weeks (Raphael *et al.*, 2001). Thus it may be concluded that debriefing is contraindicated for persons acutely bereaved, even in circumstances of traumatic deaths. What is known is that contact, support with practical arrangements including seeing the body of the deceased where this is possible, are likely to be helpful, with opportunities for follow-up in the weeks subsequently and intervention for those at high risk. For some, psychological readiness to grieve and deal with the loss of unnatural dying may only take place months later (Rynerson, 2001).

Dislocation, loss of home, and destruction of community are all potential stressors after disaster. Again the acute reactive processes have not been subjected to empirical studies which can inform early intervention; but the processes of debriefing are unlikely to address these specific stressor components.

With respect to individual trauma such as severe physical injury or assault, as noted above, studies do not support the effectiveness or value of psychological debriefing for those so exposed to such life threat.

In those potentially traumatic circumstances where violence and life threat are the result of human malevolence a further stressor exists in this. The same applies in mass violence such as terrorism or bombing, e.g., the September 11 attack on the World Trade Center in New York. Such a stressor may drive not only the search for meaning, but also for justice. It may drive fantasies or acts of retribution or revenge. These issues evolve over time but the initial experiences of shock, helplessness, horror, and then rage need to be understood in terms of individual dynamics, group process, and social construction. Again debriefing cannot answer these issues and at early stages may run the risk of scapegoating, and may lead to a focus on retribution and justice which dominates and does not enable the individual to deal with the experience in terms of his or her own psychological needs.

Making meaning is an important part of dealing with psychologically traumatic experience and loss. Individual personality and experience are potential influences. Family, group, and societal meaning are also important, as are the shared meanings of coworkers, colleagues, and those who have been through the experience together. It is suggested that formal debriefing may assist with this and it may. However, there have been recent concerns that shared meaning so derived may overshadow individual memory of what happened, and thus complicate any forensic/evidentiary processes that will follow subsequently. Nevertheless, there are strong forces for social affiliation and groups frequently come together naturally for mutual support and self-help. These may contribute over time to assist recovery as members share coping styles, but the group and its aims may also become the principal focus, putting pressure on family and personal relationships if these persons are excluded. Some models offer debriefing for families as well, but whether or how this may facilitate adaptation is not known. It is specifically important that any early intervention process is supportive of the well-being of families and children, as well as any members more directly affected.

Personality and individual coping styles are significant in adaptation as is past experience of trauma and loss and whether these were effectively dealt with or not. Other vulnerability such as a history of psychiatric disorder may increase risk. Educational level, preparation, and training to deal with trauma as well as maturity of experience may protect as may adequate access to resources, both material and social. Social support *per se* is perceived to be important. Recognition of one's experience and validation by others may be helpful although studies have not adequately addressed this. Even with the most severe exposure the majority of people do not go on to lasting morbidity. Thus it is essential that individual adaptive processes and strengths are recognized, allowed to take their course, and not interfered with. How traumatic experience and loss are coped with and adapted to may be influenced by all these variables. Individual coping styles should be recognized and supported where their influence is positive. Any debriefing process should not interfere with adaptation and should not be compulsory. It should recognize the complexities of individual differences, and indeed of individual experience of even the same shocking event. Debriefing may be harmful if it re-exposes the person who is adapting without this; if it leads to excessive rumination in those who may be predisposed to it; if it provides an attributional focus on the event when the distress experienced more realistically relates to other aspects of the person's life; if it leads to learning that is focused only on trauma and not on adaptation and hope for the future.

Another important aspect is timing. The focus on early intervention and debriefing as an intervention at this time has developed with the best of intents. There has been the hope of alleviating distress and suffering; of preventing morbidity; of enhancing well-being. Timelines of need and specificity of need vary enormously. Many people are 'not ready' when debriefing is provided in the early hours or days, and sometimes not for a time afterwards. A study of delayed 'debriefing' (Chemtob, 2000) suggested benefits. The whole matter of timing of interventions requires a much better empirical data base on the phenomenology of posttrauma reactive processes, and what may influence these, and when. It also needs empirical studies of interventions at different times, but more methodologically rigorous than those currently available (e.g., Campfield and Hills, 2001). People may not want or accept early intervention, or debriefing because of avoidance, because of preoccupation with practical realities, or because other needs predominate as they perceive them, e.g., sleep, physical health (Weisaeth, 2001).

Another major factor, which has not been taken into account, is that of culture. Weisaeth (2000) has described cultural rituals that may serve a similar purpose, e.g., in Fijian peace-keepers. But psychological trauma, PTSD, and debriefing may be alien concepts in non-Western cultures (Silove, 2000). Here there is a greater focus on survival, attachment, existential themes, security and safety, and justice where human rights abuses have occurred. Cultural prescriptions for defining problems and response should be respected and Western models not superimposed, as debriefing was for a Papuan community after a tsunami. On the other hand, such models may be adopted and shaped to a local cultural framework or be quite different even if bearing the same name. In the Philippines psychosocial programming is a framework adapted from CISD and provided to local communities, including indigenous groups. On the other hand, a brief intervention such as debriefing may be viewed as inappropriate and insensitive when applied for a recent stressor which may have minimal significance compared to generations of cultural dispossession, loss, and trauma, as with indigenous Australians (Ober *et al.*, 2000).

There are also the cultures of systems, professions, and social groups. Debriefing is the social norm for many emergency workers, but often not so for health and medical personnel. Some emergency groups give support to the concept, but have their own internal culture, for instance of 'war stories.' There has been little exploration of gender issues but much to suggest that the debriefing model has had most uptake for men who are said to be less likely to use naturally occurring social networks to deal with their experience.

The need to respond

The best of human nature and values drives the need to respond to those who have experienced trauma, loss, catastrophe, and chaos. Altruism, courage, empathy, and compassion are mobilized and should be highly valued. These processes in and of themselves can all contribute positively to well-being. Numerous psychological and psychodynamic processes also underlie the need to respond and these too should be understood. They include fears of death and loss, confrontation with personal mortality, and loss of the sense of personal invulnerability; identification with those affected; relief at survival; reawakening of earlier personal experiences; intense feelings of affiliation; a wish to undo and make good; resentment about one's own unmet need or guilt that one is unaffected when others are so profoundly. All these and many other personal factors may influence the individual response style and need to be understood.

It is also important to recognize that such processes may influence the relationship between helpers such as debriefers and those they would assist. There may be a change in personal/professional boundaries because of the intensity of the trauma, the 'high' of the helping experience, and the powerful affiliative drives. A self-awareness to monitor these complexities is helpful, without diminishing spontaneous empathy and concern.

There are many expectancies about response to those affected by trauma and disaster. Media stories reflect these expectations noting that everyone is receiving 'trauma counseling' or 'debriefing.' Social and at times legal expectancies reinforce this. Often there is little knowledge about what is meant by such terms, for whom they are appropriate, who should provide then and when. Debriefing (and trauma counseling) are seen as symbolic of an organization recognizing a worker's or person's experience and formally providing for it. This fact alone may be part of the reason debriefing is perceived as helpful, whether other benefits are measurable or not.

There is in many societies, particularly in developed countries, a convergence of would-be providers, of those who would undo what has happened and 'do good.' This in and of itself may create problems. There is the question of who is appropriately skilled and sanctioned to provide any such intervention. The necessary professional expertise and knowledge, as well as experience and accountability are part of this. This includes the need to document any intervention process and to register those receiving it. The need for systems to appraise critically and coordinate any early intervention in mental health, debriefing or otherwise, also sits alongside the need to integrate this with other posttrauma or postdisaster response.

The prevention and management of convergence is important for these helpers may also be at risk. Active planning and preparation as well as integrated formal systems to provide for response can lessen chaos and thus decrease related anxiety and perhaps arousal. This should mean that defined roles and functions for mental health responders are in place, but are not inflexible, and can be shaped relative to need.

The most difficult thing for many is to accept that debriefing, whatever it may or may not do, is not a simple or even magical solution to the complexities of human experience of trauma and disaster. Those who developed this model have always recognized this, but others have taken it up and it has spread or been proselytized as a solution to the suffering and posttrauma morbidity. It is not these things and even for those who have invested their beliefs in it, the time has come for more critical appraisal. This must involve a commitment to developing the scientific base from naturalistic studies to randomized controlled trials; from research in phenomenology to the testing of meaningful interventions; from the recognition of attribution, expectancies, and social processes to the incorporation of such understanding in response. Where knowledge is lacking, as it is, there is an ethical and moral requirement to undertake research and evaluation, not to go on with unquestioning faith or unchallengeable belief.

Conclusions

As decided at a recent consensus meeting focused on early intervention after mass violence (Ritchie, 2001), the requirement is first not to harm. Any intervention must encompass principles such as psychological first aid, ensuring safety, security, survival, shelter, and other basics. Reunion with loved ones should be facilitated, information provided, and triage carried out where disturbance is great, for instance if there is cognitive impairment, intense arousal, or behaviors of risk to the self or others. Debriefing is not effective as a one-to-one early intervention, and group debriefing is questioned. Subsequently, for those at high risk following trauma and loss, specialized counseling according to evidence from trials with trauma (Bryant *et al.*, 1998) and bereavement (Raphael *et al.*, 2001) may provide benefit for some at heightened risk, when applied weeks rather than days after the experience. Interventions should be on the basis of the necessary knowledge and skills.

Research and evaluation are critical to extend this knowledge and education and training to build on this to ensure appropriate care (Ritchie, 2001). There is clearly much to be done. Science is limited and must be extended (Raphael, 2000). Belief is profound. Wisdom dictates that there is the capacity to analyze critically, to build on what is known, to explore, to use 'common sense,' and sustain the genuineness, empathy, and compassion that are likely to be of the most profound benefit.

REFERENCES

Alexander, D. (2000). Debriefing and body recovery: Police in a civilian disaster. In *Psychological Debriefing: Theory, Practice and Evidence*, eds. J. P. Wilson and B. Raphael, pp. 118–130. Cambridge: Cambridge University Press.

Armstrong, K. (2000). Multiple stressor debriefing as a model for intervention. In *Psychological Debriefing: Theory, Practice and Evidence*, eds. J. P. Wilson and B. Raphael, pp. 290–301. Cambridge: Cambridge University Press.

Bisson, J. I., Jenkins, P. L., Alexander, J. and Bannister, C. (1997). Randomised controlled trial of psychological debriefing for victims of acute burn trauma. *British Journal of Psychiatry*, **171**, 78–81.

Bryant, R. A., Harvey, A. G., Sackville, T., Dang, S. T. and Basten, C. (1998). Treatment of acute stress disorder: A comparison of cognitive–behavioural therapy and supportive counselling. *Journal of Consulting and Clinical Psychology*, **66**, 862–866.

Caplan, G. (1964). *Principles of Preventive Psychiatry*. New York: Basic Books.

Campfield, K. M. and Hills, A. M. (2001). Effect of timing of critical incident stress debriefing (CISD) on posttraumatic symptoms. *Journal of Traumatic Stress*, **14**, 327–340.

Carlier, I. V. E., Lamberts, R. D., van Uchelen, A. J. and Gersons, B. P. R. (1998). Disaster related posttraumatic stress in police officers: A field study of the impact of psychological debriefing. *Stress Medicine*, **14**, 143–148.

Chemtob, C. M. (2000). Delayed debriefing: After a disaster. In *Psychological Debriefing: Theory, Practice and Evidence*, eds. J. P. Wilson and B. Raphael, pp. 227–240. Cambridge: Cambridge University Press.

Conlon, L., Fahy, T. J. and Conroy, R. (1999). PTSD in ambulant RTA victims: A randomized controlled trial of debriefing. *Journal of Psychosomatic Research*, **46**, 37–44.

Deahl, M., Srinivasan, M., Jones, N., *et al.* (2000). Preventing psychological trauma in soldiers: The role of operational stress training and psychological debriefing. *British Journal of Psychiatry*, **165**, 30–65.

Dunning, C. (1988). Intervention strategies for emergency workers. In *Mental Health Response to Mass Emergencies*, ed. M. Lystad, pp. 284–320. New York: Brunner/Mazel.

Eid, J., Johnsen, B. H. and Weisaeth, L. (2001). The effects of group psychological debriefing on acute stress reactions following a traffic accident: A quasi-experimental approach. *International Journal of Emergency Mental Health*, **3**, 145–154.

Flannery, R. (2000). Debriefing health care staff after assaults by patients. In *Psychological Debriefing: Theory, Practice and Evidence*, eds. J. P. Wilson and B. Raphael, pp. 281–289. Cambridge: Cambridge University Press.

Hobbs, M., Mayou, R., Harrison, B. and Worlock, P. (1996). A randomised control trial of psychological debriefing for victims of road traffic accidents. *British Medical Journal*, **313**, 1438–1439.

Horowitz, M. J., Wilner, N. and Alvarez, W. (1979). The impact of event scale: A measure of subjective stress. *Psychosomatic Medicine*, **41**, 209–218.

Kennardy, J. A. and Carr, V. J. (2000). Debriefing post disaster: Follow-up after a major earthquake. In *Psychological Debriefing: Theory, Practice and Evidence*, eds. J. P. Wilson and B. Raphael, pp. 174–181. Cambridge: Cambridge University Press.

Lindy, J. D., Green, B. L., Grace, M. and Tichener, J. (1983). Psychotherapy with survivors of the Beverly Hills Supper Club Fire. *American Journal of Psychotherapy*, **37**, 593–610.

Litz, B. T., Gray, M. J., Bryant, R. A. and Adler, A. B. (2002). Early intervention for trauma: Current status and future directions. *Clinical Psychology: Science and Practice*, **9**, 112–134.

Marshall, S. L. A. (1947). *Men Under Fire: The Problem of Battle Command in Future War*. New York: William Morrow.

Mayou, R. A., Ehlers, A. and Hobbs, M. (2000). Psychological debriefing for road traffic accident victims. *British Journal of Psychiatry*, **176**, 589–593.

Mitchell, J. T. (1983). When disaster strikes: The critical incident stress debriefing. *Journal of Medical Emergency Services*, **8**, 36–39.

Mitchell, J. T. and Everly, G. S. (2000). Critical incident stress management and critical incident stress debriefings: Evolutions, effects and outcomes. In *Psychological Debriefing: Theory, Practice and Evidence*, eds. J. P. Wilson and B. Raphael, pp. 71–90. Cambridge: Cambridge University Press.

Ober, C., Peeters, L. Archer, R. and Kelly, K. (2000). Debriefing in different cultural frameworks: Responding to acute trauma in Australian Aboriginal contexts. In *Psychological Debriefing: Theory, Practice and Evidence*, eds. J. P. Wilson and B. Raphael, pp. 241–253. Cambridge: Cambridge University Press.

Orner, R. J. and Schnyder, U. (2003). *Reconstructing Early Intervention after Trauma: Innovations in Survivor Care*. Oxford: Oxford University Press.

Pitman, R. K., Sanders, K. M., Zusman, R. M., *et al.* (in press). Pilot study of secondary prevention of post traumatic stress disorder with propranolol. *Biological Psychiatry*.

Prigerson, H. G. and Jacobs, S. C. (2001). Traumatic grief as a distinct disorder: A rationale, consensus criteria, and a preliminary empirical test. In *Handbook of Bereavement Research: Consequences, Coping, and Care*, eds. M. S. Stroebe, R. O. Hansson, W. Stroebe and H. Schut, pp. 613–645. Washington, DC: American Psychological Association.

Raphael, B. (1977). The Granville train disaster: Psychological needs and their management. *Medical Journal Australia*, **1**, 303–305.

(2000). Debriefing: Science, belief and wisdom. In *Psychological Debriefing: Theory, Practice and Evidence*, eds. J. P. Wilson and B. Raphael, pp. 351–359. Cambridge: Cambridge University Press.

Raphael, B. and Martinek, N. (1997). Assessing traumatic bereavement and posttraumatic stress disorder. In *Assessing Psychological Trauma and PTSD*, eds. J. P. Wilson and T. M. Keane, pp. 587–612. New York: Guilford Press.

Raphael, B., Minkov, C. and Dobson, M. (2001). Psychotherapeutic and pharmacological intervention for bereaved persons. In *Handbook of Bereavement Research: Consequences, Coping and Care*, eds. M. S. Stroebe, R. O. Hansson, W. Stroebe and H. Schut, pp. 373–395. Washington, DC: American Psychological Association.

Raphael, B., Singh, B., Bradbury, L. and Lambert, R. (1984). Who helps the helpers? The effects of a disaster on the rescue workers. *Omega*, **14**, 9–20.

Ritchie, E. C. (2001). Summary of consensus statement. *Consensus Workshop on Mass Violence and Early Intervention Conference*, Virginia, USA, October 29–November 1, 2001.

Robinson, R. (2000). Debriefing with emergency services: Critical incident stress management. In *Psychological Debriefing: Theory, Practice and Evidence*, eds. J. P. Wilson and B. Raphael, pp. 91–107. Cambridge: Cambridge University Press.

Rose, S., Brewin, C. R., Andrews, B. and Kirk, M. (1999). A randomised controlled trial of individual psychological debriefing for victims of violent crime. *Psychological Medicine*, **29**, 793–799.

Rose, S., Wessely, S. and Bisson, J. (1998). Brief psychological interventions ("debriefing") for trauma-related symptoms and prevention of post traumatic stress disorder. In *Cochrane Database of Systematic Reviews*, 2nd edn. Oxford: Update Software.

Rynerson, E. K. (2001). *Retelling Violent Death*. Philadelphia, PA: Brunner-Routledge.

Shalev, A. Y. (2000). Stress management and debriefing: Historical concepts and present patterns. In *Psychological Debriefing: Theory, Practice and Evidence*, eds. J. P. Wilson and B. Raphael, pp. 17–31. Cambridge: Cambridge University Press.

Silove, D. (2000). A conceptual framework for mass trauma: Implications for adaptation, intervention and debriefing. In *Psychological Debriefing: Theory, Practice and Evidence*, eds. J. P. Wilson and B. Raphael, pp. 337–350. Cambridge: Cambridge University Press.

Singh, B. S. and Raphael, B. (1981). Postdisaster morbidity of the bereaved: A possible role for preventive psychiatry. *Journal of Nervous and Mental Disease*, **169**, 203–212.

Solomon, Z., Neria, Y. and Witztum, E. (2000). Debriefing with service personnel in war and peace roles: Experience and outcomes. In *Psychological Debriefing: Theory, Practice and Evidence*, eds. J. P. Wilson and B. Raphael, pp. 161–173. Cambridge: Cambridge University Press.

Stokes, J. (2001). Response to Summary of consensus statement. *Consensus Workshop on Mass Violence and Early Intervention Conference*, Virginia, USA, October 29–November 1, 2001.

Stuhlmiller, C. and Dunning, C. (2000). Concerns about debriefing: Challenging the mainstream. In *Psychological Debriefing: Theory, Practice and Evidence*, eds. J. P. Wilson and B. Raphael, pp. 305–320. Cambridge: Cambridge University Press.

Ursano, R. J., Fullerton, C. S., Vance, K. and Wang, L. (2000). Debriefing: Its role in the spectrum of prevention and acute management of psychological trauma. In *Psychological Debriefing: Theory,*

Practice and Evidence, eds. J. P. Wilson and B. Raphael, pp. 32–42. Cambridge: Cambridge University Press.

Watts, R. (2000). Debriefing after massive road trauma: Perceptions and outcomes. In *Psychological Debriefing: Theory, Practice and Evidence*, eds. J. P. Wilson and B. Raphael, pp. 131–144. Cambridge: Cambridge University Press.

Weisaeth, L. (2000). Briefing and debriefing: Group psychological interventions in acute stressor situations. In *Psychological Debriefing: Theory, Practice and Evidence*, eds. J. P. Wilson and B. Raphael, pp. 43–57. Cambridge: Cambridge University Press.

Weisaeth, L. (2001). Acute posttraumatic stress: Nonacceptance of early intervention. *Journal of Clinical Psychiatry*, **62** (Suppl. 17), 35–40.

11

Clinical intervention for survivors of prolonged adversities

Arieh Y. Shalev, Rhonda Adessky, Ruth Boker, Neta Bargai, Rina Cooper, Sara Freedman, Hilit Hadar, Tuvia Peri, and Rivka Tuval-Mashiach

Introduction

Remaining an efficient clinician during massive adversities is a major professional challenge. Several factors contribute to such challenge (Table 11.1): First and foremost, the number of traumatized survivors can be such that intensive therapeutic interventions might not be possible. Indeed, such therapies may further impoverish an overstretched pool of community resources (Norris *et al.*, 2001). Second, therapists and clients may be equally affected by the traumatic situation, and this may either reduce or enhance one's professional efficiency. Third, adversities may continue, and potential clients may not be free to process, practice, or otherwise enjoy what therapies normally offer. Psychological defenses that interfere with recovery at the aftermath of traumatic events (e.g., numbing, avoidance, denial, stoic acceptance) might be adaptive when adversity continues. A social discourse favoring courage and sacrifice may further confound clients and their therapists (Rivers, 1918). Thus, if disclosure of traumatic experiences is salutogenic under normal conditions (Pennebaker and Seagal, 1999), this may not be the case *during* prolonged adversities. Descriptive war literature suggests, in fact, that *bonding without disclosure* is the preferred behavior of soldiers between missions (Manning, 1930). Help-seeking behavior of traumatized survivors might be impaired or inappropriate (e.g., because of avoidance, mistrust, mistaking symptoms to be normal, fear of the potential consequences of psychiatric consultation, etc.). Consequently, if client-generated help-seeking is the key for receiving treatment, then clinicians may not see many of those who need help. Finally, it is extremely difficult to differentiate pathological from normal responses during continuous adversity. Clinicians who are trained to identify disproportionate, tenacious, or disabling responses may find it difficult to tell what is appropriate or timely following major loss, or during

Table 11.1 Impediments to providing clinical treatment during mass trauma

Too many clients and few therapists

Individual or group therapies may deplete community resources

Professional efficiency of therapists who are also under stress

Clients are not 'after' but rather 'within' a traumatic situation

Too early to 'open up'?

Ineffective help-seeking by those mostly affected

Concrete needs are prominent

Difficulty to discern pathological from normal responses

Professionals cannot replace natural helpers

Secondary stressors and lack of social support are the strongest predictors of stress disorders

displacement or destruction. Early symptoms tend to be volatile, polymorphous (Yitzhaki *et al.*, 1991), and reactive to additional stress.

Beyond observation and diagnosis, some clinical techniques may be inappropriate during continuous adversities. For example, therapists are trained to respond emotionally to their clients' experiences and impressions. During repeated contacts with recent survivors, however, therapists can be overwhelmed by their clients' experiences, often to the point of closing up and avoiding further work with victims. Should therapists be better protected from the effect of interacting with horrified and shattered clients? Can they afford to deploy their usual level empathic sharing? The following vignette illustrate the burden, on a therapist, of a client's recent experience.

Following a terrorist bomb attack a female survivor was brought to an emergency room, overwhelmed by emotion to the point of dissociation. Her father was with her, sitting at her bedside, functioning well, apparently. When the therapist approached the couple, the father, as a way of explaining the traumatic experience, showed her a jacket that he wore during the explosion, on which one could clearly see small morsels of human flesh. After seconds of shock, the therapist, a medical doctor, managed to continue her intervention, eventually advising the father to put away the jacket, and tending to the daughter's extreme distress. This resulted, however, in nightmares and continuous distress in the therapist, which fortunately resolved with time and by sharing with colleagues.

It is difficult, therefore, to remain an effective clinician during prolonged adversities. The crucial question, however, is whether clinicians and therapists, using clinical skills and techniques, have much to offer during such scenarios. Part of the answer is that even major events have degrees, levels, topography, and timeline.

In other words, despite instances of extreme misery, there are also isles or larger territories of relative low exposure and stability. At such places – or indeed in most places (Levy, 1996) – human interaction, including therapies, is extremely helpful. Additionally, mass violence often concerns specific subgroups (e.g., soldiers directly involved in combat amongst deployed armed forces; core victims of major terrorist incidents within cities). Such heterogeneity leaves professionals and other resources with significant capacity to help those primarily affected. Experience further shows that clients with psychological problems do come to treatment facilities during continuous adversities, often in larger numbers than those physically injured (Bleich *et al.*, 1992). Most importantly, a growing body of evidence suggests that even within rolling adversities, such as wars, early treatment may mitigate the effect of exposure in those who break down (Solomon, 1993).

Clinicians, however, have to acquire specific knowledge and new skills in order to effectively perform under such circumstances. These encompasses observation, diagnosis, and underlying theory. Additionally, versatility and flexibility are required, such that interventions meet the client's needs, consider his or her resources, appraise eventual ongoing stressors, follow clients' progression and recovery, and monitor the quality of support offered by natural helpers. Goals and priorities of therapy during mass trauma should also be restated. Rather than 'treating' psychopathology, one's task is mainly to optimize recovery. Rather than intervening alone, or within specialized 'clinics' one's overall impact relies on being linked with family and community resources. Rather than emphasizing weakness and vulnerabilities, one must work with clients' strength and resourcefulness. Rather than expecting recovery and return to normal, when normal living conditions have been shattered successful and honorable survivorship is often as much as on can achieve (Shalev *et al.*, 1993a; see also Nuttall and Coetzee, 1998).

This chapter addresses the what clinicians may do within the traditional context of therapist–client encounter. It does not address other functions that clinicians may have, such becoming consultants to community leaders, or appearing in the media as risk communicators. In order to remain focused, this chapter emphasizes the effect of an ongoing trauma, and does not extend to reactivation of prior experiences or mental disorders. Traumatic grief is another overlapping area which clearly deserves to be fully developed elsewhere. Finally, we do not address the treatment of prolonged mental disorders, but rather those distressful and disabling conditions that occur during or immediately after disasters.

Caveats and basic assumptions

Little empirical evidence supports the long-term effect of early psychological interventions. Consequently, this chapter is limited in its capacity to offer evidence-based recommendations. Yet, the treatment of repeated trauma cannot wait for controlled

Table 11.2 Proposed principles of early interventions

Interventions are aimed to optimize recovery, rather than treat diseased states of mind
Flexible use of treatment techniques in ways that match needs and situational constraints
Support of clients' own coping resources and recovery strategies
Uncontrollable states of mind are prime targets
A shift from observing symptoms to identifying underlying mental processes
A shift from quantifying expressions of distress to assessing their efficacy in, recruiting
    support, sustaining rewarding interpersonal contacts and initiating self-exposure that leads
    to resolution
Interventions address three confluent factors: stressors, reactions and resources

experiments to be carried out. Thus, somewhat naively we assume that reducing distress and enabling better personal functioning and rewarding human interaction should affect the long-term outcome traumatic exposure. Much of the knowledge presented below has been gained during years of studying and treating recent survivors in emergency rooms and clinical settings. Such experience has also taught us that some survivors do develop chronic mental disorders despite being treated immediately, intensely, and continuously. Given such a humbling lesson, this chapter does not pretend to teach therapists how to cure trauma, but rather advises them how to optimize their approach to the recently traumatized. It goes without saying that this advice should be submitted to further empirical confirmation.

What are the central claims of this text? First, we recommend a generic approach, in which ingredients of interpersonal therapy, crisis intervention, supportive therapy, and cognitive–behavioral therapy are used in a way that matches needs and situational constraints. Second, we propose that early clinical interventions should mainly enhance and activate clients' own resources and recovery strategies. We additionally suggest that uncontrollable states of mind, whether anxious, depressive, dissociative, or agitated, should be the prime targets of therapies, because these conditions interfere with self-regulation, social interaction, and recovery. Deficient social support and secondary stressors at the aftermath of a trauma are potent risk factors for posttraumatic stress disorder (PTSD) (Brewin *et al.*, 2000). We also propose that clinicians must become acquainted with available resources and ongoing stressors and help the client manage utilize and manage both. Finally we propose a shift of attention from mental symptoms to underlying mental processes and from evaluating the intensity of responses to following their progression (Table 11.2).

We suggest that in situations of prolonged or catastrophic distress, clients' conditions are affected by three major factors: (1) Stressfulness and novelty of external reality, (2) inner and external resources, and (3) inner states of mind, involving arousal, affect, and cognition. We propose, therefore, that all therapies of recent survivors assess these three dimensions, address that which might be going wrong, and use any of these confluent domains to affect the two others. For example, following the loss of living relatives, the absence of supportive listening may seriously increase survivors' distress and disarray, and thereby lead to distorted self-appraisal and perception of others. Such a situation can be addressed by either providing a substitute to sympathetic listening (e.g., a therapist, a friend, a peer-victim) but also by affecting physiological and emotional distress (e.g., by medication) such that the patient is in better self-control and better able to find substitutes to sharing and disclosing (e.g., volunteering, helping others who are more severely affected).

Between dogma and excessive flexibility

Clinical interventions during continuous adversity suffer from two inherent problems: (1) a trend to standardize the interventions, often by recommending protocols or doctrines, and (2) a tendency to use entirely intuitive *ad hoc* responses. A salient example of the former is the doctrine of frontline 'forward' treatment during military conflicts. Implemented systematically during World War II, the Korea campaign and the Vietnam War, a rigid implementation of this doctrine is illustrated by following vignette (Camp, 1993, p. 1005).

In November 1971, Corporal A, a 20-year-old infantryman, who had been assigned in Vietnam for 5 months, was transported by helicopter to an Army evacuation hospital along with other combat casualties. Upon his arrival he was observed to be mute, grunting incomprehensibly, and posturing. He was quite disorganized and could not communicate with his examiners. He was easily startled by noise and walked with a slow, shuffling gait. When he sat in a chair, he rocked with his eyes closed and occasionally mumbled 'Mamma.' The results of his physical examination were otherwise normal.

On the psychiatric unit, Corporal A was given a shower and was 'put to sleep' with chlorpromazine (dose not available; chlorpromazine or CPZ is an antipsychotic agent). When he woke up, 18 hours later, he seemed alert, coherent, and rational. He was issued a fresh uniform and received instructions about the quasi-military ward routine. The staff told him that he was recovering from overexposure to combat and that he could expect to be returned to his military unit soon. In the group therapy meeting, Corporal A emotionally described how he had been serving as a fire team leader when six of his friends were killed and mutilated by enemy fire; he had become agitated and began screaming while loading their bodies into a helicopter. He talked despondently of his revulsion at the killing and was regretful that he had 'gone to pieces.' He felt torn because he always sought to be 'good' and wanted to be good soldier, but it wasn't his 'makeup' to kill. He said that he could not return to the field. The record notes that the psychiatric staff responded to his feelings 'with reality testing and ego support of his duty and mission.' That night he was informed that he would be returning to his unit the following day and he was again given chlorpromazine.

Several aspects of this intervention are not above critique. The use of antipsychotic medication may be inappropriate and the resulting sedation may falsely create an impression of recovery. The soldier's complaints and desires are clearly ignored and responded to by diametrically opposing decisions. The power to enforce these decisions stems from military authority, rather than medical evidence. One hardly observes compassion – on indeed any therapeutic interaction other than sedation and persuasion. However, for those practicing in Vietnam this method seemed effective, particularly when the treating team did not see the casualty for follow-up. Not surprisingly, military psychiatrists who initially endorsed this model (e.g., Colbach and Parrish, 1970) subsequently published a rebuke (Colbach, 1985). In the latter one reads as follows: 'In many ways I was a failure in actually reaching out to these fellows and touching them and alleviating their suffering' (p. 265). Camp (1993) further addresses this topic: 'combat psychiatrists are influenced by powerful, potentially competing values systems but cannot realistically assess some of the most important factors that affect the balance of harm and benefit associated with their treatment decisions.'

Protocols are tempting by their simplicity and apparent clarity. Another example of protocol-driven treatment is the somewhat uncritical implementation of the so-called critical incident stress debriefing (CISD) across situations and populations affected by traumatic events. CISD had an appealing rationale, which was to enable a revision of the recent event, allow 'ventilation' of emotions, validate individual experiences and share them with others, and receive knowledge about the normalcy of the response and about the nature of the resulting symptoms (Shalev, 2000). Additionally CISD sessions followed a simple protocol, which could be implemented and replicated without difficulty. Conflicting results, however, have started to appear in the literature during the last decade (e.g., Raphael *et al.*, 1995; Kenardy *et al.*, 1996) and in some cases debriefing seems to have increased the likelihood of developing prolonged stress disorders (Bisson *et al.*, 1997) One session debriefing is currently known to have inconsistent effects (Rose *et al.*, 2001).

Beyond these salient example other views and concepts can be rigidly implemented at the early aftermath of a traumatic event. Examples of prevailing schemata, at risk of becoming a dogma, include the belief that 'survivors should speak up, verbalize, and disclose their traumatic experiences;' the assumption that 'pharmacological treatment interferes with normal recovery' or indeed, the belief that 'cognitive–behavioral therapy (CBT) is the recommended treatment for recent survivors.' All three statements have some empirical basis (Gelpin *et al.*, 1996; Bryant *et al.*, 1998, 1999) yet probably not enough to justify an uncritical use across situations and individuals.

On the other hand there is a risk of therapeutic abstention or of totally intuitive, nonspecific interventions. Such trend may be exemplified by a recent *Guideline for*

Response to the Recent Tragic Events posted on the internet following the September 11 events in the United States (Foa *et al.*, 2001). The text reads as follows:

If someone wants to speak with a professional in this immediate aftermath period, a helpful response will be to:

a) listen actively and supportively, but do not probe for details and emotional responses. Let the person say what they feel comfortable saying without pushing for more.

b) validate a normal natural recovery.

Outcome studies of Psychological Debriefing (PD) are mixed. Overall, they do not support the efficacy of a one-session intervention shortly after the trauma in decreasing psychological disturbances after a trauma beyond natural recovery. Some studies found that in the long run, a single-session of PD may hinder natural recovery.

Accordingly, we do not recommend intervention in this initial aftermath period.

. . .

Individuals who continue to experience severe distress that interferes with functioning after three months are at higher risk for continued problems. These individuals should be referred for appropriate treatment.

While these views might have been a cautious reaction to overzealous interventions, waiting for 3 months could be excessively long. Some survivors are clearly dysfunctional and distressed at the early aftermath of traumatic events, and do present themselves to clinical facilities. Additionally, prospective studies of recent survivors suggest that some of the biological alterations that are typical to PTSD incubate during the first few months that follow a traumatic event (Shalev *et al.*, 2000). We propose that such advice be modified to suggest that all uncontrollable and disabling responses to traumatic events deserve evaluation and eventual treatment. The specifics of such intervention should be decided for each individual case.

Should all those expressing symptoms of posttraumatic stress disorder be treated?

Traumatic events regularly elicit transient expressions of distress, which often resemble PTSD symptoms. Recent surveys further show that disabling symptoms may occur among subjects exposed to media reports of a major trauma (Schuster *et al.*, 2001; Galea *et al.*, 2002). What are the clinical implications of these widespread symptoms? Should all those expressing distress be treated? If not, how does one recognize those who do require treatment?

A recent survey of population under continuous stress may help elucidate some of these points. The survey concerned a suburb of Jerusalem which between October

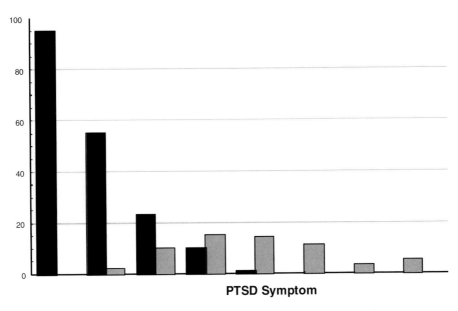

Figure 11.1 Bimodal distribution of PTSD symptoms among 177 civilians living under terrorist threat in suburbs of Jerusalem in 2001 (63 expressing the full PTSD syndrome; 223 not expressing the full syndrome).

2000 and July 2001 (when data was obtained) was subject to continuous and repeated terror in the form of roadside sniper shootings, stoning of cars, and other incidents. Several people were killed or injured on the road and, later, within the suburb. The study sample consisted of 177 middle-class dwellers, of an average age of 40.5 ± 13. Most (83 percent) were married and had children. Seventy percent had college education and 55 percent rated their income as above average. The average number of traumatic incidents experienced by a subject was 6.2. Terror seriously disrupted their life routines, affecting working hours, travel to and from work, contact with relatives living in central Israel, and leisure activities. Twenty-five percent of the sample endorsed sufficient PTSD symptoms to meet a full diagnosis of the disorder (as by the PTSD symptom scale; Foa and Tolin, 2000). Importantly, the remaining 75 percent tended to express very few PTSD symptoms. Figure 11.1 illustrates a bimodal distribution of PTSD symptoms in this sample.

   PTSD symptoms of intrusive thoughts, emotional reactivity to reminders of traumatic events, sleep disturbances, irritability, exaggerated startle and hyperalertness were frequently endorsed (i.e., in up to 80 percent of the sample) (Fig. 11.2). Problems concentrating, avoidance of thoughts, reliving of the trauma, nightmares, numbing, and distancing were less frequently expressed. Loss of interest, avoidance of activities, and traumatic amnesia were the least frequently expressed.

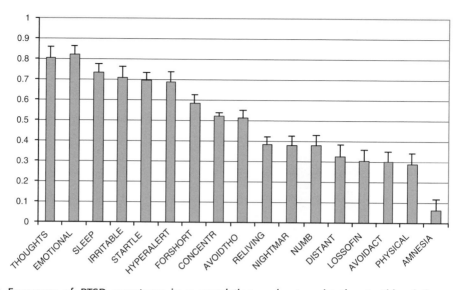

Figure 11.2 Frequency of PTSD symptoms in a population under terrorist threat. Abbreviations: THOUGHTS, intrusive thoughts about the traumatic event; EMOTIONA, heightened emotional responses to reminders; SLEEP, difficulty falling asleep; IRRITABLE, irritability; STARTLE, exaggerated startle response; HYPERALE, hyperalertness; FORSHORT, sense of foreshortened future; CONCENTR, difficulty in concentrating; AVOIDTHO, avoidance of thoughts related to the traumatic event; RELIVING, reliving of the traumatic event; NIGHT-MAR, nightmares; NUMB, numbing of responses; DISTANT, distancing; LOSSOFIN, loss of interest; AVOIDACT, avoidance of action; PHYSICAL, physiological responses to reminders of the traumatic event; AMNESIA, inability to remember (parts of) the traumatic event.

But symptoms do not tell the whole story. An evaluation of specific fears has shown an excess of realistic fears, (e.g., driving, coming home late at night) but no excess of fears from situations that were not specific to this suburb (e.g., being in crowded places). Moreover, despite threat and repeated incidents, most people held their jobs and remained involved in community and religious activities. Very few sought help.

Several conclusions can be drawn, regarding the presence of PTSD symptoms in entire communities. First, PTSD symptoms are unequally distributed amongst exposed subjects. Second, despite their frequent expression PTSD symptoms may not as disabling as in clinical cases. Third, fears may be situation-specific whereas in clinical cases they 'inappropriately' generalize (Keane *et al.*, 1985). Fourth, symptoms of numbing and dissociation are infrequently expressed. A threshold for defining a case for treatment is therefore necessary. The presence of incapacitating distress, pervasive avoidance, numbing, and dissociation may characterize a person in need for clinical intervention.

Symptoms among help-seeking survivors

Among help-seeking survivors, dissociation, depression, and the syndrome of acute stress disorder (ASD) are important risk indicators of PTSD. ASD consists of typical symptoms of PTSD (re-experiencing, avoidance, and hyperarousal) and dissociative symptoms (numbing, detachment, reduced awareness of one's surroundings, derealization, depersonalization, and dissociative amnesia). Symptoms of ASD occur within a month of exposure, last for at least two days, cause clinically significant distress, and significantly interfere with the individual's functioning or impair the individual's ability to pursue necessary tasks. The occurrence of ASD is associated with high prevalence of subsequent PTSD. However, many survivors who do not meet diagnostic criteria for ASD develop PTSD. Indeed, a subset of ASD symptoms (numbing, depersonalization, sense of reliving the trauma, and motor restlessness) strongly predicts subsequent PTSD, while other symptoms, including most dissociation symptoms, do not (Harvey and Bryant, 1998). ASD, therefore, is an extreme response, involving higher risk of subsequent PTSD. It is not the only way to develop PTSD. For example, Brewin *et al.* (1999) have shown that intense intrusive memories are as good predictors of PTSD as ASD. Dissociative responses immediately following trauma and depressive symptoms during the week that follows trauma have equally been linked with higher risk of subsequent PTSD (Shalev *et al.*, 1996; Fullerton *et al.*, 2000).

A common denominator of these early syndromes remains their incapacitating nature (as in DSM-IV criteria for ASD) and their pervasive presence and domination of other mental activities. Indeed, what clinical observations often reveal is the extent to which survivors who express a cluster of symptoms are utterly governed by their symptoms or, in contrast, experience them intermittently or partially. Conducting clinical interviews with injured survivors of terror, Shalev *et al.* (1993b) found intrusive recollections in all, yet patients differed by the extent to which these symptoms interfered with their ability to communicate with others, with their ability to relax and allocate attention to additional tasks and with core physiological functions such as sleep, bodily tension, and autonomic arousal. Additionally, Shalev (2002) argued that because early PTSD symptoms are seen in most survivors they must have an adaptive role. Early symptoms may help recruit support (by emitting a cry for help), enhance communication with others (by telling the story time and again), and promote a progressive reappraisal of one's recollections of the trauma (via repeated contemplation). When these are overwhelming, uncontrollable, and involve extreme physiological arousal they may, in contrast, consolidate the link between fear and traumatic recall, thereby lead to extended avoidance, redundant repeated recall, and ultimately to PTSD. Brewin *et al.* (1996) suggested another adaptive role of intrusive recall at the early aftermath of trauma, i.e., of transforming fear-driven, stimulus-bound, and intrusive memory traces of traumatic experiences into verbally and electively accessible episodic memories.

It ensues that clinicians should consider the extent to which early expressions of distress successfully recruit support, enhance communication and lead to reappraisal and resolution. They should be concerned by those patients in which the early symptoms become redundant, truncated, fearfully avoided, or associated with extreme anxiety or sadness. In situations of repeated terror, clinicians should additionally assess the extent to which ongoing threat reactivates prior traumatic experiences.

Responses and their clinical management

Responses to traumatic events evolve with time, from initial, survival-driven efforts through adjustment, realization of loss, adaptation, and return to normal life. Clinical interventions, accordingly, will have different goals and use different techniques at each phase. Importantly, the clinical management of survivors must be embedded in the general rescue and management efforts provided by nonclinicians, natural helpers, and community resources. Moreover, while clinical considerations should address symptoms and complaints, they must also consider the presence of concurrent stressors and the availability of inner and external resources. Since distress is ubiquitous, under continuous stress, the evaluation of clinical symptoms should specifically emphasize their disabling effect, that is, their eventual interference with normal recovery. The idea that recovery is the expected outcome in most cases implies that clinicians consider their interventions as designed to enable and optimize recovery. This will often be done by identifying and monitoring those factors that interfere with recovery. Among the latter, persistent stress and lack resources are prominent. Table 11.3 outlines four successive phases of the response to traumatic events and examines stressors, typical responses, resources, generic interventions, and clinical interventions. The table also provides milestones for evaluating one's work. The following text further extends the information provided in the table.

The impact phase

A frequent misperception of behavior under severe stress involves assuming generalized panic and uncontrollable, disorganized behavior. With the exception of few, survivors' immediate responses are goal-directed and purposeful. The main goal of behavior is survival, but survival often encompasses self *and* relatives. Many survivors find themselves caught in immediate fight–flight responses, either challenging the threat or escaping. In so doing, survivors are also 'stimulus-bound' in that they are very responsive to cues, often without taking time to reflect and modulate their responses. Survivors often imitate and follow what others are doing, or instantaneously react in one way or another. Thus, when one survivor ducks for cover, others will tend to duck as well. Altruistic behavior is often seen. Affective and affiliative bonds often dictate protective gestures sometime at an increased risk for oneself.

Given the stressfulness of the impact phase, survivors find it difficult to modify a course of action, and seem to be caught in what they initially start to do. Thus, an initial escape response may be followed through and accomplished, despite appeals for help by others. This may later become a source of endless regret and self-blame. Thus, however successful one's immediate behavior might be, the advent of overwhelming exposure, and unexpected, dominating reactions leaves many survivors with unanswered questions that they have to 'digest' and accommodate. Survivors at the periphery of major events may flow in, in an attempt to help, and subsequently be overwhelmed by scenes of horror and death. Exposure to grotesque sights, sounds, and smells, even when there is no further threat (e.g., following a bomb explosion) is strong enough to provoke severe, often paralyzing, distress. Thus, beyond their threatening dimension, stressful events constitute informational load, overwhelming by unexpected and incongruous novelty. Our experience with survivors of suicide bombs taught us that incongruous novelty (e.g., body parts, decapitated bodies) is a major trigger of early intrusive recollections. The latter may start within an hour of the exposure.

Survivors emotional responses may also be defensively blunted or dissociative (Marmar *et al.*, 1994; Shalev *et al.*, 1996; Ursano *et al.*, 1999). Dissociation during trauma (e.g., feeling disconnected, on 'automatic pilot,' experiencing time distortion or moments of forgetfulness) may be protective in the short run, (Shalev *et al.*, 1998). Dissociative symptoms during exposure predict subsequent stress disorders, but the literature is unclear on whether this is truly dissociation, or rather an extreme responses to stress. Specifically, time distortion is the most frequently endorsed dissociation symptom (e.g., Shalev *et al.* 1998; Ursano *et al.*, 1999), but time distortion is a generic stress response which might be unrelated to other dissociation symptoms. Clinicians at emergency rooms, however, face another and more severe form of dissociation, i.e. frank, severe, and paralyzing dissociative episodes resembling stupor and shock. The latter may not remit spontaneously, and are often associated with extreme physiological arousal. These extreme responses must be promptly addressed, often by medication.

Generic interventions during the impact phase of disasters include protection from threat, reduction of the randomness of situations and events (e.g., by helping to locate family members and relatives), and provision of basic needs (i.e., food, shelter, and information). Clinicians should use soothing human contact, help verbalize events and responses, reassure, listen, and assist those who come to soothe

Table 11.3 General management and clinical treatment following mass trauma

Stressor	Responses	Resources	Management	Goals and milestones
Impact phase (few hours)				
Threat	Mental processes	Inner	Generic	Generic
Incongruous novelty (exposure to grotesque)	Survival	Early coping responses	Protection from threat	Protection from danger achieved
Loss	Handling of incongruency and chaos	External	Reduction of randomness and uncertainty	Stressfulness of new reality reduced
Uncertainty	Frequent responses	Helpers	Reduction of secondary stressors	Proper information about reactions, resources and relatives provided
Exposure to extreme human behavior	Fight–flight	Family and significant others	Provision of basic needs	Contacts with significant others established
Humiliation, degradation	Blunted/defensive reactions		Resources	Community resources contacted and involved
Physiological strain	Freezing/surrender/ dissociation		Increase controllability of situations and inner states of mind	Clinical
	Distressful intrusive recollections		Renew contact with significant others	Emotions are controllable
			Maintain dignity and self-respect	Sensorium is clear and dissociative states dealt with
			Clinical intervention	Survivor and helpers informed about symptoms and reactions
			'Psychological first aid'	Survivor and natural helpers informed about treatment resources
			Soothing human contact	
			Reassurance, validation of psychological responses	
			Tranquilizers?	

Rescue and stabilization phase (0–2 days)

	Mental processes	Inner resources	Generic	Generic
Repeated exposure to primary stressors	Adjustment	Beliefs, values, hope, active coping	Protection from secondary stressors	Secondary stressors minimized
Secondary stressors: relocation, separation, injury, pain	'Accommodation'	Healing narrative	Provision of needs	Safe recovery environment established and supported
Realization of loss	Help-seeking	Attachment bonds	Reduction of randomness and uncertainty	Basic needs identified and catered for
Intensity and controllability of one's own reactions	Frequent responses	Active role in healing	Resources	Family and community resources activated
	Posttraumatic syndrome: intrusive thoughts, numbing/avoidance, arousal	External resources	Support families during grief and mourning	Clinical
	Grief responses	Concrete healing environment: shelter, food	Optimize family environment.	Uncontrollable arousal eliminated
	Reappraisal of the traumatic event and of one's early responses	Human contacts: family, friends, and other natural helpers	Optimize medical care	Early responses do not interfere with:
	Reactivation of prior vulnerabilities	Professional helpers	Optimize social support	(a) rewarding human contacts
		Social attribution, shared narratives, hope	Clinical	(b) required task performance
			Educate about early responses	(c) controllability of emotional states
			Identify and alleviate dysregulated states of mind	(d) realistic and positive self-perception
			Help the helpers	Intensity of responses decays with time
			Promote sharing and disclosure	
			Provide surrogate human contacts for those in need	

Table 11.3 (*cont.*)

Stressor	Responses	Resources	Management	Goals and milestones
Early responses (0–4 weeks)				
Repeated exposure to primary or secondary stressors	Mental processes	Inner resources	Generic	Generic
Resources loss, financial/material burden	Adaptation	Attractiveness of normal life	Optimize recovery environment	Survivors and their helpers continue to receive resources and support as needed
Realization of physical and mental disability	Assimilation	Bonding and love	Secure access to medical and psychological care	Clinical
Being left alone by helpers	Reappraisal	Hope and positive attribution	Support depleted family resources	Effective help seeking
Intolerable, distressful states of mind	Frequent responses	Healing narrative (individual and social)	Clinical	enabled and resources made available and publicized
	Exploration versus avoidance	External resources	Alleviate distressing and disabling PTSD and related symptoms	Specific syndromes identified and treated
	Aggregation versus isolation	Supportive others	Alleviate depression	
	Persistent PTSD and depressive symptoms	Nurturing recovery environment and social network	Address negative self-appraisal and blame	
	Emotional numbing	Availability and accessibility of help and assistance	Reduce avoidance of situations, places, and thoughts	
	Adverse health practices, alcohol and substance abuse		Help in the search for meaning and reappraisal	

Return to life	Mental processes	Inner resources	Generic	Detection, monitoring, and management of sources of distress
Additional stressors	Reparation	The above, and	Reduction of cues and situations reminding of the trauma	Detection and evaluation of distressed, dysfunctional individuals
Loss of resources, community, and family structures	Integration, habituation or sensitization	Acceptance of change, ability to reframe views and goals	Help in redefinition of self and working capacity	Diagnosis and proper treatment of identified cases
Demands related to social and vocational reinsertion	Frequent responses	External resources	Symbolic, community driven rituals and commemoration	Rehabilitation and reinsertion of disabled survivors
Physical disability	Engagement or avoidance	Skilled and experienced clinicians	Clinical	
Redefinitions of self and others	Acceptable survivorship versus depression; PTSD, substance abuse		Diagnosis and specialized management of syndromes and responses.	
Ongoing physical and mental syndromes	Fully formed, tenacious mental disorders		Cognitive–behavioral therapy	
			Pharmacotherapy	

and support the survivor. They may use tranquilizers to stop prolonged dissociative episodes. As in other phases of the response, the clinicians' role is mainly to address uncontrollable states of mind and enable rewarding interaction with natural helpers (e.g., relatives, friends, coworkers). Clinical criteria for discharging subjects from helping facilities include controllability of emotions, end of dissociative states, and contact with natural helpers. Survivors and helpers should be informed about the possibility of further reactions and about treatment resources in the community. As a rule, survivors should not be discharged without accompanying persons, should not be sent back to potentially stressful situations, and should have been linked with a source of care and continuous support.

Immediate 'rescue' phase

Immediately following disasters, affected survivors find themselves in new life situations (e.g., being injured, displaced, having endured a major loss), to which they have to adjust, using whatever resources they find and whatever coping mechanisms they have previously acquired and practiced. Such process has been referred to as 'accommodation' (Piaget, 1963). Primary stressors may continue (e.g., repeated terror attacks) and secondary stressors are often present. The latter include relocation, separation, injury, pain – indeed any factor that makes the situation uncontrollable, unpredictable, and demanding. Realization of losses may be extremely painful. The intensity of one's own reactions can also worry patients, make them believe that they are losing their minds. Such misinterpretation of early symptoms contributes to subsequent PTSD (Ehlers and Steihl, 1995). Individuals with previous traumata, and those who have suffered from mental disorders are particularly vulnerable (Brewin *et al.*, 2000).

Many survivors express the full PTSD syndrome at this stage (as in 94 percent of rape survivors). Depressive symptoms are also frequent, and independently contribute to subsequent PTSD (Freedman *et al.*, 1999). Traumatic recollections come to mind time and again and sharing them offers a chance of re-evaluation. However, to the extent that traumatic recollections are extremely distressful, avoided, or truncated, they may become repetitive and self-perpetuating. Beliefs, values, hope, active coping, and strong attachment bonds are the survivor's primary resources at this phase.

Once the basics are assured (e.g., provision of basic needs, medical care, contact with natural helpers), clinicians should mainly identify survivors who suffer from dysregulated and uncontrollable responses, identify the source of such responses (e.g., prior vulnerability, extreme form of exposure, secondary stressors, deficient resources, or particularly strong reaction), and try and reduce them. Cautious use of tranquilizers may be recommended, as long as their effect is monitored and followed

(Table 11.4). Rarely will a professional helper have to become surrogate source of human interaction, replacing relative and natural helpers. Such case include lonely patients (e.g., immigrants) or patients with dysfunctional or severely traumatized families. In most cases clinicians are called to help the helpers, soothe, inform and educate, help sharing and disclosing, and mediate between families and treatment agencies. Successful treatment at this stage does not necessary consist of eliminating symptoms and other expressions of distress. Instead, removal of uncontrollable states of mind and optimization of resources are more realistic goals. In so doing clinicians should evaluate the extent to which the early responses interfere with necessary task performance, prevent rewarding human interaction, and lead to negative self-perception (Pearlin and Schooler, 1978). Clients' progress is better evaluated longitudinally.

Early responses

Once out of danger and stabilized, survivors start to 'learn from experience,' that is, they start to assimilate and adapt to life following trauma. The extent of material and human loss, for example, becomes obvious, but the full implications of such loss are not yet clear. Delayed secondary stressors may operate (e.g., complication of surgery), and those may send survivors back to extreme 'survival-driven' responses. Rescue agencies often leave the scene at such time, and continuity of care may become a problem. Some survivors continue to suffer from extreme mental responses.

Survivors either explore and become involved in the new situation, or start avoiding issues and solutions. Identified cohorts of survivors may lose their cohesion (e.g., as individuals go back to their homes) and loneliness and isolation might be seen. Bereaved survivors are still emotionally numb and confused. Some survivors drink excessively or inadvertently turn to medication. Yet the attractiveness of life, emotional bonding, love, and hope start to exercise their healing effect, assisted by supportive others, professional and nonprofessional helpers. Lack of such resources may become critical at this stage. Some survivors may find it difficult to seek help, or tend to defer, cancel or miss consultations. The availability and access to treatment facilities is crucial, and steps should be taken to destigmatize self-referral.

PTSD symptoms and depression are now clear and obvious, and clinicians may wish to consider their specific treatment. Yet fully protocolized treatment packages may not be needed at this stage. Advice, information, and help in planning one's recovery path may suffice for many clients. Others can enjoy a partial implementation of cognitive techniques (e.g., challenging negative self-perception or generalization of fear) or guided self-exposure to reminders of the traumatic event. The search for meaning may be poignant, as in the following vignette:

Table 11.4. Pharmacotherapy at the early stages of the response to traumatic events

Stage	Treatment goals	Treatment options[a]	Documented effect	Justification for clinical use[a]
Impact phase (first hours)	Reduce uncontrollable distress and dissociation	Benzodiazepines, other tranquilizers	Anxiolytic effect	Anecdotal. Long-acting BZs and those with antipanic effect may facilitate psychosocial interventions
	Prevent fear conditioned responses	Propranolol	Reduces bodily responses to reminders of traumatic events in recent survivors	Preliminary
Immediate response (First days)	Prevent 'kindling' and memory consolidation	Clonidine, Carbamazepine	Partial effect in prolonged PTSD	Theoretical
	Alleviate depression	Antidepressants	Documented effect in depressive illness and PTSD	No controlled studies in acute response to trauma. Good evidence in depressive conditions of any origin
	Alleviate anxiety, insomnia, agitation	Clonidine, BZs, other tranquilizers	Improved sleep, reduced distress	Preliminary. BZs may increase the odds of developing PTSD
	Severe or repeated dissociative episodes	Major tranquilizers	Some effect on dissociative episodes in chronic PTSD	Preliminary. Long-term use not justified
Short-term response (First weeks)	Alleviate PTSD and depressive symptoms	SSRIs, TCAs, MAOIs,	Good in prolonged PTSD	Preliminary
	Reduce agitation, hyperarousal	Mood stabilizers	Partial effect	No documentation in acute PTSD
	Prevent neuronal damage	e.g., Tianeptine	Experimental evidence of neuroprotective effect under stress	Theoretical

[a] BZs, benzodiazepines; SSRIs, selective serotonin reuptake inhibitors; TCAs, tricyclic antidepressants; MAOIs, mono amine oxidase inhibitors.

> *When the terrorist bomb exploded, in the midst of the crowd one sister was sitting at a table while the other, the younger one, was dancing in the midst of the crowd. They had lost contact and our patient painfully pulled herself out of the rubble. She never saw her sister again. She nonetheless continued to look for her – in nightmares and ruminations, but also through seeking information from everyone present about the sister's last moments. Where was she? Had she been seen by someone? Slowly, there was guilt; unreasonable, yet penetrating. The quest for meaning became frantic: 'Could I have stepped on her body on my way out of the chaos?' Then sorrow came, photos were sorted and shown. 'How rebellious had she been,' 'How lively,' 'How full of life.' And then another change of tone: 'I must live for her.' 'I can't let her down by being weak and defeated.' Life has become a continuation of another life. Enabling survivor role restored.*

Return to life

Life does not return to normal before weeks and months have passed. Yet, within few weeks, survivors are called to regain many of their functions, i.e., go back to work, become a nurturing parent, resume social activities. None of this is easy or natural. Loss of resources may be poignant. Superficial adaptation to concrete tasks may mask ongoing grief, or shattered life. This is a time where diseased survivors are salient, because they 'can't make it back.' This is also a time for definite clinical diagnoses and treatment. Cognitive–behavioral therapy (CBT) and pharmacotherapy are the two main options (Table 11.3) – but couple therapies, supportive groups, or planned recreational activities may help. When trauma is repetitive, classical therapies have to be modified as in the following example.

Carrying cognitive–behavioral therapy during continuous adversities

During ongoing conflict, treatment approaches may need to be modified, in order to take into account the context in which the patient, and therapist are living. Our experience of treating patients with PTSD following terrorist attacks with cognitive behavior therapy illustrates this point.

Having used a standardized CBT protocol (Foa and Rothbaum, 1989) very successfully, we experienced specific problems with these patients. Avoidance symptoms are assumed in cognitive–behavioral models to decrease the fear symptoms typically experienced by the patient when confronted by a reminder of the trauma. In a context of ongoing conflict, avoidance is experienced by many people who have no PTSD, nor direct exposure to a terrorist attack. In this group avoidance is indicative of safety behavior. For instance, many people avoided the city center, where there had been repeated terror attacks, unless they had no alternative. This led to changes in carrying out CBT. In standard CBT, a list of avoidant behaviors is constructed, and patients begin *in vivo* exposure to these feared situations in a gradual fashion. In the context described here, we divided this list into two:

those situations that were clearly safe and generally not avoided, and those that were considered dangerous and where avoidance had become the norm (e.g., city center). Patients were encouraged to carry out *in vivo* the former list, but not the latter.

Additionally we conceptualized the avoidance of the PTSD patients and that of the general population differently, in terms of the underlying cognitions. People with PTSD were thinking 'If I go there will definitely be another attack, and this time I will definitely die,' whereas non-PTSD were thinking 'The risk is very small, but I really don't need to go and buy a book – it is not worth the risk.' Since habituation via *in vivo* exposure was impossible, we carried out cognitive therapy regarding the above cognitions, and this proved very successful. Often, patients would persist with the avoidance behaviors, but this was based on a more accurate perception of reality.

Almost all of the PTSD patients we treated experienced another similar trauma during treatment, either through direct exposure or indirectly via media broadcast, and conversations. This severely interfered with therapy: one of the goals in CBT is for the patient to realize that the trauma was a discrete event, belonging to the past (Ehlers and Clark, 2000). Re-exposures, however, confirmed patients' perceptions of present and future danger. We addressed this by firstly encouraging the patients to actively avoid indirect exposure, for instance, not watching the detailed television reports of a terrorist attack. In addition, we stressed a 'coping' model, where some avoidance was reframed as positive safety behavior. Most importantly, we assumed that the endpoint of therapy was not one characterized by no fear, but 'normal fear', given the daily stresses and dangers of living in a city under threat of violent conflict.

Survivors who do not seek help

Many affected survivors do not seek help. Others drop out of clinical facilities following an initial contact (Whittlesey *et al.*, 1999). A survey of former prisoners of war from the 1973 Yom Kippur War in Israel revealed survivors who despite manifest symptoms of PTSD did not receive help for 18 years (Solomon *et al.*, 1994). Not seeking help following traumatic events may lead to chronic and disabling condition. Additionally when trauma occurs during professional activities, failure to provide help may lead to litigation and claims of neglect. Reaching out for potentially affected survivors may be a reasonable strategy to adopt, yet the yield of such approach has not been evaluated. Group sessions involving survivors of specific events may identify subjects at risk, and this strategy is applied following major terrorist acts in Israel. Monitoring the mental health of police officers or armed services personnel may also become a recommended routine.

It is nonetheless true that some survivors prefer not to receive help. Survivors may see their condition as normal and their suffering as an expected outcome of exposure. Survivors may be reluctant to be seen by mental health practitioners because of the stigma that is associated with having a mental disorder. Survivors may be afraid of losing their job or seeing their career affected by being diagnosed with a mental disorder. Survivors may be struggling with significant adversities, or expecting additional exposure, during which time opening up or admitting vulnerability may be beyond their capacity. Some survivors attempt a first contact and find clinicians' responses unsatisfactory. Finally, there are cultural barriers to seeking help from clinicians, some of which are related to alternative healing opportunities, such as community gathering or religious relief; others stem from gaps between popular and high cultures, and yet others stem from a institutional or national cultures of denial and closure. Thus, reluctance to seek help is a complex issue, which can not be seen as reflecting denial or refusal. Solutions to this problem are complex and may involve publicity, education, risk communication, and getting closer to communities of survivors. Therapists from within affected communities may help to close the gap between potential clients and clinicians. Most importantly, clinicians should be aware of the fact that survivors quickly classify them as either relevant or irrelevant, in which case they will never see them again. They should, therefore, try to qualify as competent helpers, mainly by generously and humanely sharing and giving, but also by professionally identifying stressors, responses, and needs.

Between recovery and survivorship

Whilst recovery is a frequent outcome of traumatic events, lack of complete recovery can not always be equated with disease. For some survivors, the traumatic experience has been such that it is unforgettable. Others suffer incurable losses. Entire communities may be relocated, entire families slaughtered. Community resources may take a generation to be restored. Persecution may last for decades. Entire regions may have to be abandoned because of irradiation. Famine may prevail. Refugees and asylum seekers may endure continuous stress and humiliation. Slavery, forced prostitution, random and systematic torture have been seen. Western psychiatry has been criticized as 'medicalizing' and 'pathologizing' posttraumatic conditions (Bracken *et al.*, 1995); catering for PTSD where community destruction prevails and ignoring the impact of ethnic, political, and economic factors. While this discussion is, indeed, beyond the scope of this text, it is certainly true that for some individuals, even within affluent communities, survivorship becomes a mode of life; a second and new identity. Clinicians who treat survivors (e.g., of cancer, see Baider *et al.*, 1997; Holland *et al.*, 1999) have learned to avoid such ambitious therapeutic aims as cure or recovery. Survivorship is indeed a new equilibrium, in which freedom, well-being, or self-fulfillment are traded off for other goals, (e.g., protecting children from adversity or poverty, leading a respectable life, becoming an outspoken witness of evil, etc.). Another mode of survivorship includes projection of hate, fantasies of revenge, and acting out and endless pursuit of real or symbolic compensation. Clinicians should be sensitive to survivors who wish to assume a trajectory that does not focus on individual healing. In such case they may have to consider the ethical boundaries of their profession, and their duty to care, and be aware and explicit when their responsibilities as clinicians are made impossible. Clinicians should always be concerned when survivorship serves to justify aggression, scapegoating, and violence and to contribute to diffusing such trends.

Closing the narrative

Narrative theory postulates a link between healthy mental life and a congruous, coherent, and meaningful life story or 'narrative.' Novel life events are also experienced as coherent and interpretable and are ultimately embedded in one's narrative. Traumatic events may disrupt such continuity, and they do so at two distinct levels (Wigren, 1994). First, the narrative of the traumatic event may be partial, incoherent, or discontinuous. Second, one's whole life story may be disrupted, such that life before and after trauma is not the same.

Survivors always have a story to tell about their trauma. Initially emotional and distressful, this narrative evolves and develops, through reflection and interaction with others, until it stabilizes and is not questioned any longer (Shalev *et al.*, 1998). Memories are then accepted as the true narration of the trauma (Loftus, 1993). The resulting narrative may have different qualities. It may be 'closed,' 'rigid,' or otherwise nonreflective and compulsive. It can also be truncated, often because remembering stirs extreme negative emotions. When survivors find it impossible to narrate the event, their capacity to create a meaningful story of the trauma, and later integrate it in their wider life narrative, may be impaired. In contrast, being able to tell or write a coherent story of a traumatic event may lead to integration and better coping (Amir et. al., 1998; Pennebaker and Seagal, 1999). The process of reaching a stable narrative may be limited in time, following which additional information may be discarded and second thought avoided. The time frame within which the narrative stabilizes or 'closes' is unknown at this point.

In addition to having a story about the trauma, survivors have a story about their lives, within which a potentially traumatic event may be either be an episode, or a breaking point, a rupture. An essential feature of the latter is a split of one's life story into that which preceded the traumatic event and lost since and that which follows the trauma. The former is often mourned – and sometimes idealized – and the latter is often a story of ongoing pain and misery. Indeed, traumatized survivors do develop symptoms and changes in temperament, arousal, and world views. Those who develop PTSD are, in fact, ill. Yet the relationship between the traumatic hiatus on one's life narrative and the development of a mental condition such as PTSD may also be circular, one dimension feeding another. Thus trauma therapists may wish to address the narrative as much as the underlying and ongoing symptoms in an attempt to reverse the consequences of a traumatic event.

Conclusions

Remaining an effective clinician, during mass adversities, is an art to be further developed and explored. However, there is no reason to abstain from clinically treating those in need, indeed it would be neglectful not to do so. For many survivors clinical interventions are necessary but not sufficient. Clinicians should therefore recognize that their work may not be enough, and become active partners in a network of supportive agents. Their work is particularly complex, because it addresses survivors and their helpers, and includes a wide range of interventions. Importantly, clinicians may find it easier to work in groups, within which they can share experiences and responsibilities, find personal support, and restore their capacity to address trauma and its consequences.

Clinical work with recent survivors is also gratifying and rewarding. When recovery occurs it is often very spectacular. The quality of patient–therapist interactions is often enhanced by the relevance of the trauma to both. Attachment bonds can be intense and meaningful. Learning from survivors adds to one's appraisal of human dignity and resourcefulness. Most importantly, clinical work in an 'open field' challenges many of the misperceptions that the sealed therapeutic office generates. It is a humbling, but also an edifying experience.

REFERENCES

Amir, N., Strafford, J., Freshman, M. S. and Foa, E. B. (1998). Relationship between trauma narratives and trauma pathology. *Journal of Traumatic Stress*, **11**, 385–392.

Baider, L., Perry, S., Sison, A., Holland, J., Uziely, B. and DeNour, A. K. (1997). The role of psychological variables in a group of melanoma patients: An Israeli sample. *Psychosomatics*, **38**, 45–53.

Bisson, J. I., Jenkins, P. L., Alexander, J. and Bannister, C. (1997). Randomised controlled trial of psychological debriefing for victims of acute burn trauma. *British Journal of Psychiatry*, **171**, 78–81.

Bleich, A., Dycian, A., Koslowsky, M., Solomon, Z. and Wiener, M. (1992). Psychiatric implications of missile attacks on a civilian population: Israeli lessons from the Persian Gulf War. *Journal of the American Medical Association*, **268**, 613–615.

Bracken, P. J., Giller, J. E. and Summerfield, D. (1995). Psychological responses to war and atrocity: The limitations of current concepts. *Social Science and Medicine*, **40**, 1073–1082.

Brewin, C. R., Dalgleish, T. and Joseph, S. (1996). A dual representation theory of posttraumatic stress disorder. *Archives of General Psychiatry*, **50**, 294–305.

Brewin, C. R., Andrews, B., Rose, S. and Kirk, M. (1999). Acute stress disorder and posttraumatic stress disorder in victims of violent crime. *American Journal of Psychiatry*, **156**, 360–365.

Brewin, C. R., Andrews, B. and Valentine, J. D. (2000). Meta analysis of risk factors for posttraumatic stress disorder in trauma-exposed adults. *Journal of Consulting and Clinical Psychology*, **68**, 748–766.

Bryant, R. A., Harvey, A. G., Dang, S. T., Sackville, T. and Basten, C. (1998). Treatment of acute stress disorder: A comparison of cognitive–behavioral therapy and supportive counseling. *Journal of Consulting and Clinical Psychology*, **66**, 862–866.

Bryant, R. A., Sackville, T., Dang, S. T., Moulds, M. and Guthrie, R. (1999). Treating acute stress disorder: An evaluation of cognitive–behavior therapy and supportive counseling techniques. *American Journal of Psychiatry*, **156**, 1780–1786.

Camp, N. M. (1993). The Vietnam War and the ethics of combat psychiatry. *American Journal of Psychiatry*, **150**, 1000–1010.

Colbach, E. M. (1985). The post-Vietnam stress syndrome: Some cautions. *Bulletin of the American Academy of Psychiatry and Law*, **13**, 369–372.

Colbach, E. M. and Parrish, M. D. (1970). Army mental health activities in Vietnam: 1965–1970. *Bulletin of the Menninger Clinic*, **34**, 333–342.

Ehlers, A. and Clark, D. M. (2000). A cognitive model of posttraumatic stress disorder. *Behavior Research and Therapy*, **38**, 319–345.

Ehlers, A. and Steihl, R. (1995). Maintenance of intrusive memories in posttraumatic stress disorder: a cognitive approach. *Behavioural and Cognitive Psychotherapy*, **23**, 217–249.

Foa, E. B., Hembree, E. A., Riggs, D., Rauch, S. and Franklin, M. (2001). *Guidelines for Response to the Recent Tragic Events in the US, September 2001.* http://www.ncptsd.org/facts/disasters/fsfoa_advice.html

Foa, E. B. and Rothbaum, B. O. (1989). Behavioural psychotherapy for post-traumatic stress disorder. *International Review of Psychiatry*, **1**, 219–226.

Foa, E. B. and Tolin, D. F. (2000). Comparison of the PTSD Symptom Scale-Interview Version and the Clinician-Administered PTSD scale. *Journal of Traumatic Stress*, **13**, 181–191.

Freedman, S. A., Peri, T., Brandes, D. and Shalev, A. Y. (1999). Predictors of chronic PTSD: A prospective study. *British Journal of Psychiatry*, **174**, 353–359.

Fullerton, C. S., Ursano, R. J., Epstein, R. S., *et al.* (2000). Peritraumatic dissociation following motor vehicle accidents: Relationship to prior trauma and prior major depression. *Journal of Nervous and Mental Disease*, **188**, 267–272.

Galea, S., Ahern, J., Resnick, H., *et al.* (2002). Psychological sequelae of the September 11 terrorist attacks in New York City. *New England Journal of Medicine*, **346**, 982–987.

Gelpin, E., Bonne, O., Peri, T., *et al.* (1996). Treatment of recent trauma survivors with benzodiazepines: A prospective study. *Journal of Clinical Psychiatry*, **57**, 390–394.

Harvey, A. G. and Bryant, R. A. (1998). The relationship between acute stress disorder and posttraumatic stress disorder: A prospective evaluation of motor vehicle accident survivors. *Journal of Consulting and Clinical Psychology*, **66**, 507–512.

Holland, J. C., Passik, S., Kash, K. M., *et al.* (1999). The role of religious and spiritual beliefs in coping with malignant melanoma. *Psychooncology*, **8**, 14–26.

Keane, T. M., Zimmering, R. T. and Caddel, J. M. (1985). A behavioral formulation of post-traumatic stress disorder in Vietnam veterans. *Behavior Therapy*, **8**, 9–12.

Kenardy, J. A., Webster, R. A., Lewin, T. J., *et al.* (1996). Stress debriefing and patterns of recovery following a natural disaster. *Journal of Traumatic Stress*, **9**, 37–49.

Levy, P. (1996). *Survival in Auschwitz*. London: Macmillan.

Loftus, E. F. (1993). The reality of repressed memories. *American Psychologist*, **48**, 518–537.

Manning, F. (1930). *The Middle Part of Fortune*. London: Penguin Books.

Marmar, C., Weiss, D., Shchlenger, W. and Fairbank, J. (1994). Peritraumatic dissociation and posttraumatic stress in male Vietnam theater veterans. *American Journal of Psychiatry*, **151**, 902–907.

Norris, F. H., Byrne, C. M., Diaz, E. and Kaniasty, K. (2001). *50,000 Disaster Victims Speak: An Empirical Review of the Empirical Literature, 1981–2001*. Report prepared for the National Center for PTSD, White River Junction, VT.

Nuttall, S. and Coetzee, C. (1998). *Negotiating the Past: The Making of Memory in South Africa*. Oxford: Oxford University Press.

Pearlin, L. I. and Schooler, C. (1978). The structure of coping. *Journal of Health and Social Behavior*, **22**, 337–356.

Pennebaker, J. W. and Seagal, J. D. (1999). Forming a story: The health benefits of narrative. *Journal of Clinical Psychology*, **55**, 1243–1254.

Piaget, J. (1963). *The Origins of Intelligence in Children*. New York: WW Norton.

Raphael, B., Meldrum, L. and McFarlane, A. C. (1995). Does debriefing after psychological trauma work? *British Medical Journal*, **310**, 1479–1480.

Rivers, R. W. H. (1918). The repression of war experience. *The Lancet*, February 2, 173–177.

Rose, S., Bisson, J. and Wessely, S. (2001). Psychological debriefing for preventing post traumatic stress disorder (PTSD). In Cochrane Database of Systematic Reviews. Oxford: Update Software.

Schuster, M. A., Stein, B. D., Jaycox, L. (2001). A national survey of stress reactions after the September 11, 2001, terrorist attacks. *New England Journal of Medicine*, **345**, 1507–1512.

Shalev, A. Y. (2000). Stress management and debriefing: historical concepts and present patterns. In *Psychological Debriefing: Theory, Practice and Evidence*, eds. and J. P. Wilson and B. Raphael, pp. 17–31. Cambridge: Cambridge University Press.

(2002). Acute stress reactions in adults. *Biological Psychiatry*, **51**, 532–543.

Shalev, A. Y., Peri, T., Canetti, L. and Schreiber, S. (1996). Predictors of PTSD in injured trauma survivors: A prospective study. *American Journal of Psychiatry*, **153**, 219–225.

Shalev, A. Y., Peri, T., Rogel-Fuchs, Y., Ursano, R. J. and Marlowe, D. (1998). Historical group debriefing following exposure to combat stress. *Military Medicine*, **163**, 494–498.

Shalev, A. Y., Pitman, R. K., Orr, S. P., Peri, T. and Brandes, D. (2000). Auditory startle in trauma survivors with PTSD: A prospective study. *American Journal of Psychiatry*, **157**, 255–261.

Shalev, A. Y., Galai, T. and Eth, S. (1993a). 'Levels of trauma': Multidimensional approach to the psychotherapy of PTSD. *Psychiatry*, **56**, 166–177.

Shalev, A. Y., Schreiber, S. and Galai, T. (1993b). Early psychiatric responses to traumatic injury. *Journal of Traumatic Stress*, **6**, 441–450.

Solomon, Z. (1993). *Combat Stress Reaction*. New York: Plenum Press.

Solomon, Z., Neria, Y., Ohry, A., Waysman, M. and Ginzburg, K. (1994). PTSD among Israeli former prisoners of war and soldiers with combat stress reaction: A longitudinal study. *American Journal of Psychiatry*, **151**, 554–559.

Ursano, R. J., Fullerton, C. S., Epstein, R. S., *et al.* (1999). Peritraumatic dissociation and post-traumatic stress disorder following motor vehicle accidents. *American Journal of Psychiatry*, **156**, 1808–1810.

Whittlesey, S. W., Allen, J. R., Bell, B. D., *et al.* (1999). Avoidance in trauma: Conscious and unconscious defense, pathology, and health. *Psychiatry*, **62**, 303–312.

Wigren, J. (1994). Narrative completion in the treatment of trauma. *Psychotherapy: Theory, Research, Practice, and Training*, **31**, 415–423.

Yitzhaki, T., Solomon, Z. and Kotler, M. (1991). The clinical picture of acute combat stress reaction among Israeli soldiers in the 1982 Lebanon war. *Military Medicine*, **156**, 193–197.

12

Collaborative care for injured victims of individual and mass trauma: A health services research approach to developing early interventions

Douglas Zatzick

Introduction

Natural or human-made disasters, motor vehicle crashes, and violent trauma all entail the threat of physical injury. In the United States 37 million individuals visit emergency departments each year after sustaining traumatic injury (Bonnie *et al.*, 1999). Each year, approximately 2.5 million Americans incur injuries so severe that they require inpatient hospitalization (Bonnie *et al.*, 1999).

Trauma exposure when coupled with physical injury confers a higher risk for the development of posttraumatic stress disorder (PTSD) (Helzer *et al.*, 1987; Abenhaim *et al.*, 1992; Green, 1993). Between 10 and 40 percent of American civilians admitted to the hospital after sustaining traumatic physical injury may go on to develop PTSD (Mayou *et al.*, 1993; Shalev *et al.*, 1996b; Harvey and Bryant, 1998; Holbrook *et al.*, 1999; Ursano *et al.*, 1999; Zatzick, Kang *et al.* 2001). In trauma survivors PTSD is often complicated by comorbid, depressive symptoms (Blanchard *et al.*, 1995; Holbrook *et al.*, 1999; Shalev *et al.*, 1998) and medically unexplained somatic complaints (Engel *et al.*, 2000). Also, between 20 and 55 percent of trauma survivors hospitalized on surgical wards meet diagnostic criteria for current or lifetime substance abuse or dependence (Rivara *et al.*, 1993; Soderstrom *et al.*, 1997).

In physically injured civilians (Holbrook *et al.*, 1999; Michaels *et al.*, 1999; Zatzick *et al.*, in press a), veterans (Zatzick *et al.*, 1997), and refugees (Mollica *et al.*, 1999), PTSD makes a unique contribution to posttraumatic functional limitations and diminished quality of life above and beyond the impact of injury severity and comorbid medical conditions. In a randomly selected cohort of injured motor vehicle crash and assault survivors PTSD was the strongest independent predictor of a broad profile of functional impairment 1 year after the injury (Zatzick *et al.*, in press a). Epidemiological investigations suggest that posttraumatic stress disorders are associated not only with marked individual suffering and functional impairment but also substantial societal costs (Greenberg *et al.*, 1999; Kessler, 2000). Thus, early interventions for injured trauma survivors that reduce the likelihood of developing enduring posttraumatic disturbances may be essential components of public health efforts targeting injury control (Bonnie *et al.*, 1999).

Trauma centers provide care for injured civilians after individual and mass events

In the United States the trauma care system is the service delivery sector in which injured patients receive treatment. A trauma care system is an organized and co-ordinated effort in a defined geographic area that is designated to deliver care to injured trauma victims (Bonnie *et al.*, 1999). This care begins immediately after the injury and includes paramedic and ambulance service, emergency department triage, and inpatient surgical hospitalization. Trauma centers are acute care hospitals that are designed to treat emergent medical complications related to physical injury. Level I trauma centers are designated and equipped to care for the most severely injured patients, while level II–IV centers are designed to treat less severely injured patients and to triage to level I facilities.

Thus, in the United States trauma centers are the health care institutions that will care for patients who are injured after individual and mass events. As an example, in the wake of the September 11 attack on the World Trade Center 6497 civilians were triaged primarily to two dedicated trauma centers within New York City. Approximately 7 percent ($n = 474$) of these civilians were so severely injured that they required inpatient admission (Greater New York Hospital Association, 2001).

To date the major goals of trauma care systems have been to prevent fatalities, and to triage patients who are more severely injured to the most appropriate and cost-effective level of trauma care within a region (Bonnie *et al.*, 1999). Few guidelines for the operation of trauma care systems include comprehensive or even cursory approaches to the evaluation, referral, and treatment of injured patients who suffer from posttraumatic stress disorders (American College of Surgeons Committee on Trauma, 1999).

Efficacious treatments for posttraumatic stress disorder exist

A growing body of efficacy research suggests that individuals with posttraumatic psychological symptoms may respond to psychotherapeutic and psychopharmacological treatments (Solomon *et al.*, 1992; Shalev *et al.*, 1996a). Randomized clinical trials of cognitive–behavioral psychotherapy have established the efficacy of this

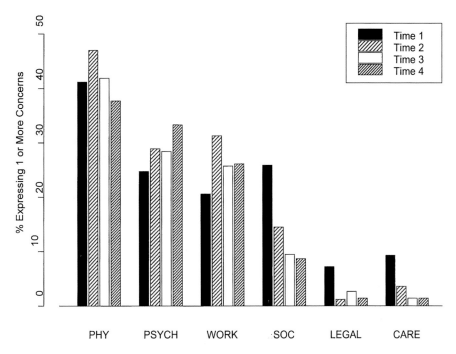

Figure 12.1   The percentage of patients expressing one or more concerns from each domain over the course of the year post injury. PHY, physical health domain; PSYCH, psychological domain; WORK, work and finance domain; SOC, social domain; LEGAL, legal domain; care, medical domain. Time 1 = surgical inpatient hospitalization ($n = 97$), time 2 =1 month post injury ($n = 83$), time 3 = 4 months post injury ($n = 74$), time 4 = 12 months post injury ($n = 69$). (From Zatzick *et al.*, 2001 a.)

psychotherapeutic modality in the treatment of PTSD (Solomon *et al.*, 1992; Foa *et al.*, 1995; Bryant *et al.*, 1998). Both the selective serotonin reuptake inhibitor class of antidepressants and the tricyclic antidepressants may be effective in treating PTSD (Connor *et al.*, 1999; Brady *et al.*, 2000; Hidalgo and Davidson, 2000). Guidelines based on this body of efficacy research have recently been formulated (*Journal of Clinical Psychiatry*, 1999).

These clinical guidelines have yet to be translated to the 'real world' treatment of physically injured trauma survivors within trauma care systems. Little clinical infrastructure exists to facilitate the translation of efficacious interventions for patients with traumatic injuries (Chesnut *et al.*, 1999) and few trauma surgery inpatients with high levels of posttraumatic psychological distress receive comprehensive mental health assessments or referrals (Danielsson *et al.*, 1999). Thus, continuity of care and care coordination may be problematic as physically injured patients move from inpatient wards to outpatient follow-up and community rehabilitation (Chesnut *et al.*, 1999; Zatzick *et al.*, 2001a) (Fig. 12.1).

Developing early interventions for injured trauma survivors treated in trauma care systems: What is mental health services research?

As a branch of psychiatric inquiry, mental health services research concerns itself with understanding how changes in the structure and processes of care delivery influence relevant individual, institutional, and societal outcomes of care. Psychiatric services research is by nature multidisciplinary, incorporating social scientific perspectives (e.g., economics, anthropology, history), and utilizing both quantitative and qualitative research methods (Zatzick *et al.*, 2001a). The overarching goal of health services research is to understand the interrelationships between the structure, process, and outcome of mental health care delivery (Starfield, 1973). Thus a mental health services research group that is designed to develop interventions for injured patients treated in trauma care systems would not only include a psychiatrist, psychologist, social workers, and other allied mental health professionals, but also acute care trauma center staff (e.g., trauma surgeons, trauma clinical nurse specialists, emergency room physicians, and injury epidemiologists), outpatient providers (general practitioners, pediatricians, and internists), and social scientists (health economists, clinical ethnographers, sociologists).

Over the past two decades psychiatric services researchers have been working to incorporate the delivery of care for depressive, anxiety, substance abuse, and chronic disorders into primary care and community settings (Katon *et al.*, 1995; Weisner and Schmidt, 1995; Wells *et al.*, 2000). Evidence-based guidelines now exist for the treatment of depressive disorders in primary care (Agency for Health Care Policy and Research, 1993).

Developing interventions for injured trauma survivors treated in trauma care systems: What is high-quality care?

The Institute of Medicine has defined quality care as care that embodies the principles of patient-centeredness, safety, effectiveness, timeliness, and equity (Committee on Quality of Health Care in America, 2001). With regard to patient-centered care, PTSD and related comorbidities occur within the broader context of trauma survivors' posttraumatic illness experience (Zatzick *et al.*, 2001a). Physically injured trauma survivors express multiple financial, social, legal, and health-related concerns; these concerns appear to evolve over the course of posttraumatic recovery (Zatzick *et al.*, 2001a). In a population-based study of posttraumatic concerns over the course of the year after injury 73 percent of patients expressed physical health concerns, 58 percent psychological concerns, 53 percent work and finance concerns, 40 percent social concerns, 10 percent legal concerns, and 10 percent medical concerns (Zatzick *et al.*, 2001a). Patients psychological concerns were diverse:

although anxiety and depressive symptoms occurred other themes such as struggles with substance abuse, realistic issues regarding personnel safety, and existential considerations in the wake of the trauma were also endorsed.

The importance of eliciting and tracking concerns is borne out when the concern data is considered along with data suggesting that a high percentage of patients with PTSD symptoms do not consider their distress serious enough to seek treatment (Kessler, 2000). Early interventions that target only the symptoms of PTSD may fail to adequately engage injured trauma survivors who endorse multiple posttraumatic concerns including, pain, financial loss, legal problems, or disruptions in social networks. The concern data suggest a working hypothesis for early interventions delivered in trauma care systems; if injured trauma survivors are to be engaged in early treatments then patient-centered intervention models must be developed and implemented. These supportive engagement techniques may in turn be expected to reduce early posttraumatic distress.

Developing interventions for injured trauma survivors treated in trauma care systems: What is collaborative care?

Collaborative care is a disease management strategy that seeks to find the optimal roles for primary care providers, specialists, and allied health professionals in the delivery of care for patients with psychiatric disorders and chronic medical conditions. Previous investigation suggests that collaborative interventions can improve clinical outcomes for patients with complex, comorbid presentations, while flexibly integrating patients' perspectives into the delivery of care (Katon *et al.*, 2001). Essential elements of collaborative care include the provision of medical support services such as case management, active sustained follow-up that promotes continuity of care delivery, and shared patient–provider treatment planning. Collaborative interventions typically employ multifaceted treatments (e.g., combining case management with psychopharmacological and psychotherapeutic interventions). Recent randomized clinical trials have documented the effectiveness of collaborative care models for patients with depressive and anxiety disorders in primary care (Roy-Byrne *et al.*, 2001).

Collaborative care for physically injured trauma survivors with posttraumatic stress disorder: Modifying the structure, process, and outcome of posttraumatic care

The theoretical basis for the collaborative care model to be piloted in the investigation is specified in Fig. 12.2. From a quality improvement perspective collaborative

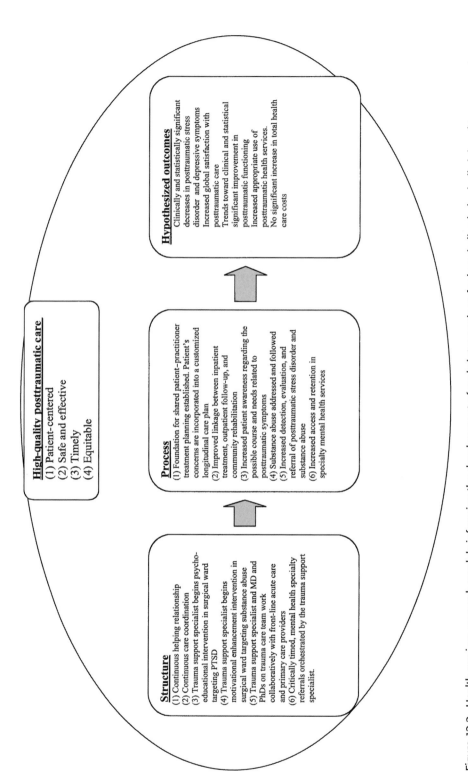

Figure 12.2 Health services research models informing the development of early interventions for hospitalized physically injured trauma survivors.

care interventions are expected to have demonstrable impacts on posttraumatic outcomes through their effect on the structure and processes of care (McGlynn *et al.*, 1988). The collaborative model introduces continuous care from a trauma support specialist, a masters-level clinician trained to evaluate, treat, and refer the spectrum of individual concerns that arise in the wake of traumatic injury. The trauma support specialist elicits, follows, and whenever possible targets for amelioration each trauma survivor's unique posttraumatic concerns. In this way posttraumatic concerns form the basis for continuous shared patient–provider treatment planning. The trauma support specialist also engages in activities such as psychoeducation, direct casework, developing natural support systems, and periodic reassessment that aim to facilitate access to services and promote a continuous recovery agenda.

Collaborative models also utilize access to specialty mental health MD and PhD expertise. Once a patient is engaged in an ongoing one on one relationship with the trauma support specialist, then more costly pharmacological and psychotherapeutic expertise can be brought in at critically time junctures or 'steps' in posttraumatic care delivery. For instance if a patient remains symptomatic with PTSD at 3 months despite the efforts of the trauma support specialist, then in order to potentially offset the development of chronic PTSD and associated functional morbidity, more intensive PTSD treatments can be delivered by MD and PhD team members.

Piloting the collaborative care early intervention in an acute care trauma center setting

Below the results of a pilot of collaborative care intervention are summarized and directions for future investigations are discussed (Zatzick *et al.*, 2001b). The overarching goal of the investigation was to develop and implement a collaborative intervention that targeted the spectrum of posttraumatic behavioral and emotional disturbances afflicting physically injured trauma survivors. The pilot study aimed to establish the feasibility of delivering the intervention and assessing outcomes in surgical wards and outpatient settings. Because of the novelty of the intervention and the few detailed accounts characterizing inpatient trauma surgical and outpatient posttraumatic health service delivery, the investigation employed clinical ethnographic methods in order to better depict the processes of care associated with the pilot intervention (Zatzick and Johnson, 1997; Hohmann, 1999). The effectiveness of the collaborative intervention was tested in a randomized design that compared intervention patients with control subjects receiving usual posttraumatic care.

Method

Participants and procedure

Patients were recruited from a Level I trauma center in inland Northern California. Patients included in the study were hospitalized motor vehicle accident or assault survivors between the ages of 14 and 65, who were English speaking. Adolescent patients were included in this effectiveness trial as they are routinely hospitalized with adults on the University of California–Davis trauma surgical service. Potential subjects were randomly selected for approach by the research associate using numerical assignments derived from a random-numbers table.

A total of 105 patients was screened for study participation. Of the 57 patients approached for the protocol, eight patients refused participation. Eleven subjects completed the interview but were discharged before they could be enrolled in the clinical trial. The 11 patients discharged prior to randomization had decreased total hospital lengths of stay (mean length of stay = 3.6, SD = 1.96), when compared to control (mean length of stay = 5.6, SD = 10.6) and intervention (mean length of stay = 10.6, SD = 9.9) subjects. There were no significant differences in age ($F(1,43) = 0.001$, $p = 0.97$), gender ($\chi^2(2) = 1.0$, $p = 0.60$), or injury type ($\chi^2(2) = 0.73$, $p = 0.69$) between the 34 patients enrolled in the intervention trial and the 11 patients who were discharged prior to randomization. Thirty-four subjects were randomized; 16 subjects were assigned to the collaborative care intervention and 18 subjects were assigned to the usual care control. The investigation achieved over 75 percent 4-month follow-up and 88 percent of patients had data from at least two time points.

Early intervention implementation

On the surgical ward each patient was assigned to a trauma support specialist who met each patient at the bedside. Three clinicians with advanced degrees and extensive experience with the surgical inpatient treatment milieu (i.e., two consultation liaison psychiatrists and one trauma clinical nurse specialist) volunteered their time as the trauma support specialists for the pilot study.

In order to establish a basis for collaborative problem definition and shared patient–provider treatment planning, the trauma support specialists were instructed to elicit and track patients' posttraumatic concerns. Thus on the surgical ward and at follow-up interviews patients were asked: 'Of all the things that have happened to you since you were injured, what concerns you the most?' Patients posttraumatic concerns were incorporated into joint problem definition and the trauma support specialists were instructed to intervene on behalf of the patients in the resolution of these concerns whenever possible. For instance, if pain was a primary concern on the surgical ward then the trauma support specialist would engage the patient's ward nurse or inpatient surgical team in a collaborative effort targeting pain control. The trauma support specialists were instructed to maintain detailed logs and field notes in order to document the spectrum of collaborative intervention activity. These data were presented to and reviewed by other members of the multidisciplinary intervention team during weekly case conferences.

Interview administration and measures

All 34 participants were administered a 1-hour interview while hospitalized. Patients were re-interviewed over the telephone at 1 month, and 4 months, after the traumatic injury. The interviews included questions regarding patients' sociodemographic characteristics and the following scales designed to assess prior trauma, current psychological distress, substance use and functional status: Post-Traumatic Stress Disorder Checklist (PCL-C), the Center for Epidemiological Studies Depression Scale (CES-D), the Peritraumatic Dissociative Experiences Questionnaire (PDEQ), the traumatic life events screen that accompanies the Composite International Diagnostic Interview (CIDI), and the PTSD module of the National Comorbidity Survey (NCS) (Kessler *et al.*, 1995). Limitations in physical functioning were assessed with a modified version of the Physical Components Summary (PCS) of the Medical Outcomes Study 12-Item Short-Form Health Survey. Alcohol and drug use at the time of the traumatic event was assessed with blood alcohol and urine toxicology screens and a single question from the Addiction Severity Index (ASI). Injury severity was abstracted from surgical records using a conversion software program that calculates the injury severity scale score from *International Classification of Disease 9th Version Clinical Modification (ICD-9CM)* diagnostic codes. Finally social support was assessed with eight items from the Medical Outcomes Study (MOS) Social Support Survey.

Statistical analyses

The main outcome variables assessed were PTSD (PCL-C) and depressive (CES-D) symptoms, at-risk drinking (ASI), and physical functioning (PCS). Outcome analyses were conducted for the both the intent-to-treat sample of 34 subjects and for those subjects with complete data on each outcome measure at all time points. For PCL-C, CES-D, and PCS scores the hypothesized effect of the intervention was tested through a mixed model repeated measures analysis of covariance (ANCOVAs) that compared mean scores on the scales across groups and at successive time points. When significant group by time interactions resulted, post hoc ANCOVAs on the change scores were computed. A literature review suggested that age, gender, injury severity, and admission alcohol and drug toxicology screen results should be included in the ANCOVA analyses as covariates. We used the χ^2 statistic and Fisher's

Exact Test to assess for group differences in self-reports of drinking alcohol to the point of intoxication. All statistical analyses were performed with the SPSS version 10.0 software (SPSS, Inc.)

Results

Characteristics of the sample

The intervention and control groups did not significantly differ on demographic, injury or clinical characteristics at the time of the surgical ward interview. Both intervention and control subjects demonstrated high levels of PTSD and depressive symptom levels while hospitalized. Approximately 20 percent of hospitalized inpatients ($n = 7$) had PCL-C scores ≥ 45 while 79 percent ($n = 27$) of patients had CES-D scores of ≥ 16. Patients' surgical ward PTSD and depressive symptom levels were highly correlated ($r = 0.70$, $p < 0.001$). Forty-seven percent of patients screened positive on admission for alcohol and/or stimulant intoxication.

Qualitative description of the intervention

Trauma support specialists spent an average of 92 minutes (SD = 54 minutes) per patient delivering the intervention over the course of the 4-month study (Fig. 12.3). Examination of trauma support specialist's logs and field notes revealed that 75 percent of the patient contact occurred between hospital admission and 1-month follow-up, while 25 percent of patient contact occurred between 1 and 4 months.

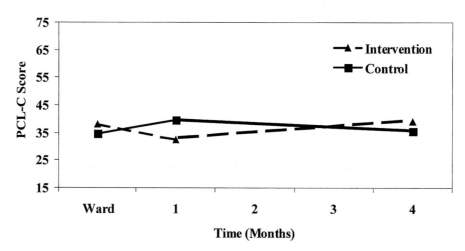

Figure 12.3 Mean adjusted posttraumatic stress disorder checklist (PCL-C) scores for intervention ($n = 16$) and control ($n = 18$) patients. Scores are adjusted for injury severity, age, gender, and surgical inpatient blood alcohol and urine toxicology screen results. (From Zatzick *et al.*, 2001 b.)

Virtually all of the surgical ward contact occurred as face-to-face counseling while after hospital discharge the vast majority of contacts were over the telephone with the patient, family members, and surgical and primary care providers. Review of study logs and field notes revealed that patients' posttraumatic concerns were frequently discussed during multidisciplinary team meetings and targeted for amelioration by the trauma support specialists.

Quantitative comparisons of the intervention and control groups

Comparisons of PTSD symptom levels between the intervention and control groups reflected the variations in the intensity of the intervention. Repeated measures analysis of covariance revealed a significant group by time interaction in the intent to treat ($F(2,54) = 4.5$, $p < 0.05$) and completer ($F(2,30) = 6.7$, $p < 0.01$) analyses. A significant group effect of gender, with women demonstrating greater symptom levels than men (intent to treat: $F(1,27) = 6.6$, $p < 0.05$; completer $F(1,15) = 4.9$, $p < 0.05$), was also observed. There were no significant main effects for age, injury severity, or admission blood alcohol or urine toxicology screens.

Post-hoc ANCOVA analyses of the intent to treat sample revealed two distinct time trends in PTSD symptom levels. From the time of the surgical ward admission through the 1-month follow-up, intervention subjects had significantly decreased PTSD symptoms when compared to controls ($F(1,33) = 6.8$, $p < 0.05$, effect size = 0.99). From the 1-month through the 4-month follow-up assessments, intervention patients' symptoms significantly increased relative to controls ($F(1,27) = 6.1$, $p < 0.05$, effect size = 1.75). These results did not vary substantially for the completer sample.

Comparisons of depressive symptom levels between the intervention and control groups revealed similar as PTSD results. One-month depressive symptom reductions were observed in the intervention group when compared to controls. The intervention group, however, demonstrated a recurrence of symptoms by the 4-month time point. Repeated measures ANCOVA comparing the intervention and control groups' functional outcome scores revealed a significant effect of time (intent to treat: $F(2,54) = 3.6$, $p < 0.05$; completer $F(2,32) = 4.7$, $p < 0.05$), but no other main effects or interactions. Also, no significant differences were found when the two groups were compared with regard to drinking to the point of intoxication.

Implications of the pilot intervention

The collaborative care intervention significantly decreased PTSD and depressive symptoms in the first month after the trauma. These statistically significant symptomatic improvements were not maintained at the final 4-month evaluation. However, the intervention appeared to be successful in both preventing the development of symptomatic distress consistent with a diagnosis of PTSD and in reducing clinically significant distress in patients with initial high symptom levels. There was no evidence that the intervention impacted posttraumatic functional limitations or patterns of alcohol consumption.

The observed reduction and subsequent recurrence of trauma survivors' PTSD and depressive symptoms followed the temporal 'dosing' of the collaborative intervention. The hospital-based interventionists were able to provide each patient with active sustained inpatient contact and telephone follow-up in the days and weeks immediately following the injury. The limitation of the hospital-based intervention became apparent after the first month post injury, when continuous follow-up could no longer be achieved and symptomatic distress in the intervention group recurred. These observations are consistent with the results of previous collaborative intervention trials that have described symptomatic recurrences in depressed patients in the absence of treatment maintenance protocols.

There are a number of important considerations in interpreting the results of this pilot investigation. The sample size in this pilot investigation was small and the results will require replication in a larger trial. There may not have been enough power to detect differences in the intervention and control groups for the alcohol and functional outcomes. The collaborative intervention was not manualized and therefore was likely to be implemented with marked variability across trauma support specialists.

Comparison of collaborative care with other early intervention approaches

Psychological debriefing involves emotional processing and review of a trauma during a circumscribed time period shortly after the event has occurred. To date the results of randomized trials of debriefing have been mixed, with reports of worse acute and long-term psychological outcomes among patients receiving the debriefing intervention (Wessely *et al.*, 1997). The current collaborative intervention differed from trials of debriefing in that trauma support specialists established an ongoing relationship with patients. Thus, a discussion and review of the trauma was an optional aspect of the intervention that could evolve over the weeks and months after the event. Future trials of collaborative interventions should document the relational processes through which patients and providers come to a shared agreement regarding the appropriate timing of traumatic catharsis and review.

Cognitive–behavioral interventionalists have delivered efficacious manualized psychotherapy protocols to select samples of trauma survivors in outpatient mental health settings over the course of 7–8 hours (Foa *et al.*, 1995; Bryant *et al.*, 1998). The current effectiveness trial differs from these investigations in that a random sampling strategy was employed to select a representative sample of patients from a population of hospitalized trauma survivors. Patients with alcohol and drug related comorbidities were not excluded from the current trial. Also, the trauma support specialists in the current study spent on average 1.5 hours with each patient.

Of note, one previous trial of a 3-month supportive counseling intervention for male motor vehicle crash survivors reported significant symptomatic and functional improvement in intervention patients (Bordow and Porritt, 1979). The collaborative intervention differed from supportive counseling in that it incorporated psychotherapeutic treatment modules that specifically targeted PTSD and substance abuse comorbidities.

Future directions: Stepped collaborative care

Taken together, these limitations and results suggest that hospital based care delivered by highly trained professionals may not be of long enough duration or great enough intensity to effect lasting therapeutic change in this population. Full-time masters-level clinicians with the ability to promptly attend to surgical inpatients as well as maintain follow-up in the community should be introduced into the trauma support specialist role.

Future larger trials may also need to incorporate a stepped approach to the delivery of collaborative care. Prior longitudinal descriptive investigations suggest that PTSD and depressive symptoms may spontaneously decrease in a less severely afflicted subsample of physically injured trauma survivors (Mayou *et al.*, 1993; Shalev *et al.*, 1996b; Zatzick *et al.*, in press b). In the stepped approach, intervention resources are allocated at gradually increasing 'doses' to patients whose symptoms do not remit after initial low intensity evaluation and treatment. Stepped protocols will also need to incorporate a psychopharmacological treatment component for patients who prefer medications and/or whose symptoms do not spontaneously remit. The stepped approach to collaborative intervention would also mandate that future intervention trials include a cost-effectiveness component, so as to inform policy discussion regarding the adoption and dissemination of the intervention model across trauma centers.

Future directions: Articulating deliberative models of the patient–provider relationship that inform early interventions

Recent commentary suggests a debate over the patient's role in medical decision-making that has been characterized as a conflict over the values of the patient and values of the provider or health care system (Emanuel and Emanuel, 1992).

In developing early collaborative interventions we have noted the tensions that exist between the patients' evolving posttraumatic concerns and the goals, values, and limitations imposed by multiple medical providers, the trauma care system, and society. The resolution of these tensions in a clinical model of the patient–provider relationship is the overarching 'meta-paradigm' (Bateson, 1979) that must inform the development of any early intervention. Mental health professionals often implicitly invoke their priority that PTSD be detected, evaluated, and treated. This paternalistic view of decision-making threatens to undermine patient autonomy and denies the patient's experience of multiple posttraumatic concerns that may take priority over specific PTSD treatment. At the other extreme a purely consumerist model of care delivery would suggest that once educated patients can make their own decision about appropriate care. This view of decision-making negates the empiric data to which clinicians are privy suggesting that PTSD may become a chronic condition that is associated with marked individual suffering and societal costs.

The collaborative care model frames posttraumatic care delivery as an ongoing *deliberation* between patient and provider in the context of a trusting relationship. A deliberation will be defined as a discussion between patient and provider that serves to help the patient determine and choose the best health related treatments/values that can be attained at a particular time point post event (Emanuel and Emanuel, 1992).

Patients' concerns, preferences, and expectations evolve over the months and week post event as do treatment recommendations. The trauma support specialist's and collaborative team's central objective is to help patients understand why certain health-related decisions and the values that underlie them are advantages to the patient. The collaborative team may therefore deliberate with the patient around multiple areas of health concern such as the long-term risk of functional impairment related to chronic PTSD, or the prevention of high-risk behaviors such as alcohol intoxication that may lead to injury recurrence.

Conclusion

In summary, no organized service delivery system exists for physically injured trauma survivors suffering from posttraumatic behavioral and emotional disturbances. The results of a pilot investigation suggest that collaborative interventions can be delivered within trauma care systems and may hold promise for reducing posttraumatic symptomatic distress. Future investigations should develop and test high-quality, cost-effective, stepped collaborative care interventions that target symptomatic and functional impairments among injured trauma survivors.

REFERENCES

Abenhaim, L., Dab, W. and Salmi, L. R. (1992). Study of civilian victims of terrorist attacks (France 1982–1987). *Journal of Clinical Epidemiology*, **45**, 103–109.

Agency for Health Care Policy and Research (1993). *Depression in Primary Care*, vols 1 and 2. Rockville, MD: US Department of Health and Human Services.

American College of Surgeons Committee on Trauma (1999). *Resources for the Optimal Care of the Injured Patient: 1999*. Chicago, IL: American College of Surgeons.

Bateson, G. (1979). *Mind and Nature: A Necessary Unity*. New York: Bantam Books.

Blanchard, E. B., Hickling, E. J., Taylor, A. E. and Loos, W. (1995). Psychiatric morbidity associated with motor vehicle accidents. *Journal of Nervous and Mental Disease*, **183**, 495–504.

Bonnie, R. J., Fulco, C. E. and Liverman, C. T. (1999). *Reducing the Burden of Injury: Advancing Prevention and Treatment*. Washington, DC: National Academy Press.

Bordow, S. and Porritt, D. (1979). An experimental evaluation of crisis intervention. *Social Science and Medicine*, **13A**, 251–256.

Brady, K., Pearlstein, T., Asnis, G. M., *et al.* (2000). Efficacy and safety of sertraline treatment of posttraumatic stress disorder. *Journal of the American Medical Association*, **283**, 1837–1844.

Bryant, R. A., Harvey, A. G., Dang, S. T., Sackville, T. and Basten, C. (1998). Treatment of acute stress disorder: A comparison of cognitive–behavioral therapy and supportive counseling. *Journal of Consulting Clinical Psychology*, **66**, 862–866.

Chesnut, R. M., Carney, N., Maynard, H., *et al.* (1999). *Rehabilitation for Traumatic Brain Injury*. Rockville, MD: Agency for Health Care Policy and Research.

Committee on Quality of Health Care in America (2001). *Crossing the Quality Chasm: A New Health System for the 21st Century*. Washington, DC: National Academy Press.

Connor, K. M., Sutherland, S. M., Tupler, L. A., Malik, M. L. and Davidson, J. R. (1999). Fluoxetine in post-traumatic stress disorder: Randomized, double-blind study. *British Journal of Psychiatry*, **175**, 17–22.

Danielsson, P. E., Rivara, F. P., Gentilello, L. M. and Maier, R. V. (1999). Reasons why trauma surgeons fail to screen for alcohol problems. *Archives of Surgery*, **134**, 564–568.

Emanuel, E. J. and Emanuel, L. L. (1992). Four models of the patient–physician relationship. *Journal of the American Medical Association*, **267**, 2221–2226.

Engel, C. C., Liu, X., McCarthy, B. D., Miller, R. F. and Ursano, R. J. (2000). Relationship of physical symptoms to posttraumatic stress disorder among veterans seeking care for Gulf War-related health concerns. *Psychosomatics Medicine*, **62**, 739–745.

Foa, E. B., Hearst-Ikeda, D. and Perry, K. J. (1995). Evaluation of a brief cognitive–behavioral program for the prevention of chronic PTSD in recent assault victims. *Journal of Consulting and Clinical Psychology*, **63**, 948–955.

Greater New York Hospital Association (2001). *The Fiscal Impact of the World Trade Center Attack on New York Hospitals, September.* http://www.gnyha.org/pubinfo/wtc/WTCFiscalImpact_20011002.pdf

Green, B. L. (1993). Identifying survivors at risk. In *International Handbook of Traumatic Stress Syndromes*, eds. J. P. Wilson and B. Raphael, pp. 135–144. New York: Plenum Press.

Greenberg, P. E., Sisitsky, T., Kessler, R. C., *et al.* (1999). The economic burden of anxiety disorders in the 1990s. *Journal of Clinical Psychiatry*, **60**, 427–435.

Harvey, A. G. and Bryant, R. A. (1998). The relationship between acute stress disorder and posttraumatic stress disorder: A prospective evaluation of motor vehicle accident survivors. *Journal of Consulting and Clinical Psychology*, **66**, 507–512.

Helzer, J. E., Robins, L. N. and McEvoy, L. (1987). Post-traumatic stress disorder in the general population: Findings of the epidemiological catchment area survey. *New England Journal of Medicine*, **317**, 1630–1634.

Hidalgo, R. B. and Davidson, J. R. T. (2000). Selective serotonin reuptake inhibitors in post-traumatic stress disorder. *Journal of Psychopharmacology*, **14**, 70–76.

Hohmann, A. (1999). A contextual model for clinical mental health services research. *Mental Health Services Research*, **1**, 83–92.

Holbrook, T., Anderson, J., Sieber, W., Browner, D. and Hoyt, D. (1999). Outcome after major trauma: 12-month and 18-month follow-up results from the Trauma Recovery Project. *Journal of Trauma*, **46**, 765–773.

Journal of Clinical Psychiatry (1999). Guidelines: The expert consensus panels for PTSD. *Journal of Clinical Psychiatry*, **60** (Suppl. 16), 3–76.

Katon, W., Von Korff, M., Lin, E. and Simon, G. (2001). Rethinking practitioner roles in chronic illness: The specialist, primary care physician, and the practice nurse. *General Hospital Psychiatry*, **23**, 138–144.

Katon, W., Von Korff, M., Lin, E., *et al.* (1995). Collaborative management to achieve treatment guidelines: Impact on depression in primary care. *Journal of the American Medical Association*, **273**, 1026–1031.

Kessler, R. C. (2000). Posttraumatic stress disorder: The burden to the individual and society. *Journal of Clinical Psychiatry*, **61** (Suppl. 5), 4–14.

Kessler, R. C., Sonnega, A., Bromet, E., Hughes, M. and Nelson, C. B. (1995). Posttraumatic stress disorder in the National Comorbidity Survey. *Archives of General Psychiatry*, **52**, 1048–1060.

Mayou, R., Bryant, B. and Duthie, R. (1993). Psychiatric consequences of road traffic accidents. *British Medical Journal*, **307**, 647–651.

McGlynn, E. A., Norquist, G. S., Wells, K. B., Sullivan, G. and Liberman, R. P. (1988). Quality-of-care research in mental health: Responding to the challenge. *Inquiry*, **25**, 157–170.

Michaels, A. J., Michaels, C. E., Moon, C. H., *et al.* (1999). Posttraumatic stress disorder after injury: Impact on general health outcome and early risk assessment. *Journal of Trauma*, **47**, 460–467.

Mollica, R. F., McInnes, K., Sarajlie, N., *et al.* (1999). Disability associated with psychiatric comorbidity and health status in Bosnian refugees living in Croatia. *Journal of the American Medical Association*, **282**, 433–439.

Rivara, F. P., Jurkovich, G. J., Gurney, J. G., *et al.* (1993). The magnitude of acute and chronic alcohol abuse in trauma patients. *Archives of Surgery*, **128**, 907–913.

Roy-Byrne, P., Katon, W., Cowley, D. and Russo, J. (2001). A randomized effectiveness trial of collaborative care for patients with panic disorder in primary care. *Archives of General Psychiatry*, **58**, 869–876.

Shalev, A. Y., Bonne, O. and Eth, S. (1996a). Treatment of posttraumatic stress disorder: A review. *Psychosomatic Medicine*, **58**, 165–182.

Shalev, A. Y., Freedman, S., Peri, T., *et al.* (1998). Prospective study of posttraumatic stress disorder and depression following trauma. *American Journal of Psychiatry*, **155**, 630–637.

Shalev, A. Y., Peri, T., Canetti, L., and Schreiber, S. (1996b). Predictors of PTSD in injured trauma survivors: A prospective study. *American Journal of Psychiatry*, **153**, 219–225.

Soderstrom, C. A., Smith, G. S., Dischinger, P. C., *et al.* (1997). Psychoactive substance use disorders among seriously injured trauma center patients. *Journal of the American Medical Association*, **277**, 1769–1774.

Solomon, S. D., Gerrity, E. T. and Muff, A. M. (1992). Efficacy of treatments for posttraumatic stress disorder. *Journal of the American Medical Association*, **268**, 633–638.

Starfield, B. (1973). Health services research: A working model. *New England Journal of Medicine*, **289**, 132–135.

Ursano, R. J., Fullerton, C. S., Epstein, R. S., *et al.* (1999). Acute and chronic posttraumatic stress disorder in motor vehicle accident victims. *American Journal of Psychiatry*, **156**, 589–595.

Weisner, C. and Schmidt, L. A. (1995). Expanding the frame of health services research in the drug abuse field. *Health Services Research*, **30**, 707–726.

Wells, K. B., Sherbourne, C., Schoenbaum, M., *et al.* (2000). Impact of disseminating quality improvement programs for depression in managed primary care: A randomized controlled trial. *Journal of the American Medical Association*, **283**, 212–220.

Wessely, S., Rose, S. and Bisson, J. (1997). A systematic review of brief psychological interventions ('debriefing') for the treatment of trauma related symptoms and the prevention of posttraumatic stress disorder. In *Cochrane Database of Systematic Reviews*. Oxford: Update Software.

Zatzick, D., Kang, S., Hinton, W., *et al.* (2001a). Posttraumatic concerns: A patient-centered approach to outcome assessment after traumatic physical injury. *Medical Care*, **39**, 327–339.

Zatzick, D. F. and Johnson, F. A. (1997). Alternative psychotherapeutic practice among middle class Americans. 1: Case studies and follow-up. *Culture, Medicine and Psychiatry*, **21**, 53–88.

Zatzick, D. F., Jurkovich, G. J., Gentilello, L. M., *et al.* (in press a). Posttraumatic stress, problem drinking and functioning 1 year after injury. *Archives of Surgery*.

Zatzick, D. F., Kang, S. M., Mueller, H., *et al.* (in press b). Predicting posttraumatic distress in acutely injured hospitalized trauma survivors. *American Journal of Psychiatry*.

Zatzick, D. F., Marmar, C. R., Weiss, D. S., *et al.* (1997). Posttraumatic stress disorder and functioning and quality of life outcomes in a nationally representative sample of male Vietnam veterans. *American Journal of Psychiatry*, **154**, 1690–1695.

Zatzick, D. F., Roy-Byrne, P., Russo, J., *et al.* (2001b). Collaborative interventions for physically injured trauma survivors: A pilot randomized effectiveness trial. *General Hospital Psychiatry*, **23**, 114–123.

Part IV

The intersection of disasters and terrorism: Effects of contamination on individuals

13

Responses of individuals and groups to consequences of technological disasters and radiation exposure

Lars Weisaeth and Arnfinn Tønnessen

Introduction

The Greek inventor Daedalus was not concerned whether his inventions helped or harmed society. Icarus, his son, joyfully ascended on the wings his father invented. As he flew closer to the sun, however, the wings melted, sending Icarus plummeting into the sea, where he drowned. Man versus nature, man against himself, and man versus technology, is the topic of this chapter.

Technology has a dual character. It is able to prevent disasters and to cause disasters. By definition, a technological disaster is the result of a failure of human-made products. These include air crashes, large-scale road accidents, train derailments and collisions, passenger ship and other maritime catastrophes including oil-rig destructions, industrial explosions, oil blowouts, large fires of all sorts, mining disasters, nuclear plant accidents, leakages of hazardous substances from toxic waste disposal, etc. In contrast to war, another type of human-made disaster, technological disaster, is not intended. In a technological disaster, a human action, or a product of human hand (a failed technology), results in the disruption of a community, and, at times, considerable death, injury, and destruction.

Technology is certainly becoming safer. Road traffic, airlines, and railways are subject to stringent safety procedures. However, the absolute number of technological disasters is increasing. As technology develops, there are simply more things that can go wrong, even if unintended and uncalculated. When something does go wrong, or a mistake is made, there has been a human error and someone is always responsible. But is there always someone willing to assume the responsibility? Whether or not someone does assume the responsibility makes a substantial difference in the psychological reactions of those affected and of the public at large.

Since the Industrial Revolution, human beings have tried to harness the forces of nature by their inventions. In all walks of life, the last 200 years has seen amazing scientific progress. The pace of development itself, at times, seems to get out of control and nature, like the Greek gods, hits back. Ever since the Greek dramas, 'hybris' (arrogance, foolhardiness, and false pride) has meant the hero's downfall: 'Do not fly too close to the sun.' The 'experts' said that the Titanic was unsinkable and that nuclear reactors would only get out of control once every 5000 years. What is foolproof?

The aim of medicine has been to prolong life at nearly all costs, but it is increasingly evident that it is more important to add life to years rather than years to life. Our attempts to escape the unavoidable suffering inherent in the fragmentary nature of our present existence give rise to most of the avoidable sufferings in life (Kingsmill, 1944). Half a century later, one can observe our love affair with technology, and wonder to what extent it gave us a false sense of mastery and serves to deny man's eternal existential problems of death and human frailty.

About 5 percent of all deaths in Western countries are violent or 'unnatural.' The vast majority are caused by accidents, primarily transport accidents. Very few of these violent deaths, about 5 percent, involve multiple deaths (more than five lives lost). Still, the large-scale accident or disaster is overwhelming when it strikes. For example, the 158 deaths caused by the ferry disaster off the Norwegian coast in April 1990 made up 30 percent of the transport-related deaths of the entire year in Norway.

The leak of poisonous gas from a Union Carbide Corporation plant in Bhopal, India, occurred in a densely populated suburb. It is now believed to have killed more than 3800 people. In addition, of the 300 000 injured, 30 000 were temporarily blinded by keratitis, and many were permanently disabled. The psychiatric morbidity has, of course, been striking (Sethi *et al.*, 1987).

How many deaths ionizing radiation and radioactive fallout from the Chernobyl reactor accident caused or contributed to will perhaps never be known for certain. However, it is known that more than 2000 children in areas of the former Soviet Union affected by fallout have suffered thyroid cancer, most probably caused by Chernobyl fallout (United Nations Scientific Committee on the Effects of Atomic Radiation, 2000) (We are aware that the correct Ukrainian and thus currently official spelling is Chornobel rather than Chernobyl, but it has been chosen to use the better-known name.).

Such incidents of mass death and injury overwhelm the emergency care services, at least in the initial phase. Helpers are likely to share the sense of powerlessness of the disaster victims. For this reason, disaster medicine and its subdiscipline, disaster psychiatry, are taught in medical schools as a part of emergency medicine.

This chapter will address recent developments which highlight the importance of technological disasters in our time. In addition, the chapter will describe both the classical technological disaster and the newer toxic type of disaster. Data from two recent technological disaster studies will be used to illustrate the major issues. The acute and long-term psychosocial responses to a classical technological disaster are presented in a study of individuals exposed to an industrial explosion. In contrast to this familiar scenario, the much more alarming and newer type of technological failure, the toxic disaster, exemplified by the Chernobyl nuclear plant accident, and its short- and long-term psychosocial consequences, is presented.

Natural versus technological disaster: A blurred distinction?

Traditionally, the two types of disaster have been (1) natural, i.e., an act of God, and (2) 'human-made.' Whereas in Western countries 'an act of God' has come to mean the power of the elements, a natural or accidental causation, in other parts of the world, divine intervention is still seen as a possible explanation for a disaster. Islamic fatalism, for example, explained the death of more than 1400 people in a tunnel during the Haj in Mecca on 3 July, 1990 as God's will.

The United Nations designated the 1990s as the decade of natural disaster reduction (World Health Organization, 1988). Does the idea of reducing natural disasters seem surprising? Consider the following. Of the 109 worst natural disasters between 1960 and 1987, 41 occurred in developing countries (Berz, 1989). Furthermore, the number of deaths caused by disasters was far greater in the developing countries: 758 850 compared to 11 441 in developed countries! In general, the number of deaths and injuries caused by disasters is closely related to a country's level of economic development. This is how technology comes in. Preparedness, prevention, and mitigation are the three key activities for coping with disasters and disaster risks. Earthquakes, windstorms, tsunamis, floods, landslides, volcanic eruptions, wildfires, and other calamities have killed nearly 3 million people world-wide over the past two decades, and have adversely affected the lives of at least 800 million more (World Health Organization, 1991). The vast majority of these lives could have been spared by better warning systems, more evacuation capacity, better building construction, etc. For example, the Netherlands has not suffered a major flood since the devastating 1953 flood, which claimed 1500 lives. One consequence of this disaster was the development of an intensive program of dam building. Technology can save lives.

If, however, technology can save lives by controlling natural hazards, failure or lack of technology increasingly is seen as responsible for deaths occurring in previously 'natural' disasters. As the world grows smaller, people in developing countries will probably alter their attitude about deaths from natural disasters, from a resigned and fatalistic outlook, to feelings of bitter despair: 'It could have been prevented.' The previous understanding and acceptance of the natural disaster through a general religious and fatalistic outlook may be lost. It is likely that this will increase the psychiatric morbidity of disasters.

In addition, disasters previously classified as natural are today considered, to an ever increasing degree, to be human-made. Mamiduzzaman Khan Choudhury, a professor of meteorology from Bangladesh, commented at a 1990 meeting where representatives from 75 countries discussed the problem of global climatic changes: 'You quarrel while we drown.' He knew that 'human-made' future climatic changes which result in a rise in sea level may drown Bangladesh; floods used to be only natural disasters. The 1991 flood in Bangladesh claimed 200 000 lives. Still, there were 300 000 fewer casualties than there would have been without technological advances. How did the survivors interpret the causes of the flood? We do not fully know as yet, but there are reports that the educated citizens discussed the deforestation of the Himalayas, the weakening of the ozone layer, etc., as possible contributory causes, while the uneducated masses felt that God was angry with them.

The earthquake in Armenia in December 1988 claimed 30 000 lives. The majority died because their houses were poorly constructed. Was this a natural disaster or a technological failure? Similarly, after the San Francisco earthquake in 1989, harsh criticism was directed towards the method of road construction that had been used. Collapsing freeways had caused a number of deaths The earthquake, however, was the same Richter magnitude as the Armenian one. The effects of an earthquake in modern times depend, to a large extent, on the breakdown of human-made products.

Will man's changing perceptions of who is responsible, or who is to blame for disasters, have any psychological consequences? In all likelihood it will. Nature can do harm, but nature has no evil intent. Man has this capability. A dramatic example of the striking difference in response between a new technological threat and a permanent but natural threat is offered by the public reactions after the Chernobyl reactor accident. After the disaster, there was strong public reaction in several countries to the radioactive fallout from the Chernobyl reactor. In contrast to this is the moderate, or even absent, reaction to the normal background radiation from radon, which is a much greater dose contributor than Chernobyl fallout. The former can be blamed on somebody, the latter is more one's own responsibility since it depended upon where you chose to build your home.

The more human causation lies behind a disaster, the more pathogenic it seems to be in terms of psychiatric morbidity. Human-made disasters are said to be more traumatic because of their unfamiliarity, unpredictability, uncontrollability, and culpability. War may be an exception to this rule, since the suffering and death in war may take on a deep sense of noble sacrifice, perhaps increasing the stress tolerance. However, these propositions require more direct study. Although there is still a dearth of comparative studies (Frederick, 1986), the few findings available point to a more virulent effect of what humans do to humans than what nature does to humans (Luchterhand, 1971) or what accidental trauma, for which no one is to blame, does to humans (Weisaeth, 1989). The human-to-human context differs from natural trauma in the pernicious and ever-present attacks on individual's integrity and self-respect. Nature does not threaten man's self-respect even if it kills him. Thus, human failure and violence are likely to produce more aggressive responses. In the words of Kai Erikson (1976), technological disasters are not necessary. They are avoidable, therefore, they produce aggression rather than acceptance. They also produce more distrust and fear of other humans than do natural and accidental traumas. Because of this, human-made disasters frequently cause withdrawal and social isolation which is more detrimental to mental health than the limited phobias of natural disasters (Weisaeth, 1989). There are no available comparative studies of responses to a technological disaster which was perceived as truly accidental, and one which was seen as due to negligence, in which to examine this further.

Risk perception research has demonstrated the values involved in the judgment of different qualities of risks. The public's ratings of risks are not a function of the average annual fatalities according to best available estimates, but rather are more dependent upon the evaluation of various attributes of the risks (National Research Council, 1989). Slovic *et al.* (1979) and Covello (1998) have presented different sets of qualitative factors of importance for the public concern associated with a risk. These factors as proposed by Covello (1998) are shown in Table 13.1.

Clearly some of these proposed factors are closely interdependent and it is not self-evident which are truly 'separate' categories. For instance, dreaded effects and catastrophic potential are closely connected, and the same goes for familiarity and understanding of process. Work by Slovic *et al.* (1979) has suggested that two main organizing dimensions are present; 'familiarity' and 'dread' may subsume all these detailed qualitative factors. The most outstanding issue with regard to a nuclear threat as in for example a radiological emergency, is that almost all of these proposed factors will be placed on the side that has been found to be associated with increased public concern. A nuclear threat might very well be described as uncontrollable, with catastrophic potential, with dreaded effects, unfamiliar with processes not understood, putting children specifically at risk, producing delayed effects and possibilities for risk to future generations; the effects are irreversible, the trust in responsible institutions might be threatened, there will be much media attention, there is a history of major accidents, the eventual exposure is involuntary, the distribution of risk and benefits are clearly inequitable, the benefits are unclear and the threat is caused by human actions or failures.

Among these 17 factors one that might be seriously discussed is that concerning statistical versus identifiable victims. In most contexts, the possibility of identifying a victim (thinking of a family member or neighbor as a victim, witnessing an

Table 13.1 Qualitative factors of importance for public concern for a risk

Qualitative factor	Decreased public concern	Increased public concern
1. Personal controllability	Controllable	Uncontrollable
2. Catastrophic potential	Fatalities random and scattered	Fatalities grouped in space and time
3. Dread	Effects not dreaded	Effects dreaded
4. Familiarity	Familiar	Unfamiliar
5. Understanding	Mechanism or process understood	Mechanism or process not understood
6. Effects on children	Children not specifically at risk	Children specifically at risk
7. Manifestation of effects	Immediate effects	Delayed effects
8. Effects on future generations	No risk to future generations	Risk to future generations
9. Reversibility	Effects reversible	Effects irreversible
10. Victim identity	Statistical victims	Identifiable victims
11. Trust in institutions	Trust in responsible institutions	Lack of trust in responsible institutions
12. Media attention	Little media attention	Much media attention
13. Accident history	No major or minor accidents	Major and sometimes minor previous accidents
14. Voluntariness of exposure	Voluntary	Involuntary
15. Equity	Equitable distribution of risks and benefits	Inequitable distribution of risks and benefits
16. Benefits	Clear benefits	Unclear benefits
17. Origin	Caused by acts of nature or God	Caused by human actions or failures

accident, looking at a photograph of a person who might well be a member of one's own social group) adds to the unacceptability of a risk when compared to the anonymous character of victims identified only by a percent proportion of a population. In the case of nuclear threat, however the fact that the victims are *not* identifiable may specifically increase public concern. The victims of nuclear release will to a large extent be unidentifiable in that pathologies will be delayed and cannot be attributed with absolute certainty, but the projected victims are still identifiable social group members. This accentuates the unacceptable aspects of mystery and uncontrollability. As radioactive fallout to some extent might expose everyone in the population to increased doses of ionizing radiation, the fact that there is no way of identifying victims even after effects have occurred adds to concern: with such invisible threat, there is no way of being certain that oneself and one's loved ones are *not* victims.

Deadly "survival" responses? Is humanity captive of its evolution?

Through 4 million years of evolution the human race has had a long and intimate relationship with nature. In order to survive, the human race has had to cope with the natural dangers of the elements, wild animals, and human enemies. One has good reasons to believe that the genetic apparatus in the survivors, the people of today, has become uniquely adapted to cope with such threats. Some survival instincts can still be seen almost daily by semirealistic phobias such as fears of closed spaces, heights, darkness, etc. These atavisms sometimes still have life-preserving effects.

It is interesting to speculate whether the capacity of humans to survive natural disasters and war is greater than their survival capacity when facing technological hazards. This hypothesis has not been systematically studied. But the fundamental question has been raised as to whether adaptive skills previously used with success in the pretechnological age have now become detrimental (Dixon, 1987). Every psychotherapist knows, and for that matter every psychotherapy patient perhaps knows even better, how extremely difficult it is for the human brain to rid itself of the effects of very early experiences. Is humankind even more at a loss when it comes to ridding itself of evolutionary effects of selection in the survival of the fittest?

While human interaction with natural hazards has been going on for several thousand generations, experiences with the breakdown of human-made constructions can hardly be longer than a few hundred generations, i.e., a few thousand years. Perhaps this is not even enough to give evolution a chance to work out its principles. Modern technology, dating back to the Industrial Revolution with power-driven machines, trains, and manufacturing industry utilizing hundreds of potentially harmful materials, is scarcely 200 years old. A few examples will illustrate how, when facing a modern technological disaster, human instinct at times costs rather than save lives.

In 1988 only six miners survived the coal-mine disaster in Borken, Germany. Fifty other miners died. The only miners to survive were those who fled *into* the mine. All who tried to run out, to escape in the open air, perished because of toxic gases at the exit (Wolfram Schüffel, personal communication).

On Saturday morning just after 09.00 on November 11, 2000, the first official day of the ski season, a disastrous fire broke out because of a defective heater in the rear driver's cabin on a funicular train leading to the Kitzsteinhorn ski slope just outside Kaprun, 50 miles southwest of Salzburg, Austria. The Kitzsteinhorn funicular railway had been operating since 1974, always with two trains running, one going up to the glacier and one going down. Each train had two driver cabins, one in the front and one in the rear. The 9-minute journey took skiers up 1500 meters to an altitude of 2400 meters.

The following chronology of events has been kindly provided by Dr Clemens Hausmann (personal communication). Because of the defect in the heater in the rear driver cabin (separated from the passengers' cabin) a small fire occurred. Some skiers noticed the small fire, but there was no means for them to communicate either with the driver or with the base station. Approximately, when the train entered the 3.2-kilometer long tunnel, the fire broke out heavily. The train stopped after 600 meters travel into the tunnel, which sloped at 45 degrees. The driver was in radio contact with the mountain station for about a minute or two. Then he left his cabin and, beginning from the upper end of the train, the driver opened the doors manually. The driver kept on this work until he lost consciousness. Several people broke the windows to escape even though there were no emergency hammers available. Survivors report that the smoke had a rapidly numbing effect. They told investigators there was no mass panic in the train. There were no shouts or cries, people just took a few breaths and broke down. All died of exposure to poisonous gases; only after that the fire, which was also fueled by the ski clothes, etc., burnt their bodies.

Approximately 80–90 people were found outside the train on the stairs leading upwards. All the 12 survivors from the train were passengers at the rear end of the train and escaped by smashing a window and then running downwards in the tunnel. It took them about 40 minutes to get down to the base station. The survivors told investigators that everybody fled away from the fire. That seemingly was their leading cue – to get away from the fire. The majority of those who managed to escape the train were killed by poisonous gases while trying to escape upwards. It should be noted that they were moving upwards, even though there was something like 2.8 kilometers to run upwards in the tunnel, and only 600 meters to run downwards. In the tunnel there were no emergency signs and no electric light. Furthermore, judging from pictures of the tunnel, the stairway was quite narrow, implying that it would have been hard having people passing each other going in different directions. Thus, if the direction of those 80–90 people found on the stairs was upwards, if would be very difficult for someone considering downwards escape to get past the upward stream of people.

There was a strong chimney effect in the tunnel. The poisonous smoke reached first the train going downwards and killed three people there, then reached the mountain station, which was being evacuated, and killed three more people. Two of those killed in the mountain station were trapped by the poisonous smoke while on the toilet. Fortunately there were not so many people in the mountain station at that time in the morning.

There were no instructions or emergency plans that related to a fire accident in the tunnel. According to Dr Hausmann nobody had ever thought that such a thing could happen there. In addition to those three at the mountain station, and the three in the train moving downwards, some 149 passengers on the up-going funicular train were killed.

What if there had been clear fire evacuation routines established? Similar to instructions about never using lifts in a house in case of a fire, it seems reasonable that in such a tunnel, the main rule in case of fire should be always to evacuate downwards in case of fire, even if it means running through point zero of the fire.

Flight behavior in the natural environment, as well as when facing human enemies, has long been man's instinctive response to dangers with which he could not cope. Uncontrolled flight, as in individual or group panic, is characterized by overwhelming fear and the compelling thought of 'getting out' and 'getting away.' The consequences of such uncontrolled escape behavior can be fatal in human-made environments like mines, and also in high-rise buildings, ships, oil rigs, etc.; the fear of engulfment precipitates premature jumping from sinking ships; fear of flames and smoke elicits jumping from high buildings.

However, it should also be underlined that in many disasters humans' prosocial behaviors are observed, and controlled escape behavior is often reported, especially as long as escape is perceived as possible. For instance after the September 11 attack on the Twin Towers of the World Trade Center, a blind worker, Michael Hingson, together with his guide dog managed to descend from the 78th floor of the North Tower. Mr Hingson in an interview with Larry King reported how many cheered him and encouraged his escape, and there were no problems with those who wanted to descend the stairs more quickly than Mr Hingson was capable of.

Perceptually, humans are not only inclined to, but have no other choice than to react to cues of danger discovered with their limited senses. In a tunnel fire, for example, individuals will react to the sight of smoke, and its irritable and seemingly choking effect, provoking extreme fear and uncontrolled flight. At the same time, the effects of poisonous gases, like carbon monoxide, will not be noticed. When designing the physical layout of a construction site, to what extent is planning for survival in, for instance, a hotel fire, based upon technical calculations of toxic elements, rather than on the stimuli which will be detected by one's senses and probably contribute more to behavior?

If smoke moves faster than 7 meters per second, which it sometimes does, you cannot survive by running away from it. But your legs will probably try. It is a biological instinct, like that of the elk that tries to outrun your car by running ahead of it. The task, therefore, may be to control one's basic survival patterns.

Many died in Bhopal because they ran ahead of the approaching gas cloud. Certainly, many who were indoors died because they failed to shut the windows. More importantly the police instructed people to run away from the area. By fleeing, many were exposed to inhalation of large amounts of toxic methyl isocyanate. The police should rather have instructed residents that lying down indoors on the floor

Table 13.2 Time phases of disaster and methods of coping

Phase	Proximity of the danger	Coping
Steady state	Distant	Preparedness
Crisis	Approaching	Crisis management
Disaster impact	Imminent/present	Survival/rescue
After-periods	Passed	Working through shock and
Shock phase		posttraumatic stress
Reaction phase		reactions
Repair phase		
New orientation		

and covering their faces with wet cloths would have provided effective protection against the gas (Shrivastava, 1992).

Controlling natural responses is not enough. Problem-solving is also needed. Under severe stress, man's basic, primitive response patterns tend to appear while learned responses tend to disappear. Drilled responses and overlearnt procedures are the most stress-resistant, while creativity which is so essential in complex problem-solving easily gives way to stereotypical responses.

If this hypothesis is correct, that in some situations there is a conflict between human natural behavior tendencies and necessary survival behavior, then education, training, and practice must be the decisive determinants of disaster response if one is to cope successfully with the dangers of human-made disaster environments (Table 13.2). By stress inoculation training (training in simulated environments) and other techniques, industrial employees have been able to increase their problem-solving capacity under stress (Hytten *et al.*, 1990). Much work remains to be done in this promising research field.

The human brain is programmed for various types of adaptive behavior that are almost automatic. Fear helps humans to discover dangers and facilitates defensive strategies like flight behavior. However, the freezing response, adaptive when facing certain animals, is hardly helpful for the pedestrian who loses his mobility when seeing a car approaching.

Through its familiarity with natural dangers, the human perceptive apparatus has become suited for the discovery of danger. This is less so with 'unnatural' dangers. Technological threats do not give the same warning. Frequently, some instrument is required to discover danger in the early phase. Knowledge and information becomes more important, and trust in information sources. In Beck's word one gets dependent upon 'Erfarung aus zweiter Hand' (this German expression is close in meaning to '*second-hand experience*') in order to learn about the risks (Beck, 1986).

Table 13.3 Psychic trauma and presumed cause with corresponding more likely effects

Presumed cause	Likely effects
Natural cause	Accepted as accidental deaths, fatalistic acceptance
	Dangerous, not evil
	Poses no threat to self-esteem (own worth)
Human failure	Blame for loss of control
	Lack of preventive measures
	Questions self-esteem
Human negligence	Blame, loss of credibility
	Challenges self-esteem
Human malice	Fight (aggression), flight (fear), surrender (shame)
	Attack on self-esteem, humiliation, narcissistic injuries, hatred, eventually revenge, cycles of violence

'The position of man is obviously extremely insecure unless he can find out what is happening around him' (West, 1955). In their study of leakages of carbon monoxide from a closed underground coal mine, Couch and Kroll-Smith (1990) found that many exposed people refused to use the measuring instruments provided by the authorities. The population outside the risk area thought the problems of the affected population were exaggerated in order to increase compensation claims.

Risk factors and dimensions of disaster trauma

Those involved with technological disaster need to know predictors of the frequency of the disaster, the disaster type and severity, and the course of the resulting psychosocial disturbances. The psychosocial impact of a disaster is affected by the cause of the disaster, the amount of geographical displacement, degree of threat to life, and degree of loss and community disruption caused by the disaster.

A proposed relationship between human agency of the disaster situation and predicted responses is shown in Table 13.3.

Risk and protective factors for disaster behavior and posttraumatic stress disorder

In 1976 a tremendous explosion hit the production plant of Norway's largest paint factory. The building collapsed and a series of new explosions followed. A huge fire destroyed the production plant and warehouses. Nearly 30 000 square meters of buildings were engulfed in flames stretching up to a height of 400 meters. The fire was fed by millions of liters of chemicals and 50 million cubic meters of air. A local windstorm was created by the combustion. The explosion shook the neighborhood and was heard many kilometers away. The threat of spreading fire and further explosions necessitated the evacuation of 1000 people. Helped by earlier rain and fortunate wind direction, 150 firefighters contained the fire within 12 hours and extinguished it after 36 hours. Six workers were killed. Of the 125 survivors, 21 had minor injuries and two had severe injuries. The community lost about 400 jobs as a result of the fire.

In terms of structural damage, this was the largest industrial disaster that has ever occurred in Scandinavia. Many aspects made this large-scale technological accident a typical example of a 'modern disaster' and a psychic 'shock trauma': the lack of forewarning (90.4 percent of the 125 employees received no kind of warning), the brief but violent impact, the circumscribed but completely damaged area, and the great material destruction but limited number of casualties. The disaster was unprecedented, unanticipated, sudden, violent, uncontrollable, and brief. Central to the disaster was the large number of people exposed to shock trauma, and the narrow escape. Many individuals were exposed to severe danger but were not physically harmed.

While the factory was still smouldering, all employees were guaranteed continuous employment and assured that they would suffer no economic losses. Within 2 weeks the company improvised new jobs. The additional (secondary) disaster stressors, e.g., unemployment, economic difficulties, and compensation issues which usually occur following disaster were less than usual.

A model summarizing these depicts risk and protective factors for PTSD in this population (Fig. 13.1). It highlights major features to be considered when planning for the mental health consequences of an industrial disaster. For a detailed description of the projects and its results, see Weisaeth (1994).

The Chernobyl nuclear accident

On April 26, 1986 at Unit 4 at the Chernobyl nuclear power plant a nuclear accident of unforeseen dimensions occurred. In contrast to the Three Mile Island accident, where the safety containment held much of the release, at Chernobyl there were extremely large releases of radioactivity to the environment. It led to substantial cross-border radioactive fallout. The graphite used for moderating the RBMK (Reaktor Bolshoy Moshchnosty Kipyaschiy, Large Power Boiling Reactor) reactor kept a fire alight and the releases going for about 10 days. About one-third of the total release from Chernobyl occurred during the first day, but there was a substantial release over the following days (Organization for Economic Cooperation and Development, Nuclear Energy Agency, 1996).

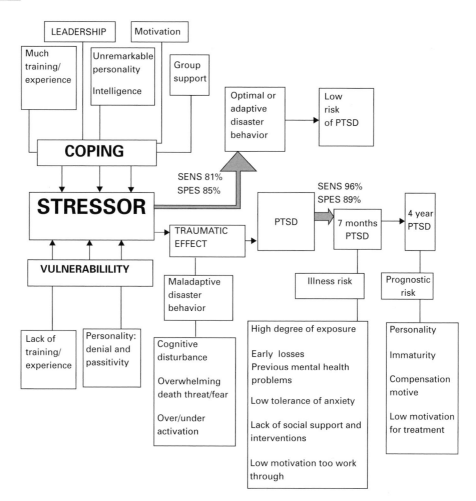

Figure 13.1   Risk and protective factors for disaster behavior and posttraumatic stress disorder in 125 survivors of an industrial explosion in 1976. SENS, sensitivity (the ability to predict those with later occurring serious PTSD; SPES, specificity (the ability to make predictions that do not include those with a fair outcome). (From Weisaeth, 1984.)

The Chernobyl nuclear power plant (NPP) is located in the Kiev region of Ukraine, 15 kilometers from the southern border of the Gomel region of Belarus and 150 kilometers from the western part of the Bryansk region in Russia. The nearest city is Pripyat with 49 000 inhabitants, 3 kilometers from Chernobyl NPP.

At the time of the accident there were 200 employees at work at reactor Units 1, 2, 3, and 4, and 1 kilometer away 300 people were working night-shift on constructing the new reactor Units 5 and 6. A plant employee working immediately above the exploding reactor was killed immediately. His body could not be recovered. Another employee was crushed by debris and badly burnt and died from his injuries within hours. More than 100 firefighters, both plant firefighters and firefighters from around the city of Pripyat, participated in the firefighting, and at around 5.00 a.m. all fires except the graphite fire in the core were extinguished.

Radiation levels were so high in the damaged part of the plant and outside that the monitoring equipment could not measure it: they all went completely off scale. The firefighters and the plant personnel had no personal dosimeters, and were very severely exposed. Within 1 hour the first of many cases of acute radiation syndrome (ARS) appeared, and during the first 12 hours 132 emergency workers were hospitalized in Pripyat suspected of suffering from ARS. During the day on Saturday a specialized emergency team was established and examined some 350 persons within the first three days identifying 299 suspected cases of ARS.

After 3 months a total of 28 had died of ARS making the total death toll 30, all of whom belong to the operating staff of the reactor and the firefighting crew. To avoid deterministic effects the city of Pripyat was evacuated on April 27 (United Nations Scientific Committee on the Effects of Atomic Radiation, 1988). However, because of the information blockade by the Soviet authorities the accident 'outside' the former Soviet Union started as a local incident in Uppland, Sweden on the morning of Monday, April 28. As an employee entered the Forsmark NPP with Chernobyl fallout particles on his shoes the alarm went out. Measurement patrols sent out reported readings that indicated elevated levels of ionizing radiation around the plant, the NPP was evacuated, and the Director at Forsmark called the local radio at 11.15 a.m. to inform them about this situation. Ten minutes later Radio Uppland made an extraordinary news broadcast about the incident at Forsmark NPP. After further analysis it was found that the measured levels of radiation had nothing to do with Forsmark NPP, and after pressure from many, ITAS-TASS at 7.00 p.m. on April 28 ran a short notice about a nuclear accident in Ukraine.

Inside the Soviet Union, on May 2 and 3 an additional 11 000 inhabitants in 14 villages in the zone 10 kilometers round Chernobyl were evacuated, while 42 000 inhabitants of 83 villages within the 30-kilometers zone were evacuated between May 4 and May 7. Furthermore from June to September an additional 57 villages in Belarus, one village in Ukraine, and four villages in Russia (Bryansk region) were resettled, resulting in a total of 116 000 evacuated individuals (Shigematsu, 1991).

The fallout from the Chernobyl accident resulted in three main spots of contamination within the former Soviet Union; they have been termed the Central, the Bryansk–Belarus, and the Kaluga–Tula–Orel spots. The central spot was formed during the initial release stage and is mainly to the west and northwest of Chernobyl, the most contaminated area being within the 30-kilometer radius surrounding the reactor where caesium-137 activity levels exceeded 1.5 MBq per square meter. The Bryansk–Belarus spot was formed on April 28–29 as the result of rainfall and is situated some 200 kilometers to the north-northeast of Chernobyl NPP. The radionuclide composition in the Bryansk–Belarus is different from that in the central spot, and as radioactive caesium is more dominating it is called 'caesium hot spot.' The levels of caesium in the most contaminated parts of the Bryansk–Belarus spot are comparable to levels of the central spot. The Kaluga–Turel–Orel spot in Russia was also formed by rainfall on April 28–29 and is situated 500 kilometers northeast of Chernobyl NPP. As it was formed from the rainfall from the same cloud that formed the Bryansk–Belarus spot it is also a caesium spot, but with somewhat lower deposition levels.

A total area of some 10 300 square kilometers with caesium-137 contamination exceeding 600 KBq per square meter was called with somewhat parallel terms as a 'restricted,' 'control,' or 'strict control zone' area. The restricted area consisted of 109 000 inhabitants of a 6400-km^2 area of the Gomel and Mogilev regions of Belarus, 52 000 inhabitants of a 1500-km^2 area of the Kiev and Zhitomor regions of Ukraine, and 112 000 inhabitants of a 2400-km^2 area of the Bryansk region of Russia. For the total of 273 000 people in something like 786 settlements in the control areas in Belarus, Ukraine, and Russia various radiation protection measures were implemented, including delivery of uncontaminated food products, measures to decrease radioactive content of their agricultural production, etc.

There is currently an ongoing discussion of whether the negative psychosocial consequences of extensive measures taken are larger that the benefits of radiation protection achieved by implementing these extensive measures (United Nations Development Program and United Nations Children's Fund, 2002).

The far-field fallout was very dependent upon the meteorological conditions. The radioactive clouds first spread to Scandinavia and then turned towards the Balkans affecting various other parts of Europe. The United Nations Scientific Committee on the Effects of Atomic Radiation (1988) has estimated that 57 percent of the collective effective dose was received in Europe outside the former Soviet Union.

It is important to note that the washout from the Chernobyl fallout plumes resulted in very heterogeneous fallout, especially as compared to the previous experience with atomic bomb test fallout. Indeed the levels of bomb fallout was also associated with washout and precipitation levels, but not with such extreme local variations as observed with the Chernobyl fallout. The previous experiences with more homogeneous bomb fallout made quite a few experts believe that the early measurements from a few areas could be valid indications for larger areas. However, with such a patchy fallout pattern this was not the case. Thus, in Norway when the central Oslo area was only slightly affected with fallout, one made conclusions about the rest of the country that later turned out to be premature.

The air currents containing most of the radioactivity drove northwest towards the Nordic countries. This was an unusual wind direction for Scandinavia with the worst possible meteorological conditions, wind and rain. Within three days, the air masses spread over mid-Scandinavia and patchy heavy rain fell.

Measurements indicated an enormous increase in the washout ratio by the rainfall. Even 1 millimeter of light drizzle brought down particles that might have otherwise passed by. The cloud also hit the mountain chain along the Swedish–Norwegian border, increasing the fallout in both countries. The wind direction later turned the air currents towards Poland, Czechoslovakia, Austria and East Germany, and the Balkans. Then the wind currents changed direction once more causing a second peak in measurements observed in Sweden, Denmark, and Norway. In Norway due to unsatisfactory information management, the second peak in measurements was not communicated clearly to the public. This was picked up by the mass media and filtering of information by the authorities was then a main news story.

The downfall precipitated a fallout of various iodine isotopes, perhaps most notably iodine-131, and of caesium-134 and caesium-137. The half-life of iodine-131 is 8 days, and caesium-134 and caesium-137 have half-lives of approximately 2.4 years and 28 years, respectively. Thus, in the short term iodine was a prime concern, while caesium contamination has been and still is the main problem in affected areas. By chance no areas of Sweden and Norway that were only sparsely populated were affected by fallout. However, in Norway some of the seminatural ecosystems affected by fallout is extensively used for sheep grazing, and Norway has spent around US 50 million on various countermeasures in order to keep the sheep meat below the intervention level for content of radioactivity. The most affected group in Norway was the indigenous group of Southern Saamis (Mehli *et al.*, 2000). Due to the lichen–reindeer–Saami pathway for radioactive caesium they were in 1996 found to have a comparable whole body levels as peasants in restricted areas of the Bryansk–Belarus spot described above (Tønnessen *et al.*, 1996). It has been estimated that in 2001, 15 years after the accident, some 70 percent of the caesium-137 is still left.

Clearly a significant part of the threat from far-field radioactive fallout is the fact that it is not detectable by our senses, leaving us dependent upon someone else (experts) to measure, interpret, and communicate the threat. For such type of threats, information from someone else is necessary for the threat to become 'alive.' Inherent in such a kind of threat will thus always be a trust relationship towards the source of this threat information. Hence, it is important to study the mass media reports of such types of risks, or as described by Ursano and colleagues: 'The knowledge itself is the stressor. The potential for information and, similarly, news reports to create distress in the listener or viewer needs further study in our media-intensive age' (Ursano *et al.*, 1995, p. 201).

A content analysis we conducted of Swedish and Norwegian newspaper of the Chernobyl 10-years commemoration coverage found ionizing radiation risk to be given voluminous coverage that was quite condensed in time (Nilsson *et al.*, 2000). This finding is similar to that of the already noted 'big bang' pattern of mass media coverage of major disasters (Nohrstedt and Tassew, 1993). The coverage was also found to be context dependent. Thus, in Sweden where a substantial proportion of electricity is generated by nuclear power, risks connected to chemical waste were portrayed more often as alarming than were those associated with domestic nuclear power. In Norway where there are no nuclear power plants, ionizing radiation risk stories were found to be more alarming than other risk stories. A comparatively unusual focus in Norwegian newspapers concerned 'military nuclear technology' related to the Kola Peninsula.

An ecological study we conducted *post hoc* of the European publics' reaction to Chernobyl far-field fallout, utilizing various Eurobarometer data sets, found a wide range of reactions across the 12 national samples in the European Community. The difference between countries is of such an order of magnitude that it is advisable to describe the responses at the national level, rather than describing a 'mean' European response. An association of a significant rank order correlation was found at the national level between the first-year effective dose estimate from Chernobyl fallout and several indicators of 'psychological fallout.' There was a significant rank order association at the national level between first-year mean effective dose estimate and (1) the proportions reporting exposure to 'a lot of' Chernobyl information, (2) the proportions reporting perceived threat from Chernobyl, (3) the proportions reporting having carried out behavioral interventions, and (4) the proportions rating the most serious Chernobyl consequence to be a serious health threat. Overall this indicated a quite proportionate response by the publics of the 12 countries included in the survey data sets (Tønnessen *et al.*, in press). The proxy used for fallout level in each of these 12 countries was United Nations Scientific Committee on the Effects of Atomic Radiation's (1988) estimates of first-year effective dose.

Without going into various specifics, the important overall finding is that of proportionate and quite reasonable public concerns and reactions. These findings are similar to those reported by Renn (1990), except the point that Greece in fact as indicated by the United Nations Scientific Committee on the Effects of Atomic Radiation's estimate of first-year effective dose was a country quite affected by the Chernobyl fallout.

It should be noted that even though the response was quite proportionate, with overall stronger public reactions in countries with more fallout, this does not indicate anything about the absolute level of reactions. Thus, nearly one out of two Europeans was found to have made behavioral changes because of Chernobyl.

An interesting difference was observed between having undertaken a behavioral change and having 'protected themselves.' Thus, in a 1996 survey in five European countries it was found that many of those reporting to have undertaken behavioral changes, such as dietary changes, did not report to have undertaken any 'protective measures' (Sjöberg *et al.*, 2000).

As part of a Scandinavian study (Mårdberg *et al.*, 1987; Lundin *et al.*, 1993; Weisaeth, 1990, 1991), we decided when the first fallout was noted in Norway on April 28, 1986 to carry out a survey to study the distant reactions to a nuclear reactor accident.

Surveys with national representative samples were carried out in Sweden, Denmark, and Norway. All surveys were carried out within the first eight weeks after the fallout. We found that the majority of persons perceived the accident as a very negative event. The public reported poor understanding of mass media coverage. Response by the authorities was judged to show poor preparation and a negative evaluation was made of the information provided by these sources. Among those suffering a higher degree of emotional trauma, intrusive memory was the major reaction (although infrequent). The data indicate that although the majority of the population was psychologically affected by the crisis in that all but a few people had some thoughts or feelings about it, only a small proportion seems to have developed stress reactions of such a severity that they needed or sought help.

Marked gender differences were found on both cognitive threat structuring variables and emotional impact variables. That women, regardless of age, were more worried than men about the threat to the physical health of the family, while the young women were more worried than the older women about sustaining long-term injuries, indicates that the worry of the caretaker and the fear of harm to a future fetus may have played a role. A similar result was found after the Three Mile Island accident (Bromet, 1998). Perhaps it can be stated that women are closer to life in the sense that they give birth to children and usually have more responsibility for feeding children. Genetic effects of radiation exposure and the increased risk to children were areas that were highly emotionally charged during the information crisis.

Through her own body a mother might poison or damage her fetus, a terribly frightening and unacceptable possibility. Øystein and Marit Krüger together with other physician colleagues interviewed 46 pregnant women in June 1986 in the county of Nor-Trøndelag of Norway (Krüger and Krüger, 1995). The study was performed by having five out of seven physicians practicing in the municipality of Levanger collect information from those attending antenatal care during the period June 10–19. The average of the four earth samples from the municipality of Levanger indicated a total (caesium-134 plus caesium-137) radioactive caesium contamination of 57.5 kBq per square meter by June 1986 (Backe *et al.*, 1987). The mothers-to-be expressed concern about malformations of the fetus. A slight increase in concern was observed for those in the first trimester as compared to the others, while parity was not related to levels of reported concern. Nine out of ten women reported having made behavioral changes to reduce exposure, the most commonly reported being to avoid locally grown vegetables (Krüger and Krüger, 1995).

The extensive changes in food and drinking habits reported by the women further convey their experience of this risk. The gender differences found regarding information about nuclear threats and reactions to these show interesting paradoxes. A larger proportion of female respondents report being involved in these issues, they report poorer knowledge, and more often a need for being informed about these issues, and still they do less to keep themselves informed, and less frequently follow mass media coverage. The gender difference in attention to mass media coverage, combined with the more frequently expressed need among women for more information, may be related to the concept of 'knowledge gap.' The gender difference is large enough to conclude that the mass mediated coverage is not compatible with the expressed need for more information. It is a particularly important challenge for the responsible authorities to preplan information material in order to facilitate rapport with the female part of the population.

An association between dysphoric feelings and the ratings of Chernobyl threat was found in the Scandinavian data set. We propose to view the relationship between reports of feeling more sad/depressed and larger impacts of Chernobyl in the perspective of the 'depressive realism' hypothesis as proposed by Alloy and Abramson (1979). They found that slightly depressed students reported less of the 'optimistic bias' so often found in risk perception research (Weinstein, 1989), and suggested them to be 'sadder but wiser' (Alloy and Abramson, 1979; Dunning and Story, 1991; Pacini et al., 1998). The depressive realism hypothesis has been criticized by some (Hancock et al., 1996), and is also considered by some not to be compatible with the cognitive theory of depression. However, David Haaga and Aaron Beck have convincingly argued that there are important differences between clinical depression and feeling 'slightly' down like the students of Alloy and Abramson, and that rather than seeing 'depressive realism' as an antagonist of cognitive theory of depression it could be used for further developments (Hagga and Beck, 1995).

Possibly those of our respondents who 'felt sad' had less 'optimistic bias,' and thus in their appraisal process more easily felt this diffuse threat from Chernobyl fallout to be of importance for themselves? To use the concepts of Lazarus's coping theory one could suggest that those slightly depressed in their primary appraisal process are more likely to assess threats as thwarting some personal goals (Lazarus, 1991).

The relationship between Chernobyl impact and previous psychological problems found in Norway disappeared when running partial correlation controlling for the 'mood' component (Weisaeth, 1991). Perhaps feeling 'not too happy' is also a state when we are less urgently in need for using rose-colored glasses to judge the world (Alloy and Abramson, 1979).

Looking at national differences in public response between Sweden, Denmark, and Norway, it should be noted that Norway and Sweden were severely affected by fallout in specific areas, while Denmark was not affected. At the time of the survey the fallout situation was not determined in Norway, while in Sweden, even though the survey was carried out earlier information was coming through much earlier that parts of the country had been quite substantially affected. Among the national differences observed we hypothesized that Swedish subjects to a larger degree had been challenged on their own shortcomings in preparedness levels. Thus, some Norwegian subjects were asked at a time when the authorities were issuing statements saying there was no need to take any measures at all because of the fallout.

The data confirm the impression from the first weeks following the Chernobyl disaster of an information crisis with a public discontented with the information and guidance provided by the authorities.

The information crisis probably resulted from a combination of factors: shortcomings in previous public education on the matter; shortage of reliable and unambiguous data on the extent and concentration of the radioactive fallout; the diffuseness of the threat and ambiguity of the risks; the complexity of the subject; the seeming contradiction between the health authorities' assurance that the radiation level was not dangerously high, and their statement that some precautions had to be taken; the experts' obvious difficulties in formulating simple information on complicated matters and statistical risks; and the media thriving on the disagreements between the experts.

The frequency with which fears of attracting some radiation injury were expressed, contrasts with the absence of manifest illness or injury cases and the low statistical risk for developing cancer as a late effect of the small increase in ionizing radiation exposure. This should be contrasted with the expected latency time for such stochastic effects, and the fact that no one for certain could exclude the possibility of the small excess risk affecting specific individuals. The threat to physical health of the radioactive fallout has certain properties that make it particularly frightening. Individuals lacked personal control over the events. There were no danger signals to monitor; everyone was dependent on outside information but the actual data were scarce and ambiguous. Exposure to ionizing radiation from Chernobyl fallout was frightening because it was involuntary, caused by another country, and carried the risk of cancer.

It is difficult to judge the clinical importance of the psychic reactions on the bases of our mainly survey data. The posttraumatic stress reactions and frequency of very pronounced sadness/depression indicate that perhaps only about 1 to 3 percent of the subjects may have developed reactions of a clinical intensity. Furthermore, with such small cell sizes our observations of proportions do not permit a generalization from these survey samples to the general population; we may only conclude that reactions of such severity were very infrequent.

Of the more classical symptoms resembling those of posttraumatic stress disorder (PTSD) intrusion was reported by a substantial proportion in our Scandinavian data set. A substantial minority reported their thoughts and feelings to be affected in such a way that 'I have to think about the accident now and then even though I don't want to': a response that could be interpreted as an intrusion phenomenon (Horowitz, 1975). About one out of three responded this way in Sweden and Norway, while one out of four so responded in Denmark. The large proportions that confirmed intrusion might be seen not in complete agreement with other observations with Chernobyl threat response (Havenaar, 1996), but perhaps well in harmony with the model by Marty J. Horowitz on intrusion (Horowitz, 1975). In his research he exposed subjects to stressful films and found intrusion to be a widespread phenomenon afterwards.

The human consequences in the Soviet Union of the Chernobyl disaster

As a result of the accident or of their work in dealing with its immediate consequences, 30 people were killed or died from acute radiation sickness and many, perhaps over half a million, received high doses of radiation.

Some of the radiation illness cases presented mainly psychiatric symptomatology in the acute phase, such as euphoria, others suffered loss of consciousness, fatigue, nausea, vomiting, etc. A number of individuals with bodily anxiety reactions had to be examined to rule out radiation illness. From what is known today one must assume that a number of the radiation sickness cases were not allowed to figure in the official statistics. As of 1991, the official number of deaths in the Soviet Union has risen to 250.

The start of the Chernobyl disaster was similar to many classical industrial disasters: mismanagement led to a crisis that could not be handled, there was an explosion that killed people and caused massive material destructions. However, one specific dimension of some toxic disasters made this event very different from an 'ordinary' explosion: the lack of boundaries. The contaminated areas in the Soviet Union alone have a population of some 4 million, more than 800 000 of whom live in regions where the contamination level is above 5 Ci per square kilometer. In the spring and summer of 1986, 116 000 people were evacuated from the danger zone. As described in a report to the UN General Assembly (United Nations Scientific Committee on the Effects of Atomic Radiation, 1988), the following three periods can be distinguished in the efforts to deal with the after-effects of the accident. The first period, from April to May 1986, involved making initial estimates of the scale of the disaster and the radiation situation, taking action to prevent a spontaneous chain reaction and radioactive emissions from the damaged reactor, identifying areas exposed to radioactive contamination, and evacuating the population and farm animals from a 30-kilometer zone. However, the May 1 outdoor celebrations in Kiev went ahead as usual; no alarming information had been issued. In the following week thousands were evacuated.

The second period, from summer 1986 to 1987, involved mapping out the contaminated areas, construction of the 'encasement' ('Sarcophagus'), decontamination of the working area of the nuclear power plant, restarting of the reactor Units 1, 2, and 3, measures to protect water resources from radioactivity, decontamination of settlements, scientific investigations, and special measures on agricultural land. Like many technological disasters, the accident at the Chernobyl NPP was not an acute, time-limited event. Rather, the nuclear plant accident started a sequence of events that will continue to unfold over several years, thereby creating a situation of chronic stress for many people.

A working group on 'Psychological effects of nuclear accidents' from the World Health Organization (1990) emphasized that whereas a great deal of scientific knowledge exists on the physical effects of radiation, much less is known about the psychological damage and how this can best be handled by the responsible authorities, by the individual health care workers, and by those affected. The group, when visiting in the summer of 1990 an area with a level of contamination of 5–15 Ci per square kilometer, was very much struck by the level of anxiety evident from the great number of people who had left the area out of fear. This had caused considerable social disruption, for example shortage of labor.

Very serious worries are now being experienced by the population in the affected areas, worries that appear to increase with time. Among the dimensions that need to be understood are the following: changes in illness behavior of the population and diagnosis by the doctors; the sociocultural dimension of displacement causing social disruption of communities; the psychological dimension of perception of risk resulting from radiation, and the part information policy plays; the socioeconomic dimension involving among others the reversal to other sources of energy; and finally pathogenic factors, relating to physiological stress reactions and to changes in lifestyle, e.g., dietary habits and the consumption of alcohol.

Awareness of individual health status has increased enormously since the disaster, and anxiety and its concomitant physiological reactions are spread far beyond the heavily contaminated areas. Shortly after the disaster, manifold subjective and objective symptoms were attributed to radiation exposure. Except for independent sources, the media had low credibility and the understanding of the consequences of exposure to radiation was incomplete in the public as well as among community physicians. Dissatisfaction with medical and administration management was considerable:

In order to cope with general anxiety and uncertainty about the possible health effects of exposure to radiation, people focus on the more tangible aspects of their physical state of health, seeking out the health care system and requesting explanations. In the absence of reliable data about the health effects of the accident, the medical profession lacks adequate explanations and responds predictably with more extensive and intensive diagnostic screening of populations and individual patients. As a result, hitherto unobserved morbidity patterns and individual variations emerge which are without explanation and which confuse the situation further. (World Health Organization, 1990)

Five years after the Chernobyl accident it was certain that there are substantial psychosocial problems in its aftermath, particularly in the Soviet Union. The interpretation of these problems differs, however. One extreme position defines the whole problem as irrational: 'The Chernobyl psychiatric disaster.' The psychiatric label 'radiophobia' has been coined to describe the human response. One should, however, be cautious in using psychiatric labels when characterizing such responses, particularly when a large proportion of the population appears to share that response. How fear-driven is the response, how irrational is the fear? Could it be understood as a protest or reflect a distrust in people?

After all, people had been misinformed about the fallout for a long time, and it is not a new observation that when credibility is lost it may never be won back. The other extreme position holds that the psychosocial responses reflect real and objective factors.

Recently the International Atomic Energy Bureau proclaimed that the radiation level was far less than had been feared and although most radiation experts exercise some caution in long-term predictions as yet, an optimistic forecast was presented as regards damage to health. According to reports at the end of 1991, half of the population living in contaminated areas experience psychological stress symptoms; eventually these stress reactions will produce psychosomatic and somatic illnesses in some number.

The problems encountered should come as no surprise. An information crisis had been predicted to occur after such accidents a long time before Chernobyl. Even in the area of the accident the major responsibility of the health services should have been to inform and calm the many thousands of frightened persons, and not merely to treat the acute radiation exposure cases. No country had foreseen the magnitude of the problems involved in handling the information issue.

Concluding comments

Modern technology has a Janus face. On the one side, technology spares lives in natural disasters through better preparedness, prevention, and mitigation of the effects of the disasters. On the other side, although technology is becoming relatively safer, there are simply more things that can go wrong. The classical technological disaster is sudden, without warning, tremendously powerful and extremely destructive within a confined area. Usually, it leaves the surrounding environment intact. However, man's increasing interference with nature has not only blurred the distinction between natural and human-made disasters, but has also broken down the geographical boundaries of the traditional technological disaster by toxic dispersion. In human-made disasters, failed technology implies a loss of control by those responsible, which contributes to the psychological trauma experienced by the population.

Technological disasters generally cause more severe mental health problems than natural disasters when they are of roughly the same magnitude. This is probably related to the greater unpredictability, uncontrollability, and culpability in technological disasters.

Compared with peacetime victims of severe violence, however, technological trauma causes less psychiatric morbidity in its victims. Some evidence indicates that the disaster behaviors, the natural responses of victims of human-made disasters, such as fight–flight, may be less adaptive than in a natural environment.

Optimal disaster behavior appears to be strongly related to an individual's level of training and experience in handling physical danger situations. In this particular industrial disaster presented here, the later occurrence of PTSD was substantially related to the immediate failure to cope. Thus, a high level of training might be the best preventive factor for later PTSD. Stress inoculation of employees in high-risk occupations has also been shown to increase resilience. The explosion itself in this industrial disaster was severe enough to produce acute PTSD in previously healthy subjects, mainly in somewhat vulnerable personalities.

Finally, the helplessness and anxiety of single individuals and the general population when confronted with the invisible danger of a toxic disaster, such as Chernobyl, are substantial. Dissatisfaction with medical advice and the public administration, as well as confusion about the real health effects, lead to substantial psychosocial problems.

REFERENCES

Alloy, L. B. and Abramson, L. Y. (1979). Judgment of contingency in depressed and nondepressed students: Sadder but wiser? *Journal of Experimental Psychology*, **108**, 441–485.

Backe, S., Bjerke, H., Rudjord, A. L. and Ugletveit, F. (1987). *Nedfall av cesium I Norge etter Tsjernobyl ulykken.* Osteras: Statens Institut for Stralehygiene.

Beck, U. (1986). *Risikogesellschaft: Auf dem Weg in eine andere Moderne.* Frankfurt am Main: Suhrkamp Verlag.

Berz, G. (1989). List of major natural disasters, 1960–1987. *Earthquakes and Volcanoes*, **20**, 226–228.

Bromet, E. J. (1998). Psychological effects of radiation catastrophes. In *Effects of Ionizing Radiation: Atomic Bomb Survivors and Their Children (1945–1995)*, eds. L. E. Peterson and S. Abrahamson, pp. 283–294. Washington, DC: Joseph Henry Press.

Couch, S. R. and Kroll-Smith J. S. (1990). Slow burn. *The Sciences*, May–June, 5–7.

Covello, V. T. (1998). Risk perception, risk communication, and EMF exposure: Tools and techniques for communicating risk information. In *Risk Perception, Risk Communication and its Application to EMF Exposure*, eds. R. Matthes, J. H. Bernhardt and M. H. Repacholi, pp. 179–213. M. H. Munich: International Commission for Non-Ionizing Radiation Protection.

Dixon, N. F. (1987). *Our Last Enemy*. London: Jonathan Cape.

Dunning, D. and Story, A. L. (1991). Depression, realism, and the overconfidence effect: Are the sadder wiser when predicting future action and events? *Journal of Personality and Social Psychology*, **61**, 521–532.

Erikson, K. T. (1976). Loss of communality at Buffalo Creek. *American Journal of Psychiatry*, **133**, 302–304.

Frederick, C. J. (1986). Psychic trauma in victims of crime and terrorism. In *Cataclysms, Crisis, and Catastrophes: Psychology in Action*, eds. G. R. Vanden Bos and B.K. Bryant, pp. 59–108. Washington, DC: American Psychological Association.

Haaga, D. A. F. and Beck, A. T. (1995). Perspectives on depressive realism: Implications for cognitive theory of depression. *Behaviour Research and Therapy*, **33**, 41–48.

Hancock, J. A., Moffoot, A. P. R. and O'Carroll, R. E. (1996). 'Depressive realism' assessed via confidence in decision-making. *Cognitive Neuropsychology*, **1**, 213–220.

Havenaar, J. M. (1996). After Chernobyl: Psychological factors affecting health after a nuclear disaster. PhD thesis, University of Utrecht.

Horowitz, M. J. (1975). Intrusive and repetitive thoughts after experimental stress. *Archives of General Psychiatry*, **32**, 1457–1463.

Hytten, K., Jensen, A. and Skauli, G. (1990). Stress inoculation training for smoke divers and free fall lifeboat passengers. *Aviation Space and Environmental Medicine*, **61**, 983–988.

Kingsmill, H. (1944). *The Poisoned Crown*. London:

Krüger, Ø. and Krüger, M. B. (1995). Pregnant women's worries and actions in a local community in response to the Chernobyl accident: A survey by general practitioners and district physicians. In *Biomedical and Psychosocial Consequences of Radiation from Man-Made Radionuclides in the Biosphere*, ed. G. Sundess, pp. 211–216. Trondheim: Tapir.

Lazarus, R. S. (1991). *Emotion and Adaption*. New York: Oxford University Press.

Luchterhand, E. G. (1971). Sociological approaches to massive stress in natural and man-made disasters. In *Psychiatric Traumatization: After Effects in Individuals and Communities*, ed. H. Krystal and W. G. Niederland, pp. 29–51. Boston: Little, Brown.

Lundin, T., Mårdberg, B. and Otto, U. (1993). Chernobyl: Nuclear threat as disaster. In *International Handbook of Traumatic Stress Syndromes*, eds. J. P. Wilson and B. Raphael, pp. 431–439. New York: Plenum Press.

Mehli, H., Skuterud, L., Mosdøl, A. and Tønnessen, A. (2000). The impact of Chernobyl fallout on the Southern Saami reindeer herders of Norway in 1996. *Health Physics*, **79**, 682–690.

Mårdberg, B., Carlstedt, L., Stalberg-Carlstedt, B. and Shalit, B. (1987). Sex differences in perception of threat from the Chernobyl accident. *Perceptual and Motor Skills*, **65**, 228.

Nilsson, Å., Reitan, J. B., Tønnessen, A. and Waldahl, R. (2000). Reporting radiation and other risk issues in Norwegian and Swedish newspapers. *Nordicom Review*, **1**, 33–49.

National Research Council (1989). *Improving Risk Communication*. Washington, DC: National Academy Press.

Nohrstedt, S. A. and Tassew, A. (1993). *Communication and Crisis: An Inventory of Current Research*. Stockholm: Swedish National Board of Psychological Defence Planning.

Organization for Economic Cooperation and Development, Nuclear Energy Agency (1996). *Chernobyl – Ten Years On Radiological and Health Impact: An Appraisal by the NEA Committee on Radiation Protection and Public Health*. Paris: Organization for Economic Cooperation and Development.

Pacini, R., Muir, F. and Epstein, S. (1998). Depressive realism from the perspective of cognitive experiential self-theory. *Journal of Personality and Social Psychology*, **74**, 1056–1068.

Renn, O. (1990). Public responses to the Chernobyl accident. *Journal of Environmental Psychology*, **10**, 151–167.

Sethi, B. B., Sharma, M., Singh, T. and Singh, H. (1987). Psychiatric morbidity of patients attending clinics in gas affected areas in Bhopal. *Indian Journal of Medical Research*, **86**, 45–50.

Shigematsu, I. (ed.) (1991). *The International Chernobyl Project: Assesment of Radiological Consequences and Evaluation of Protective Measures. Report by an International Advisory Committee*. Vienna: International Atomic Energy Agency.

Shrivastava, P. (1992). *Bhopal: Anatomy of a Crisis*, 2nd edn. London: P. Chapman.

Sjöberg, L., Jansson, B., Brenot, J., *et al.* (2000). *Radiation Risk Perception in Commemoration of Chernobyl: A Cross-National Study in Three Waves*. Stockholm: Center for Risk Research.

Slovic, P., Fischhoff, S. and Lichtenstein, B. (1979). Images of disaster: Perception and acceptance of risks from nuclear power. In *Energy Risk Assessment*, eds. G. Goodman and W. Rowe, pp. 223–245. London: Academic Press.

Tønnessen, A., Mårdberg, B. and Weisæth, L. (in press). Silent disaster: A European perspective on threat perception from Chernobyl far-field fallout. *Journal of Traumatic Stress*.

Tønnessen, A., Skuterud, L., Panova, J., *et al.* (1996). Personal use of countermeasures seen in a coping perspective: Could the development of expedient countermeasures as a repertoire in the population optimise coping and promote positive outcome expectancies when exposed to a contamination threat? *Radiation Protection Dosimetry*, **68**, 261–266.

United Nations Development Program and United Nations Children's Fund (2002). *The Human Consequences of the Chernobyl Nuclear Accident A Strategy for Recovery*. New York: United Nations Development Program and United Nations Children's Fund.

United Nations Scientific Committee on the Effects of Atomic Radiation (1988). *Sources and Effects of Ionizing Radiation*. New York: United Nations.

United Nations Scientific Committee on the Effects of Atomic Radiation (2000). *Sources and Effects of Ionizing Radiation*. New York: United Nations.

Ursano, R. J., Fullerton, C. S. and Norwood, A. E. (1995). Psychiatric dimensions of disaster: Patient care, community consultation, and preventive medicine. *Harvard Review of Psychiatry*, **3**, 196–209.

Weinstein, N. D. (1989). Optimistic biases about personal risk. *Science*, **246**, 1232–1233.

Weisaeth, L. (1984). Stress reactions to an industrial disaster. PhD thesis, University of Oslo.

Weisaeth, L. (1989). The stressors and the post-traumatic stress syndrome after an industrial disaster. *Acta Psychiatrica Scandinavica Supplementum*, **80**, 25–37.

Weisaeth, L. (1990). Reactions in Norway to fallout from the Chernobyl disaster. In *Radiation and Cancer Risk*, eds. T. Brustad, F. Langmark and J. B. Teitan, pp. 149–155. New York: Hemisphere.

Weisaeth, L. (1991). Psychosocial reactions in Norway to nuclear fallout from the Chernobyl disaster. In *Communities at Risk: Collective Responses to Technological Hazards*, eds. S. R. Couch and J. S. Kroll-Smith, pp. 53–80. New York: Peter Lang Publishing.

Weisaeth, L. (1994). Psychological and psychiatric aspects of technological disasters. In *Individual and Community Responses to Trauma and Disaster: The Structure of Human Chaos*, eds. R. J. Ursano, B. G. McCaughey and C. S. Fullerton, pp. 72–102. Cambridge: Cambridge University Press.

West, R. (1955). *A Train of Powder*. London: Macmillan.

World Health Organization (1988). *Resolution on the International Decade for Natural Disaster Reduction*. Geneva: World Health Organization.

World Health Organization (1990). *Working Group on Psychological Effects of Nuclear Accidents*. Geneva: World Health Organization.

World Health Organization (1991). *Psychosocial Guidelines for Preparedness and Intervention in Disaster*. Geneva: World Health Organization.

14

Psychological effects of contamination: Radioactivity, industrial toxins, and bioterrorism

Jacob D. Lindy, Mary C. Grace, and Bonnie L. Green

In recent years, we, in the trauma field, have given increased attention to the short- and long-term psychological effects of exposure to invisible toxic agents and pathogens in the environment, such as dioxin, radioactivity, and most recently, anthrax spores. The nuclear accident at Three Mile Island, the toxic chemical spills at Love Canal and Times Beach, the nuclear meltdown at Chernobyl, and contamination of United States mail with anthrax spores remind us that we are all potentially subject to technological and bioterrorist catastrophes. Whether by accident or design, we unfortunately are not immune from these silent and invisible pathogens which could contaminate our workplaces, our homes, and our bodies. Contamination increases risks ranging from illness and death within days to long-term pathology such as cancer, birth defects, and infertility which may not be known for years. Unlike other traumatic events which are grounded in sensory experiences, here the instigating event, the stressor, is information alone. These disasters then may hinge on what authorities say or deny. Because toxic threat cannot be seen or heard, it is tempting for authorities to deny or minimize its effects. This new type of 'disaster' is unlike its more acute, traditional predecessors, such as floods, fires, and explosions, where the physical effects on property and persons are immediate and obvious. Because of the different nature of this type of threat, it is certainly possible (indeed evidence is accumulating) that the nature of the psychological response is somewhat different from that which follows more traditional events.

The purpose of this chapter is to describe, clinically and empirically, the nature of the symptom picture that emerged following residents' receipt of information about their exposure to radioactive contamination from a nuclear weapons plant in Fernald, Ohio. We later confirmed this picture among workers at the same plant, as well as residents living near two additional contaminated nuclear plants (Rancho

Seco, California and Piketon, Ohio) The data were drawn from interviews with individuals who were active participants in a class action lawsuit, and were used for these purposes. Because the subjects were highly selected, they are not seen as necessarily representative of all individuals so exposed, particularly with regard to their extent of psychopathology. Rather, we will focus on the types of symptoms which were relatively prominent, and which of these decreased over time and which remained more chronic. Finally we shall describe some of the similarities and differences between one type of invisible disaster prominent in the mind-set of the second half of the twentieth century, information about radioactive contamination, and a more recent global threat, now part of the mind-set of the first decade of the twenty-first century, information regarding exposure to bioterrorism such as anthrax spores.

Characteristics of contamination stressors

Baum and his colleagues have written extensively about 'technological catastrophe' (Baum *et al.*, 1983a; Davidson *et al.*, 1986). Based on their work at Three Mile Island, they contrasted such events (generally what others called 'human-made' disasters) with natural disasters along several critical dimensions. Natural disasters remind us that there are certain forces over which we have no control, although some, like hurricanes, may be somewhat predictable. Technological catastrophes, on the other hand, represent a 'loss' of control of systems over which we presume to control. Further, disasters such as Three Mile Island have no clear 'low point,' i.e., a point where clearly the 'worst is over.' Exposed residents may expect that the consequences of the event will be development of disease in themselves and their children years after the exposure, providing an ongoing, chronic stressor. Confidence in future controllability of technology is also likely to be eroded (Baum *et al.*, 1983a).

Bromet (1989) separates (catastrophic and dramatic) technological events (with chronic origins) like Three Mile Island, Chernobyl, and Bhopal from 'human-made' events which are truly acute like train crashes. She also distinguishes dramatic toxic disasters from those that unfold more slowly and less dramatically, and in which residents may not be aware of their exposure until the process has been going on for quite some time. Bertazzi (1980) referred to this latter type of industrial disaster as a 'diluted disaster' which becomes apparent only because human targets happen to be in the way of toxic releases, or because, over time, environmental evidence crops up that something is wrong.

A further characteristic of these slowly unfolding technological disasters is that fears may be elevated by agencies that seem to be unresponsive or concealing facts, so that people come to believe that there is a hidden, but serious, threat (Hallman and

Wandersman, in press). Also, the announcement of the discovery of the contamination is frequently the first awareness residents have that a disaster has occurred (Edelstein and Wandersman, 1987).

Bertazzi (1989) suggested that all industrial accidents (including more 'overt' events) have the following characteristics:

1. Uncertainty (fear of unknown health damage along with a strong feeling of lack of protection).
2. Insecurity about housing and jobs (e.g., fear of contamination of homes).
3. Social rejection (discrimination based on perceived contamination).
4. Media siege.
5. Cultural pressure (public pressures on how to behave, political issues such as whether exposed women should have abortions, etc.).

Since 1994, a number of studies of psychological consequences of toxic contamination have occurred. These include spilled natural products such as refined oil (Arata *et al.*, 2000), metals and metalic compounds such as molybdenum (Momcilovic, 2000), asbestos (Barak *et al.*, 1998), chemical products such as sulfuric acid (Cone, 1996), catacarb (Bowler *et al.*, 1998), gases such as carbon monoxide (Dhara, 1994), sarin (Yokoyama, 1998), and mustard gas (Schnurr, 2000), byproducts of nuclear reactions, accidents, and waste (Quastel, 1997; Viel, 1997; Korol, 1999; Kronic, 2000), and mixed exposure to a range of toxic agents within a theatre of war including pesticides, dioxin, burning oil wells, and possible agents of biological warfare (Procter, 1998; Enserink, 2001). Within these populations studied there are those with documented exposure, and those with potential exposure. Among the samples are adults and children, men, and women in locations worldwide, with a variety of demographic and cultural variables. At the time of possible exposure some were in a military environment preparing for or carrying out military action, others were civilians totally unprepared for these invisible dangers. The exposed populations learned, sooner or later, of a variety of possible health consequences. Some agents were immediately lethal; others caused cancer or damaged the body's capacity to fight illness as well as to reproduce. Some would likely affect a single organ system; some might have any number of health consequences.

Most of these toxic agents are invisible, and lack any reliable sensory warning of danger. In all these situations, the individual's assessment of danger is a function of information and the assessment of the accuracy of that information.

Psychological responses to contamination stressors

What kind of psychological effects accompany this unique type of stressor? Bromet (1989) described four sets of studies that were conducted by a variety of research groups following the Three Mile Island radiation leak. Homogeneous samples were studied as well as specific groups, such as workers at the plant, mothers of small children, psychiatric patients, and children. The mothers, perhaps most attuned to health risks to their children and most aware of potential damage to reproductivity, seemed to be the most affected group of all, showing higher levels of depression, anxiety, hostility, and somatization than controls. When the reactor was restarted, this group showed distress scores elevated over all previous levels (Dew *et al.*, 1987). Neither workers nor children showed elevated symptom rates. Bromet concluded that:

> 1) Contrary to early findings of the President's commission, long-term studies *have* revealed persistent elevations in psychological distress, but 2) the levels are by and large at the high end of the normal range and functioning... appears not to have been impaired... (Bromet, 1989, p. 130)

Baum and his colleagues (Baum *et al.*, 1983c; Davidson *et al.*, 1986) followed Three Mile Island residents over time. While their work was summarized by Bromet (1989), it will be discussed separately because it provides specific information regarding symptoms and their course. These studies showed that at about $1\frac{1}{2}$ years post accident, subjects had elevated scores on the following SCL-90 scales relative to controls: anxiety, alienation, and somatic distress (Baum *et al.*, 1983c). The highest scores for the Three Mile Island subjects were in the areas of somatization and obsessive–compulsive thoughts (labeled 'concentration' by the study group), which covers repeated unpleasant thoughts that won't leave your mind, trouble concentrating, etc.

By 5 years post event (Davidson *et al.*, 1986), most of these scores actually increased, with obsessive thoughts remaining high relative to other scales, but with hostility and suspiciousness showing particularly dramatic increases (scores were among the highest). Long-term effects were also evident in a task of concentration (proofreading) and in physiological measures. Also, Three Mile Island residents showed higher levels of norepinephrine and cortisol than controls.

This group also studied residents within a 1-mile radius of a toxic waste landfill in a mid-Atlantic state about a year after the announcement that the site was among 10 of the most potentially hazardous in the country (Davidson *et al.*, 1986). Subjects in this group had depression, anxiety, fear, and suspiciousness symptom levels elevated over those of the Three Mile Island residents at 5 years. They also were more distressed than nonexposed controls. Both the Three Mile Island and the toxic landfill groups showed elevated scores on the impact-of-event scale, particularly on intrusive symptoms (e.g., 'I thought about it when I didn't mean to'; 'I had dreams about it'). Intrusive symptoms were more prominent than avoidance symptoms (e.g., 'I tried to remove it from memory'; 'I stayed away from reminders of it') in these samples.

A study of residents exposed to dioxin and floods at Times Beach, Missouri, focused primarily on diagnosis (Smith *et al.*, 1986). This study found poorer psychological health in residents exposed directly to the disasters than in indirectly or nonexposed samples. Furthermore, flood and dioxin exposure together caused more problems than either disaster alone. The most common diagnostically related symptoms for the residents directly exposed to dioxin were somatization and depression. With regard to 'new' (since disaster) symptoms, somatization and depression far surpassed other types of symptoms in terms of their frequency.

Asukai and Maekawa (2002) describe an eerie scene when deadly sarin gas was released in five Tokyo subway cars in 1995. Eleven people were killed and 5500 people were affected. They quote a firefighter on the scene: 'Something had happened but people remained silent around the site; I have never experienced such a scene; just victims' coughing heard in the perplexing silence.' Twenty percent of the hospitalized survivors whom they followed at 1 month reported intrusive and avoidant symptoms at the posttraumatic stress disorder (PTSD) level. They also describe long-term psychological effects regarding apprehension about health (including genetic risk to children) and lingering symptoms of intrusion and avoidance. Lifton (1999) described the mind-set of the apocalyptic terrorists involved in the sarin gas release, foreshadowing the terrorist attacks on the United States in 2001.

Coping with radioactive contamination

In terms of individuals' attempts to 'cope' with this type of event, Baum, Fleming, and Singer (Baum *et al.*, 1983b) examined the types of coping styles that were used by residents of Three Mile Island. High use of emotion focused coping was associated with significantly lower levels of stress (distress), while problem focused coping was associated with higher levels of distress. The authors hypothesized that these paradoxical relationships held because there was little that individuals could do to alter the situation. Thus, regulation of one's emotional response might be a realistic way of exerting some control in a basically uncontrollable situation. Further, self-blame was associated with less stress, and it was also associated with the subject's perception of control over things that happened to them.

The Fernald disaster

The revelations about possible contamination following exposure to radioactive leaks into the air and groundwater at the Fernald, Ohio Feed Materials Production Center followed the pattern noted by several investigators cited above. Although some information was released earlier, in October of 1984, the media focused on information that the facility was negligent in the disposal and storage of toxic waste. Many residents learned about the danger from the plant for the first time at

Table 14.1 Contamination
stressors at Fernald

Lack of warning
Diffuseness of impact
Information as stressor
Chronicity of threat
Economic features
Stigma

this point. During congressional hearings in 1985, the Environmental Protection
Agency reported that Feed Materials Production Center was the worst emitter of
radioactive materials in the nation (Carpenter, 1986). It was later learned that the
government intentionally withheld information about contamination for decades.
These revelations were shocking to many residents who had lived in the area for
years, or had moved there to build their dream homes because they liked the pastoral
nature of the area: hills, trees, cows grazing. Most were not even aware that the Feed
Materials Production Center, with the red-and-white checkered towers, processed
nuclear feed, rather than animal feed, so the information was doubly distressing.
Information about the extent of radioactive leakage from this nuclear weapons
production facility was released gradually, often preceded by denials, disclaimers,
or minimization about the extent of exposure. In 1987, residents and landowners
living within a 5-mile radius of the plant were named as plaintiffs in a class action
against the company that managed the plant. The authors served as expert witnesses
in the portion of the case that related to claims of 'emotional distress' and examined
a small subset of the class. The data reported upon in this chapter were collected in
November of 1987.

As we listened to the residents we were evaluating, we were struck by differences
between these invisible stressor experiences and those of survivors we had previously
studied from visible traumatic events, a slag dam collapse, a supper club fire, and
the Vietnam War (Table 14.1). More recently we observe a parallel set of differences
in stressors among reactions to invisible versus visible forms of terror: on the one
hand reactions of those exposed to anthrax and on the other, of those exposed to
the September 11 World Trade Center destruction and attack on the Pentagon.

Characteristics of the stressor event

Lack of warning

For those near Fernald, there was no warning of the increased hazard. Indeed, only
retrospectively were residents aware of previously released radioactivity, or that their

water well contained dangerous radioactive elements. By and large, there was no odor, sight, or sound which could alert them to hazard. Faced with this situation, the residents became sensitized to those warning systems, accurate or inaccurate, upon which they had to rely: increased dust; the sound of a siren, presumably from the plant at Fernald; an unusual metallic odor; increasingly sophisticated monitoring devices.

Information as stressor

Unlike the vivid picture of overwhelming and multisensory experiences of a tornado, earthquake, or flood, the Fernald disaster took place against a quiet, seemingly normal backdrop. Only a news report or information from a neighbor identified this situation as a disaster, and the resident as one who had been exposed to it. Information, *per se*, was the initial stressor. Additional information served as secondary stressors. The residents felt that they had to rely on the authoritative sources of information yet at the same time they feared and distrusted them. The resident was understandably concerned, lest the information be inaccurate out of self-interest.

Diffuseness of impact

The danger of this type of radioactive contamination is chronic and diffuse, that is, it has already been active, continues to be active, and for the foreseeable future continues to present danger. Residents were being exposed long before they were aware of this. The continued storage of radioactive material and likelihood if its seepage into surrounding land and water created a situation where the exposure might well continue into the future.

Chronicity of threat

As noted by Baum *et al.* (1983a), nuclear disasters have no 'low point' where the worst is over; future threat is ongoing. Increased exposure to radioactive materials increases the likelihood of the development, many years later, of a variety of illnesses, including cancers and leukemia, decreases the effectiveness of the immunologic system, and increases the likelihood of radioactive exposure to genes, affecting rates of miscarriages, birth anomalies, and fertility. The medical consequences are described as probabilities, not certainties, and society places the burden of uncertainty on the inhabitant.

Lifton (1967) described this uncertainty in the 'hibakusha' (survivors of the atomic bomb in Hiroshima) he interviewed many years after their exposure. While the severity of exposure clearly differs between the two incidents, the quality of the feeling is similar: 'survivors feel themselves involved in an endless chain of potentially lethal impairment, which, if it does not manifest itself in one year – or in one generation – may well make itself felt in the next' (Lifton, 1967, p. 130).

Fernald residents had to cope with the ongoing fear of a contaminated habitat. Some residents reported being careful not to use water from the tap for drinking. Some were cautious about the amount of time they spent outside exposed to the air. They worried about dangers to children and grandchildren, and about the longevity of their ancestral line.

Aspects of cognitive processing

Impaired problem-solving

Once aware of the problem, some residents formed groups, gained representation, and sought out expert advice. But usual problem-solving skills were frustrated as more information simply made worries greater while introducing disagreement by experts and confusion regarding course of action.

Aspects of the recovery environment

Economic features

The loss in market value of the residents' property is an understandable consequence of the above dangers, and becomes a secondary stressor. The inability to receive a fair price for their homes meant, practically speaking, that many residents felt 'trapped' in this potentially contaminated place.

Fears of radioactive contamination of the crops which grew on residents' properties created a secondary level of problems. Danger existed for those who relied on the sale of small crops to supplement their income. The crops identified as coming from the Fernald region might not be bought. At the same time, if the crops were successfully raised and sold, the resident was left with a gnawing sense of guilt at having potentially exposed others.

Stigma

As noted by Bertazzi (1989), contemporary society is frightened of and, to some extent, unkind towards innocent victims of radioactive contamination. Because we fear the unknown, we tend to stigmatize those who have been contaminated. Again, referring the 'hibakusha' of Hiroshima, Lifton (1967) argued that outsiders, when observing those who were exposed to contamination, saw the survivors as tainted with death. This perception caused them to experience a threat to their own sense of continuity and immortality, and to 'feel death anxiety and death guilt activated within themselves' (Lifton, 1967, p. 170). In defending against this guilt and anxiety, others may turn upon the exposed residents in an attempt to distance themselves from the threat. For example, residents at Fernald reported, with distress, jokes about their 'glowing in the dark.'

The Fernald study

In light of the special characteristics of these stressors and on the basis of exploratory interviews with six Fernald residents, review of the depositions of the nine representatives of the class action, and notes on past interviews with residents at Three Mile Island (about 12), we hypothesized a spectrum of symptomatology which would be similar to, yet distinguishable from, PTSD that would manifest itself in the quantitative measures. Like PTSD, the syndrome we would expect following possible radioactive contamination at Fernald would be set in motion by events which are outside of the range of normal, or expectable, human experience. The pathology would likely arise due to failure of successfully processing the intrusive cognitive problems that were presented by the stressor. Unlike PTSD, however, the stressor in this case was ongoing, future oriented, somatically based, and not confined to a single past event that could be processed by the senses.

Based on the characteristics of the stressor and research by other investigators, we expected several types of responses including obsessive/intrusive thinking related to worries about future illnesses along with attempts to avoid such thoughts. Because of the type of perceived risk, we expected somatic concerns to be high relative to other symptoms, although general anxiety symptoms were expected to be prominent as well. Finally, the way in which residents were informed about the leaks (i.e., the attempts to hide exposure, etc.) was expected to produce symptoms of suspiciousness/mistrust. We were interested in whether a unique cluster of symptoms defining a specific syndrome would emerge from the clinical observations and the research instruments.

Method

Participants

The 57 plaintiffs who had previously filled out questionnaires and interrogatories were identified by their lawyers as the respondent pool for first wave of interviewing. Not all of these 57 people were seeking restitution for 'emotional' distress. Their names, addresses, and phone numbers were provided to the Traumatic Stress Study Center at the University of Cincinnati for the purpose of scheduling interviews. Preceding phone calls by interviewers was a letter that was sent by the law firm to each of the 57 plaintiffs informing them of the involvement of the Traumatic Stress Study Center and explaining the interview that was being requested. Residents were encouraged, but not required, to participate. Each of the six interviewers were given the names of six to eight residents to interview. Interviews were usually conducted in the resident's home and averaged approximately $1\frac{1}{2}$ hours in length.

Interviews and instruments

Four advanced clinical psychology students, the research coordinator for the Traumatic Stress Study Center, and an experienced survey research interviewer served as interviewers for this project; four were female, two were male. All but one had worked on previous research studies at the Center doing field interviews of a similar sort to the one employed in this investigation. Extensive training in the administration of the interview protocol was completed before the interviewers entered the field. We used the psychiatric evaluation form (PEF) (Endicott and Spitzer, 1972), impact-of-event scale (IES) (Horowitz *et al.*, 1979), symptom checklist-90R (SCL-90R) (Derogatis, 1983), and the coping strategies inventory (CSI) (Tobin *et al.*, 1989). See Figs 14.1 and 14.2 for results.

Information about the subjects' stressor experiences was collected via a structured interview format. For complete methodology see Green *et al.* (1994, pp. 154–176).

Results

Fifty residents of Fernald were interviewed. Of the 50 cases, the average age of subjects was 46.78 (range 29–69). Men represented 58 percent of the sample; while women represented 45 percent. Ninety percent of the residents were married; they had an average of 2.5 children. With regard to education, 74 percent had completed high school. All but five residents owned their own homes and had lived in them for an average of 9.8 years. Occupationally, the majority of subjects, if they worked, were either blue-collar workers or in business, and most were working full time. The average family income was $39 000.

Specific stressors

The subjects lived an average of 1.6 miles from the plant, and approximately two-thirds of the sample lived within a 1-mile radius. Slightly over a quarter of the sample reported some illness. About half reported the illness of an acquaintance or family member that they thought could be related to the contamination. No one thought that they had cancer caused by the plant, but 35 percent thought that other friends, relatives, and acquaintances had contamination-related cancer.

Contents of worries and dreams

In order to assess the content of mental phenomena, we asked the residents during their interview to address their specific concerns, i.e., what did they worry, ruminate, or dream about that was related to the plant. Of the 40 subjects with completed data on these items, most subjects (95 percent) named a worry of some type. The most common of these (overlapping) concerns were fear of illness in self (45 percent) or

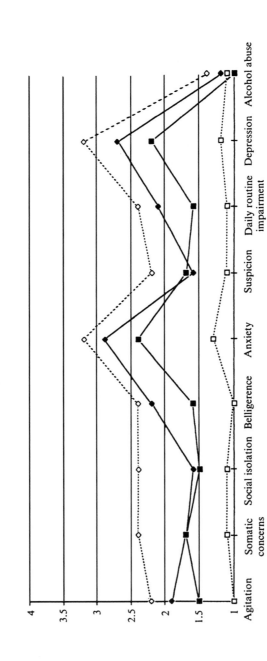

Figure 14.1 Average clinical ratings on selected scales of the PEF for Fernald residents and comparison samples.

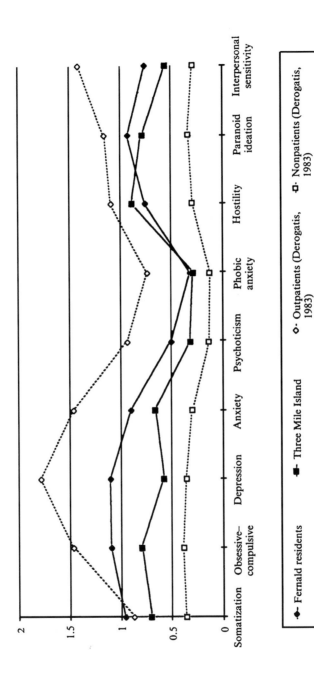

Figure 14.2 Average current self-report symptoms on the SCL-90R for Fernald residents and comparison samples.

family (48 percent), and fears about contamination (43 percent). Many residents also worried about housing or property devaluation (30 percent). Less often, residents mentioned distrust of authorities and concerns regarding fertility, ineffective warning systems, and safety of their children.

Regarding dreams, 43 percent of the sample reported a frightening dream of some sort. These dreams usually involved being endangered in some way and/or being chased or trapped, or a family member being in danger. Examples include: 'alarm at the plant going off,' 'dream about dying,' 'the plant blowing up,' 'locked in a vault with rising water,' 'tragedy in the family,' 'wife dying,' and 'baby dying.'

Case reports

The following are two case vignettes. They are residents who were seen by one of us (JDL) during the course of evaluating the plaintiffs for the lawsuit. The presentations and concerns are characteristic of the individuals we interviewed.

Mrs K

Mrs K was a 35-year-old married mother of two daughters, aged 9 and 6. She and her husband, both college-educated, built their dream house in rural Ohio, within commuting distance of Mr K's executive position in a Cincinnati firm. Mrs K told a friend they were moving to a location that was not far from the 'Ralston grain plant,' referring to the checkered tower of the 'feed' processing plant. Three years prior to being seen, she and her husband had learned through the news media that the plant at Fernald processed radioactive material, not grain; that venting of radioactive materials was occurring; and that radioactive waste which had been generated as far back as the Manhattan project in the 1940s, was inadequately stored and seeping into the community water system.

Mrs K became an active citizen participant with other neighbors in speaking with, and engaging, scientific experts on the extent of the danger. She and her immediate family underwent total body radiation counts. She unsuccessfully sought adequate monitors. The couple invested in an extensive purifying system. They explored selling their house, but learned they would have to inform the buyer of the risks from Fernald. Selling the house under these circumstances would have been a catastrophic financial loss.

During this period she became anxious, irritable, and preoccupied with fears of the possibility of her children developing leukemia. To a lesser extent, she also worried about her husband and herself. Each ache, pain, and fever stirred intense worry which she told herself was irrational, but which she could not contain. Sleep was restless and dreams were ominous but indistinct. She began to repeat tasks, double check the stove, and overprotect her children. Hearing from the school nurse that her child was ill set off a panic attack, and she had an auto accident on the way to pick her up. The 6-year-old daughter began sleeping in the parents' bed after her unsettling experience in the body radiation chamber. Although test results were not abnormal, anxiety worsened after the testing procedure. Abruptly, Mr K ordered Mrs K and the rest of the family not to seek further information about the plant, because each time they learned something new, everyone got worse. They were not to speak of the Fernald danger any more in the home. She noticed after this that tension grew between the two of them. Further, taking the worries of Fernald on by himself, her husband performed worse at work and for the first time was passed over for a promotion. Mrs K was now giving up the idea of having more children because of the risk of genetic danger to an unborn child. She felt desperately trapped in the four walls of her dream house; dreading the present and fearful of the future.

Mr J

Mr J was a 65-year-old retired assistant manager at the local dry goods store. Mr and Mrs J lived on 3 acres near Fernald as had their families for generations. Only their children had moved to the city. Mr J had developed congestive heart failure about 8 years earlier. Along with bronchitis, high blood pressure, and rare episodes of alcohol abuse, he was not a picture of perfect health. But, while these ailments made life annoying, he did enjoy his large vegetable garden which supplemented his income, the company of his wife, and visits from their grandchildren.

Mr J grasped only the rudiments of the scientists' explanations regarding radioactive contamination from Fernald. He learned of it directly from the neighbor whose water well was contaminated. He thought this must explain those albino animals, and the poor crops. He remembered when the Fernald plant opened, and never gave a second thought to its safety.

He cried easily as he explained this breach in trust with the Government. While not having served in combat, Mr J was a veteran and deeply patriotic in his views. His wife articulated even better how betrayed he felt. Joy seemed gone from Mr J's life. He no longer knew where he would sell his crops; and worried that the persons who bought them might be contaminated. Neither he nor his wife thought that the grandchildren should visit, fearing contamination, and indeed they had stopped coming. Unbidden thoughts, restless sleep, depression, and alienation characterized his psychic life. Each spot on the skin got inspected nightly for cancerous growth. Each morning as water from the shower struck his skin, he thought about radioactive particles. Each time he drank a glass of water the same thoughts intruded. Mr J could not remove obsessive thinking of the effects of Fernald from his mind.

Discussion

Being informed that one lives in an area contaminated by radiation is a unique type of stressor experience. Radiation cannot be seen, felt, tasted, or smelled. There is no agreement among experts about what the effects of such exposure are, and authorities often have their own interests in mind when providing information about such effects. By the time one finds out about the exposure, it has already taken place (although it may continue), and it is never quite clear whether or not one was harmed. Fears arising from such exposure may be labeled unreasonable (blaming the person exposed), while at the same time the person may be stigmatized by acquaintances.

From a psychological perspective, any one of these elements is likely to lead to uneasiness or preoccupation at best, because of the vagueness, all-pervasiveness, and chronicity of the threat. (Erikson, 1990) captured the essence of the potential response to this intangible stressor when he distinguished the 'dread' associated with toxic contamination from the fear of natural disasters. The comments of residents he interviewed, living near a toxic dump, were remarkably similar to those at Fernald.

Research designed to assess the psychological effects of contamination is increasing. With few exceptions, however, it has tended to focus on the extent of impairment rather than the particular constellation of symptoms that make up the psychological reaction to this type of event. However, there are data available, particularly from the work of Baum and colleagues on Three Mile Island (Baum *et al.*, 1983a, b, c), that addresses this question. In general, the findings from the present report coincide well with findings from Three Mile Island even though the two events were dissimilar in several ways, including the acuteness of the onset an the length of exposure.

Limitations of study

As noted earlier, the conclusions that can be drawn from our empirical findings are limited in several ways. First, the subjects participated as part of the process of a lawsuit and there is no reason to believe that the individuals who agreed to make themselves available from the designated class for the study were necessarily typical of class members in general. Second, we did not have a control group for this particular study. Thus, the findings presented do not attempt to draw conclusions about the extent of impairment. Rather, we have focused on the constellation of symptoms and the interaction of symptoms and stressors in the particular individuals we did see to suggest hypotheses about the nature of the impact of this particular type of event. Further, subjects provided retrospective data on their psychological condition which is another reason that it needs to be viewed with caution. For all of these reasons, findings which coincided with other studies were given most credence and all of the findings are clearly tentative until replicated on more extensive and general samples. We wish mainly to stimulate thinking about the nature of the reactions to this chronic and vague stressor.

Symptom constellation and duration

Generally speaking, the overall profile of the Fernald group, and the Three Mile Island group as well, were not unlike profiles of outpatients (although not as elevated), with relatively (compared to other types of symptoms) high levels of the general symptoms of anxiety, depression, and impairment of daily routine. However, individuals with radioactive exposure are also high (relative to their own scores on other measures, and to 'normals') on somatic symptoms and concerns, obsessive thoughts, and suspicion and mistrust of others. It is this latter group of symptoms that may distinguish the reaction to toxic exposure, particularly 'human-caused' exposure. As noted earlier, subjects worry about what physical harm may have been done to them, that they can't seem to get thoughts and worries about the exposure out of their minds, are not trusting of others (neighbors/authorities), and feel alienated from the rest of the world. These symptoms make sense given the diffuse and vague nature of the stressor and the chronic, unknown, and future threat. Similar symptom pictures emerged in the three additional populations we studied between 1989 and 1994: former workers at the Fernald plant, residents at Piketon, Ohio, and residents at Rancho Seco, California. Somatic concerns, obsessive thinking, anxiety, and depression were characteristic of all. Suspicion and mistrust of others applied to the additional groups as well, although this was less marked in the Rancho Seco group, perhaps because this facility was governed locally and not part of a sequestered, secret, federal nuclear arms program.

Further, there is evidence from Three Mile Island and our Fernald subjects that these latter symptoms are ongoing over relatively long periods of time. Davidson *et al.* (1986) showed continued high levels of obsessive thoughts in their Three Mile Island subjects between $1\frac{1}{2}$ years and 5 years, with hostility (including feelings of fear of losing control) and suspiciousness becoming especially pronounced. In the Fernald sample, anxiety, depression, and impairment of their daily routine improved (decreased) for most subjects between their 'worst' time (in terms of knowledge/revelations about the plant and their symptoms) and the time they were evaluated for the present study. However, similar to the Three Mile Island findings, there were no changes in the areas of somatic concerns, social isolation, and suspicion. These areas remained elevated. While neither study was a rigorous longitudinal one, the findings are strikingly similar and clearly suggest that at least some individuals exposed to nuclear radiation continue to be obsessively worried about their health and the future, and are suspicious and untrusting of others. Davidson *et al.* (1986) noted continued effects on physiology and cognitive capabilities over this period as well. Once more, we found these symptoms lasting many years in our studies of Fernald workers, and Piketon and Rancho Seco residents as well.

Fernald residents' attempts to cope with this particular threat were primarily trying to avoid it and to wish it away. Avoidance of thoughts of the events surrounding the plant were particularly high, as expressed on both the impact-of-event scale and the coping inventory. This coping activity fit well, both as a response to the high level of intrusion/obsessive thoughts and in terms of the actual situation. No active coping strategy can undo the threat; therefore, not thinking about it may make the most sense. Residents also used other disengagement strategies; social withdrawal (also noted in the other measures) and wishful thinking (e.g., 'I hoped a miracle would happen,' 'I wished that the situation would go away or somehow be over with'). These coping strategies are not usually associated with healthy functioning. We found this spectrum of coping styles repeated with residents at Piketon and Rancho Seco.

Relation of Fernald study to exposure to bioterrorism

In the recent concern worldwide regarding focal exposure to bioterrorism in the form of anthrax spores, we find preliminary support for the relevance of many of the clinical principles which we have observed in unaware citizens who were informed that they have been exposed to radioactive contamination.

Characteristics of the stressor event

As in toxic contamination stress, the stressor is information. While one may observe a white powder, it is the scientific examination of this substance by experts which provides the data that one has or has not been exposed to lethal anthrax spores. Since it is information which is so central, efforts to hide or deny betray trust and exacerbate symptoms. As in radiation exposure, the risks are potentially lethal, although in this case immediate rather than long term. Unlike radiation exposure there is known treatment for the exposure which is capable of preventing both immediate and long-term sequelae. As in toxic contamination stress, the source of danger is created by humans rather than naturally occurring events. Here, however, the willful destruction of innocent lives by terrorists carries an even more heinous quality than flaws, sometimes intentionally hidden, in the handling of highly dangerous industrial and military materials.

Symptoms

While it is too early to generalize about psychological symptoms, and our data come from selected interviews with survivors and mental health professionals who have been working with survivors rather than systematic data, it does appear that irritability, somatic preoccupation, mistrust, hypervigilance, indecisiveness, and worries which tend to be excessive are central. Where authorities have acted quickly, decisively, and accurately, those exposed tend to cope better. Where authorities contradict themselves, change course, especially suspecting danger where they earlier promised none, and expected people to perform duties in areas which they later said were dangerous, psychological stress is greater.

Coping strategies

Because treatment options do exist for anthrax exposure, problem-solving techniques are more useful than other coping strategies like denial or spirituality. But where authorities avoid or deny danger and access to preventive intervention is denied, a similar kind of hopeless dread develops which can overwhelm usual coping strategies.

Dreams

As in exposure to radioactive contamination, dreams do not take on the physical and sensory traumatic detail of the event of exposure so much as being characterized by a tone of dread, a poisoned atmosphere, or ominous danger.

Recovery environment

To date those exposed to anthrax do not report the isolation that those exposed to radioactive contamination feel. This aspect of the condition could change if there were more lethal cases. It is interesting to note, however, that while the call for and the response by mental health outreach has been vigorous at the sites of violent terrorist destruction, they have been less vigorous in the case of those possibly exposed to anthrax. Stigma and alienation is a latent danger in those who are informed they may have been exposed to anthrax.

Case report 3

Mr HD is a 36-year-old married government employee who was alarmed to learn that one of his coworkers, while working at a location which he often frequented, was exposed to contaminated mail there and tested positive for anthrax. He had at first dismissed the idea of danger because authorities whom he trusted told him he was at no risk. Now, after his coworker tested positive, the same authority reversed his position, explaining that his workplace had been contaminated and he was not allowed in. He was frightened watching the workers in decontamination suits maximally protected in the same work area in which he had had no protection. Irritability first took the form of feeling inconvenienced and preoccupied that his favorite family pictures, an old pipe, and some important papers were impounded there. He was informed he should take cipro for 60 days, but worried about side effects, and about women colleagues who had to choose between cipro and the safety of their pregnancy. Later he became aware of feeling intensely angry, betrayed, and frightened. He became hyperattentive to any kind of danger, noted fluctuations in his energy level, and was preoccupied when he cleared his throat (fearing a cough was coming on.) He worried lest his clothes might have become contaminated and that he had inadvertently brought anthrax spores home to his family. Both he and members of his family had dreams of being poisoned, endangered, or captured. He noted that he and others seemed to be more irritable, and that they coped with that irritability by taking on more responsibility and working harder. This was especially so because he took his work as a public servant quite seriously, while recognizing that the very nature of his work made him the target of terrorist attacks. He believed that others, not similarly affected, did not understand the severity of his distress. At times he had an image of himself dying from anthrax.

He was aware that counseling had been made available to friends who worked near the terrorist plane crashes and destruction of September 11, while none appeared for him or his coworkers nor did he, on his own, seek any. He worried intensely, was anxious, depressed, irritable, suspicious, and somatically preoccupied.

Toxic contamination stress

From a clinical perspective, we would like to propose that the various toxic stress reactions described in this chapter be considered as a specific subtype of PTSD, and to note briefly its similarities and differences both from other diagnoses and from traditional PTSD, along with its hypothesized dynamics and associated features. This proposal represents an hypothesis based on our beginning clinical work, and on our own and others research findings to date. More research is clearly needed.

Toxic contamination stress (TCS) is similar enough to PTSD to be considered within its rubric. Like PTSD, toxic contamination stress is set in motion by events which are outside the range of normal, expectable human experience. Like PTSD, pathology arises in the failure to be able to process successfully the intrusive cognitive problems which the stressor presents and which would be stressful to most persons. The stressor, in this case, however, is ongoing and future oriented. It is not confined to physical events themselves which can be processed by the senses and, therefore, the pathology is less likely to include traumatic nightmares and re-enactments.

Like adjustment reactions of adulthood, which may follow common stressful life experiences like divorce, job loss, etc., TCS may occur to anyone, regardless of predisposition, and, like these reactions, often contains features of depression and anxiety. But, unlike the adjustment reaction, this syndrome is not necessarily self-limited; it is not healed by a shift in philosophical perspective. It mimics, in ways that adjustment reactions do not, the features of an obsessive–compulsive disorder in which the intrusive thoughts that are an important feature of PTSD recur in unbidden form.

Like PTSD there is a cycling of mental activity. As persons are informed of radioactive contamination of their living space or workspace, a set of unsatisfactory cycles of mental activity, involving intrusion and denial, begins to occur. The subject, at one phase, struggles with the temptation to worry. His first line of defense is to cut the worry off before it begins. He seeks to sequester the problems so that they will not interfere with daily function. Once information has spread regarding harmful effects of toxic exposure, for those, for example, who live in the backyard of a nuclear waste dump, denial has already been pierced by actual findings of increased thorium, uranium, etc. and can no longer be totally effective. Efforts expended in turning away decrease the energy available for pleasurable activity, and are accompanied by a low-grade agitation and depression. The presence of any new health-related symptom, any unusual odor or metallic taste, a piece of information from a community meeting or a newspaper article, all act to catalyze worry.

In another phase of the syndrome, an action-oriented phase, residents or workers acknowledge the hazards and decide that they must cope. They inform themselves of the nature of the contamination so far reported, and the consequences. They attempt to clear their homes and workplaces of the noxious agent and inform themselves about ways to monitor future and ongoing danger. But how can they truly clear their habitat from contamination? And where can they go to feel safe? The normally successful coping method of confronting difficulties actually increases intrusive symptoms, and as these coping strategies become less effective, residents may become more anxious, depressed, and hopeless. Residents and workers may also become angry and frustrated, particularly with public officials and spokespersons for the site of the contamination. They may become alienated from their neighbors who are attempting to deny or minimize the problems.

Similarities and differences with bioterrorist contamination

While falling within the broader classification of PTSD, toxic contamination stress encompasses many types of toxic contaminants in addition to radioactivity, such as toxic chemicals, particulate matter, and toxic gases, as well as agents of bioterrorism (anthrax spores). Unique characteristics of different toxic events affect the population at risk, the health consequences to those exposed, the clarity of information about criteria for exposure, the ability to create safety, and the presence or absence of definitive medical treatment for the exposure. Further each toxic agent in a given context will be more or less comprehensible within the world view of those affected (for example, industrial neglect versus acts of terrorism or war), and the resulting recovery environment may vary from positive to alienating and stigmatizing.

While being exposed to radioactive contamination and to bioterrorist anthrax spores have much in common (e.g., information as stressor, difficulties processing new invisible dangers, somatic, and obsessive and paranoid features, as well as anxiety and depression), they also have differences of note: anthrax infection may cause death within days while radioactivity causes long-term risk to health. Anthrax exposure is amenable to definitive medical prevention while health effects of radioactivity can only be monitored medical risks without definitive prevention.

Implications for intervention

Treatment implications for residents near contaminated nuclear facilities and for those exposed to anthrax spores who show the spectrum of symptoms outlined above are not yet clear. Psychotherapy can neither remove the source of contamination nor the potential effect of contamination already experienced. The subject's primary concern is to find a safe place to work and live. Re-establishing trust on the basis of reliable and responsible communication from authorities is an essential first step. As in other ongoing traumatic situations, like spouse abuse, or rape threat when the offender is at large, the first task is to remove or contain the noxious agent. Thus, it may be that social, legal, or military action may be necessary to reduce ongoing threat, and where possible, relocation to a safe environment may be the most reasonable first effort to prevent further damage. A supportive treatment relationship by mental health professionals may reduce unnecessary distress. Clinicians need to learn more about this syndrome as, sadly, our technological society will likely have much more of it in coming years.

Acknowledgment

The authors wish to acknowledge the contributions of Dr Ellen Gerrity, of the National Institute of Mental Health, currently working on a detail on Capitol Hill on mental health legislation.

REFERENCES

Arata, C. M., Picou, J. S., Johnson, G. D., *et al.* (2000). Coping with technological disaster: An application of the conservation of resources model to the Exxon Valdez oil spill. *Journal of Traumatic Stress*, **13**, 23–39.

Asukai, N. and Maekawa, K. (2002). Psychological and physical health effects of the 1995 Sarin attack in the Tokyo subway station. In *Toxic Turmoil: Psychological and Societal Consequences of Ecological Disasters*, eds. J. Havenaar, J. Cwikel and E. Bromet, pp. New York: Plenum Press.

Barak, Y., Achiron, A., Rotstein, Z., *et al.* (1998). Stress associated with asbestos: The trauma of waiting for death. *Psycho-Oncology*, **7**, 126–128.

Baum, A., Fleming, R. and Davidson, L. M. (1983a). Natural disaster and technological catastrophe. *Environment and Behavior*, **15**, 333–354.

Baum, A., Fleming, R. and Singer, J. E. (1983b). Coping with victimization by technological disaster. *Journal of Social Issues*, **39**, 117–138.

Baum, A., Gatchel, R. and Schaeffer, M. A. (1983c). Emotional, behavioral, and physiological effects of chronic stress at Three Mile Island. *Journal of Consulting and Clinical Psychology*, **15**, 565–572.

Bertazzi, P. (1989). Industrial disasters and epidemiology. *Scandinavian Journal of Work Environmental Health*, **15**, 85–100.

Bowler, R. M., Hartney, C. and Ngo, L. H. (1998). Amnestic disturbance and posttraumatic stress disorder in the aftermath of a chemical release. *Archives of Clinical Neuropsychology*, **13**, 455–471.

Bromet, E. (1989). The nature and effects of technological failures. In *Psychosocial Aspects of Disaster*, eds. R. Gist and B. Lubin, pp. New York: Wiley Press.

Carpenter, T. (1986). *Fernald Fact Sheet Summary*. Washington, DC: Government Accountability Project.

Davidson, L., Fleming, I. and Baum, A. (1986). Post-traumatic stress as a function of chronic stress and toxic exposure. In *Trauma and Its Wake*, vol. 2, ed. C. Figley, pp. New York: Brunner/Mazel.

Derogatis, L. R. (1983). *SCL-90 R Version: Manual I*. Baltimore, MD: Johns Hopkins University Press.

Dew, M. A., Bromet, E., Schulberg, H. C., *et al.* (1987). Mental health effects of the Three Mile Island nuclear reactor restart. *American Journal of Psychiatry*, **144**, 1074–1077.

Edelstein, M. R. and Wandersman, A. (1987). Community dynamics in coping with toxic contaminants. In *Neighborhood and Community Environments*, eds. I. Altman and A. Wandersman, pp. New York: Plenum.

Endicott, J. and Spitzer, R. (1972). What! Another rating scale? The Psychiatric Evaluation Form. *Journal of Nervous and Mental Disease*, **154**, 88–104.

Erikson, K. (1990). Toxic reckoning: Business faces a new kind of fear. *Harvard Business Review*, January–February, 118–126.

Enserink, M. (2001). Gulf War illness: The battle continues. *Science*, **291**, 812–817.

Green, B. L., Lindy, J. D. and Grace, M. C. (1994). Psychological effects of toxin contamination. In *Individual and Community Responses to Trauma and Disaster: The Structure of Human Chaos*, eds. R. J. Ursano, B. G. McCaughey and C. S. Fullerton, pp. 154–176. New York: Cambridge University Press.

Hallman, W. and Wandersman, A. (in press). Perception of risk and toxic hazard. In *Psychosocial Effects of Hazardous Waste Disposal on Community*, ed. D. Peck. Springfield, IL: Charles C. Thomas.

Horowitz, M., Wilner, N. and Alvarez, W. (1979). Impact of Event Scale: A measure of subjective stress. *Psychosomatic Medicine*, **41**, 209–218.

Korol, M. S., Green, B. L. and Gleser, G. C. (1999). Children's responses to a nuclear waste disaster: PTSD symptoms and outcome prediction. *Journal of the American Academy of Child and Adolescent Psychiatry*, **38**, 368–375.

Lifton, R. J. (1967). *Death in Life: Survivors of Hiroshima*. New York: Random House.

Lifton, R. J. (1999). *Destroying the World to Save It*. New York: Metropolitan Books.

Momcilovic, B. (1999). A case report of acute human molybdenum toxicity from a dietary molybdenum supplement: A new member of the 'Lucor metallicum' family. *Archives of High Radiation Toxicology*, **50**, 289–297.

Quastel, M. R., Goldsmith, J. R., Cwikel, J. G., *et al.* (1997). Lessons from the study of immigrants to Israel from areas of Russia, Belarus, and Ukraine contaminated by the Chernobyl accident. *Environmental Health Perspectives*, **105** (Suppl. 6), 1523–1527.

Schnurr, P. P., Ford, J. D., Friedman, M. J., *et al.* (2000). Predictors and outcomes of posttraumatic stress disorder in World War II veterans exposed to mustard gas. *Archives of Environmental Health*, **53**, 249–256.

Smith, E., Robins, L., Przybeck, T., Goldring, E. and Solomon, S. (1986). Psychosocial consequences of disaster. In *Disaster Stress Studies: New Methods and Findings*, ed. J. Shore, pp. 49–76. Washington, DC: American Psychiatric Press.

Tobin, D. L., Holroyd, K. A., Reynolds, R. V. and Wigal, J. K. (1989). The hierarchical factor structure of the Coping Strategies Inventory. *Cognitive Therapy and Research*, **13**, 343–361.

Viel, J. F., Curbakova, E., Dzerve, B., *et al.* (1997). Risk factors for long-term mental and psychosomatic distress in Latvian Chernobyl liquidators. *Environmental Health Perspectives*, **105** (Suppl. 6), 1539–1544.

Zilberg, N. J., Weiss, D. S. and Horowitz, M. J. (1982). Impact of Event Scale: A cross-validation study and some empirical evidence supporting a conceptual model of stress response syndromes. *Journal of Consulting and Clinical Psychology*, **50**, 407–414.

15

Relocation stress following catastrophic events

Ellen T. Gerrity and Peter Steinglass

The thing is, it makes you realize how fast and easy you can lose everything you've worked a long time to get. You find out that life goes on and that maybe there are more important things than money and possessions. These can be swept away in an instant. Family and friends, your happiness in life, is where it's all at.

Introduction

Natural disasters account for much of the damage and destruction of homes and businesses in the United States. During the years 1975–94, natural hazards killed over 24 000 people and injured at least four times that many (Mileti, 1999). During these same two decades, dollar losses to property and crops from natural hazards and disasters were between $230 billion and $1 trillion (based on 1994 dollars standards). These events include climatological hazards (events that originate in the earth's atmosphere, such as drought, dust storms, extreme cold and heat, floods, hurricanes, tornadoes), as well as earthquakes and volcanic eruptions. Although there were several catastrophic events during this period, most of the financial losses occurred in events too small to qualify for federal assistance and most of the financial costs were not insured; thus losses were borne for the most part by the survivors.

Measuring financial loss is itself very difficult because no single national database exists that utilizes consistent criteria for measuring such losses, and thus these figures must be derived from several sources. Even more importantly, these dollar figures do not take into account the value of such losses that are not directly related to market value, and excludes the most poignant losses such as lost memorabilia, destruction of historic monuments, environmental degradation that is never restored, indirect costs such as downtime for businesses and lost employment, and the short- and long-term cost of psychological trauma.

Tucker County, West Virginia, one of the communities in our family research study, was only one of the 29 West Virginia counties declared a disaster area as a result of a major flood in 1985. The dollar damage to homes, agriculture, businesses, and public property in Tucker County was estimated at $66.3 million. More than 400 families were displaced, and about 90 percent of the businesses sustained major damage or were totally destroyed (Bittinger, 1985; Teets and Young, 1985, 1987).

Home loss affects millions of people each year as a result of disaster experiences. Homes can be destroyed instantly – by a tornado, flood, or war – or more gradually, through the seepage of toxic waste or the impersonal progression of urban change or economic downturns. The ultimate outcome is the same: the home is gone and the family must come to terms with the loss and its consequences. Although much has been written regarding the impact of disasters on individuals and communities, the specific focus on home loss is relatively rare, particularly with regard to its effect on family adjustment. Often this loss is accompanied by profound disruption, which affects the internal fabric of family life, social networks, community ties, work routines, financial income, and in the most extreme cases, the physical and psychological health or life of family members.

Because the home has enormous psychosocial and practical importance in the lives of families, the loss of a home as a result of a catastrophic event can have a lasting impact on a family. This chapter is devoted to what the loss of a home means to families, and in what ways some families manage to cope with this loss, while others are destroyed by it. Included is a review of relevant psychological and sociological literature on loss of home as a background for this discussion. Interview excerpts about family coping strategies from our research study are presented, including ones that highlight some of the mental health consequences for families relocated as a result of a natural disaster. These passages are from families who had experienced 100 percent home destruction as a result of the severe flood in West Virginia. The positive and negative coping styles of families are also addressed, based on various theoretical approaches. Finally, the implications for mental health interventions and future research directions are discussed.

Our family interviews were part of a study conducted by the Center for Family Research of the George Washington University Department of Psychiatry during the years 1985–9. The study was funded by the National Institute of Mental Health and focused on how families respond to residential relocation caused by a major natural disaster and how their responses affect the subsequent psychosocial recovery process for family members. During the four years of this study, the project team collected data on site in three communities that experienced a natural disaster resulting in temporary or permanent relocation of substantial numbers of families in the community. In West Virginia, interview participants were members of 40 families, including a husband, wife, and one or two children between the ages of 8 and 21. Three sets of data were collected over an 18-month period, and included self-report questionnaires, a semistructured family interview, a structured diagnostic interview (the Diagnostic Interview Schedule), and direct behavioral assessments of family interaction (Steinglass and Gerrity, 1990a, b).

To begin, a description of one family's experience is presented in greater detail, to help place the experience in a more personal context for the reader. In this and other examples, family names have been changed as a safeguard to their identity.

The Webster family

The Webster family had owned their home in a small town in West Virginia for 10 years. Larry Webster was self-employed as a carpenter, while Kathy Webster worked part-time in her in-laws' clothing store and had most of the daily responsibility for raising their four children. Their situation was similar to many of the families locally: although they were not wealthy, their expenses were minimal, and their financial status was fairly secure. Their home was paid for, other expenses were few, and little was spent on entertainment, travel, or personal luxuries. Like most families in their town, they had no flood insurance.

The floodwaters rose suddenly following several days of rain caused by Hurricane Juan, with the flood level cresting at 21 feet at 3.00 a.m. on November 5, 1985. The family left the house, escaping the floodwaters by moving to higher ground. They clung together during the long night, fearful about their home, their friends, neighbors, and relatives, and their future.

What they saw the next day was shocking. Their home was completely gone. The depth and force of the flood had washed it off its foundation and away. Although the house was later found downstream, most of the remaining contents were water-soaked and unsalvageable. Over the next several weeks, the family made numerous trips to the destroyed home to confront the painful task of sorting through what remained of their possessions.

The Webster family moved three times during the following months, first to stay with Larry's parents, then to a trailer provided by the Federal Emergency Management Agency, and finally to their new home. As months passed, family roles and responsibilities shifted. Larry had lost all of his carpentry tools in the flood, and thus his livelihood. Jobs were in short supply in the town, and he remained unemployed. He filled his time repairing and cleaning his parents' store, which had also been severely damaged in the flood. Kathy worked 50–60 hours each week in the store helping with the cleaning and the customers, while struggling with the responsibilities for the care of her family. Worries about the future were heightened by delays in the response from government agencies responsible for disaster relief.

Family strain between children, parents, and grandparents intensified as the two families tried to live together in one house. The children became withdrawn and school grades started to drop. Arguments became more frequent. When government disaster loans became available, the long process of building their new home began. Rebuilding was fraught with obstacles such as severe weather, unreliable contractors, unexpected expenses, and lack of help. These obstacles contributed to daily tension and caused the reconstruction to be repeatedly postponed. Moving from living with relatives into the trailer brought some relief, allowing the family more autonomy, but also forced the family to live in crowded conditions, and to struggle further with complicated government regulations.

The problems experienced by the Websters were very similar to those other disaster survivors. The suddenness of the disaster and the consequent impact on family life forced the family to face unforeseen difficulties and fears that they might not survive as a family. The loss caused immediate changes in the most personal family routines and interactions, as well as serious adjustment problems as the long-term implications of the loss became clear. But to fully understand what the loss of home can cause, we will examine what the 'home' itself can mean to a family.

Meaning of 'home'

Since Marc Fried's 'Grieving for a lost home' appeared in 1963, the potentially powerful effects of home loss on individuals, families, and neighborhoods became a focus of much social science research. Fried had documented the depth and quality of the loss experience as one that closely resembles profound grief, and for some people, had long-term negative effects on adjustment. For these individuals, 'home' meant much more than the physical or social environment. The home was integral to the sense of self, so much so, that when it was lost, a reorganization of the self became necessary. For many of these individuals, home represented an extension of the self, identity with family, and a symbol of the future. Without the home, all of these things were threatened. In later works (1982a, b, 1984, 2000), Fried continued to explore the loss and relocation experience of these and other families, expanding his investigation of the symbolic and aesthetic properties of the home.

Early studies of home loss, described in further detail in Gerrity and Steinglass (1994), showed how strong a bond exists is related to the extent to which the needs of the individual or the family are met, the quality of the environment, and, more importantly, how invested a family was in staying within a specific community when the loss was experienced. Defining what 'quality' means is elusive, however, as it is subjectively determined. How satisfied someone may be with a new environment, even if it appears objectively better, may in fact depend upon how much it is similar to the old environment and may even be a motivation for rebuilding a home on the original, but now hazardous property.

The perception of personal choice as an essential element to what home means is presented in Rapoport's (1985) thoughtful review of the meaning of the home environment. Rapoport makes the case that 'if an environment is not chosen, it is not home' (p. 256). A crisis situation, by definition, often eliminates most of the conditions that enable one to choose freely, while demanding immediate actions that may have a long-term impact on long-term future adjustment. And in most instances, available choices after sudden home loss continue to be greater for those who had more freedom of choice prior to the loss, for financial or other reasons (Bolin, 1989; Gerrity and Steinglass, 1994).

While an unchosen and truly novel housing environment can become a home, efforts are needed to make this happen, by transforming the key physical and social elements into something personally meaningful (Saile, 1985; Gerrity and Steinglass, 1994). Sudden change can destroy any or all of these qualities, many of which might have been preserved if the change had been slower or more controllable. These qualities can apply to sudden destruction and other larger social units, such as neighborhoods and work environments, as well (Fullilove, 1996; Schabracq and Cooper, 2000).

In most of the work concentrating on home and attachment, theorists generally agree that individuals can become attached to their sociophysical environment, at varying levels of connection. This attachment has important implications for both adjustment and loss (Bolin, 1989; Gerrity and Steinglass, 1994; Wiesenfeld and Panza, 1999). Within disaster research, investigators have examined this issue closely.

Home destruction due to a catastrophic event

In disaster research, it has generally been assumed that home destruction which results n involuntary relocation will be associated with substantial short- and long-term evidence of psychosocial maladjustment, or even major psychopathology (Erikson, 1976a, b; Rossi *et al.*, 1983; Gerrity and Steinglass, 1994). One well-known example is the extensive study of the 1972 Buffalo Creek flood (Gleser *et al.*, 1981). The flood was caused by the sudden bursting of an earthen dam that released a tremendous mass of water and debris into Buffalo Creek Valley in West Virginia. This disaster led to massive property loss, substantial loss of life, and the destruction of the community life. As often occurs after disasters, little effort was made to relocate survivors based on prior communal ties or extended family relationships.

The results of this study suggested almost uniform short- and long-term psychopathology in adults and children. The mental health teams reported short-term reactions in adults, including psychic numbing, sluggishness in thinking and decision-making, anxiety, grief, despair, and severe sleep disturbances. Long-term responses (2 years post disaster) included physical complaints, survivor guilt, listlessness, apathy, decreased social interaction, and chronic depression. Although this research study had serious scientific limitations (i.e., no comparison group, the interviews were litigation plaintiffs, and interview data were largely clinical and not based on standardized research instruments), these findings were compelling enough to warrant further investigations. Current studies of Buffalo Creek are documenting long-term effects while utilizing comparison groups and standard measures (Grace *et al.*, 1993; Green *et al.*, 1994, 1996, 1997; Green, 1995).

Community-oriented researchers have incorporated into their studies such community level factors as cohesion and community responsiveness, believing individual suffering to be absorbed by qualities inherent in the community response (Quarantelli, 1978, 1985). Difficulties arise in separating the effects of home destruction from the multitude of other stressors, which occur after catastrophic events. Trauma research studies have attempted to consider social context and personal attributes (e.g., family and social community) as well as characteristics of the disaster (Solomon *et al.*, 1993; Gerrity and Steinglass, 1994; Garrison *et al.*, 1995; Green and Solomon, 1995; Kaniasty and Norris, 2001). In this regard, one of the most interesting studies of the mental health impact of relocation is a study of the long-term effect of Cyclone Tracy, which struck the Australian community of Darwin on Christmas Day in 1974 (Milne, 1977). The disaster totally destroyed an estimated 5000 of the 8000 homes in the community. During the 10 days following the disaster, the community population was reduced from 45 000 to 10 500 people, largely as a result of a massive evacuation to communities that could provide medical assistance and shelter. The findings of this study indicated that that those participants who had stayed in Darwin, rather than being evacuated, fared best in their postdisaster recovery. Evacuees who never returned to Darwin fared worst. Milne proposed that disaster survivors who stay within a familiar community, with an intact social support network, survive much better in the long run than do those who leave their communities.

Other researchers have focused specifically on the issue of relocation as well. Studies of the Armenian earthquake showed that women who were relocated after the earthquake had significantly higher depression scores than women who were not relocated (Najarian *et al.*, 2001), but that children who were relocated and those who were not had equally high levels of depression and posttraumatic stress disorder (Najarian *et al.*, 1996). A similar study of relocated men following an Italian earthquake showed higher levels of distress among men who were permanently relocated with accompanying social disruption, as compared to men who were temporarily relocated and then returned to their original community (Bland *et al.*, 1997). Shelter residents who had lost their homes were studied in the aftermath of Hurricane Andrew in Florida (Sattler *et al.*, 1995). Findings suggested that the loss of home and property were related to depression and psychophysiological distress. Long-term effects of relocation were examined among immigrants to Israel who had relocated there following the 1986 Chernobyl accident (Cwikel *et al.*, 1997). The 2-year follow-up study compared immigrants from the exposed areas with immigrants who had come from outlying areas. Although all respondents in the two groups experienced the stressors of emigration, some psychological distress associated with the emigration is waning, as the new immigrants are absorbed into Israeli society. However, there still remains some independent effect on health associated with the experience of the Chernobyl accident itself.

Another major body of work has developed in recent years that focuses on the effect of relocation on those who are forced from their homes as a result of war or political upheaval (Marsella *et al.*, 1994). The growing number of refugees, many of whom have been exposed to multiple and extreme trauma as well as loss of home, are vulnerable to mental and physical illnesses (Jaranson and Popkin, 1998; Gerrity *et al.*, 2001). A few of these studies have focused on the specific effect of exile on the adjustment of refugees (Solomon, 1995; Sundquist and Johansson, 1996; Ajdukovic and Ajdukovic, 1998; Richman, 1998; Silove, 2000). These studies show that the loss of home and community can have a unique and often negative impact on the already difficult adjustment and recovery process of adults and children exposed to war-related trauma and torture. They often face unique issues of loss, confrontation with an alien culture, loss of control, challenges to identity, even the death or unexplained disappearance of family members. Sundquist and Johansson (1996) point out, however, that these negative consequences must be weighed against the realities of remaining in a dangerous, war-torn culture that may no longer be the home the individuals once knew, and may also have few community resources such as food, shelter, or safety, which could mitigate other stressors.

It is clear that within the context of research on families, the loss of home takes on special significance. When the home is lost, the family is exposed in an extraordinary way to their larger physical and social environment, one that is often dangerous during and in the aftermath of catastrophic events. During these times, researchers have an opportunity to examine how families function during times of crisis, to document the range and variability of family response, and to investigate useful forms of support and intervention that will contribute to recovery (Raphael, 1986; Steinglass and Gerrity, 1990a, b; Gerrity and Steinglass, 1994).

Families and loss of home: A conceptual framework

How the experience of the family is understood is largely dependent on the theoretical and conceptual foundation of the research. Our research was most strongly

Table 15.1 Theoretical approaches to family research on home loss

Theoretical approach	Key elements	Key citation
Family systems theory	Organization Morphogenesis	Steinglass (1987)
Social construction theory	Family paradigm	Reiss (1981)
Attribution theory	Personal versus universal Helplessness	Abramson *et al.* (1980)
Stress and coping theory	Appraisal Emotion-focused coping Problem-focused coping	Lazarus and Folkman (1984)

influenced by four perspectives: family systems theory (Steinglass, 1997); social construction theory as applied to families (Reiss, 1981); attribution theory (Abramson *et al.*, 1980); and cognitive approaches to stress and copying models (Lazarus and Folkman, 1984) (Table 15.1). How these approaches related to the disaster experience and home loss, is briefly reviewed.

Family systems theory

Family systems theory is built on the assumption that families, as open systems, maintain their internal constancy through a continuous exchange and flow of information with their larger environment (Steinglass, 1987). Such operating principles as constancy, adaptiveness and change, order and organization, subsystems, boundaries, and permeability all contribute to an understanding of how a family may function during a crisis. The organization within the family itself, as well as the interaction of the family and the environment, are of particular importance, at times more important than the influence of specific characteristics. According to this theory, a family may begin to malfunction after a crisis because the family system itself is unable to cope with the sudden change, rather than because of the specific impact of the new experience. Within the family system, individual members are constrained and shaped in their behavior by the nature of their relationships with others in the system.

Furthermore, core constructs within family system theory help to provide an understanding of the family crisis of home destruction. In a functional family system, the membership is made up of 'those individuals whose constancy of contact and relationships produce predictable patterns of functional behavior' (Steinglass, 1987, p. 36), which can be relied upon for system 'organization' and maintenance. After a severe crisis, family members could rely on one another to behave in predictable patterns during the adjustment and resolution of the crisis period because of this 'organization.' A second concept central to family systems theory, 'morphogenesis,' has to do with change and growth. Morphogenesis is the process by which a system responds to an event that is disrupting family stability, and which may lead to changes in the organization. First-order changes may generate realignment of family elements; second-order change (often occurring after a serious crisis) may involve complete restructuring of the system. The better the quality of information within the family system, and the more clearly it is communicated from one member to another, the greater the capacity of the family to grow and function effectively following a crisis.

Social construction theory

A second approach to understanding families in crisis has been developed by Reiss and his colleagues (Reiss, 1981). At the core of the Reiss model is the construct of the 'family paradigm.' Reiss proposes that, just as individuals develop social constructions about the world in which they live, families as groups also develop such constructions. These shared underlying assumptions about reality, in combination, make up a family's 'paradigm.' In general, families can be distinguished in three ways: (1) in their conception of safety or danger about the world; (2) in their belief about whether the world treats the family as a group or as isolated individuals; and (3) in the extent to which the families experience the environment as novel or familiar.

Social construction theory proposes that a family's coping response to stress is determined by the family's cognitive and emotional appraisal of the event, by the efficacy of the family's own response, and by the relationship of the event to the family's concept of its development (Reiss and Oliveri, 1980). Based on this theory, in one instance a family might initially respond to sudden home destruction by viewing the loss as a family issue, taking responsibility for responding to the event, and focusing on current, not past, family issues arising from the experience. Alternatively, another family may focus on its 'victimization,' leaving individual members isolated in their experience, and make little effort to respond to this new information.

Attribution theory

Within attribution theory, the concepts of personal and universal helplessness are relevant to the process by which survivors of catastrophic events seek to understand why such an event has occurred to them. The concept of 'universal helplessness' is characterized by the belief that an outcome is independent of all of one's own responses as well as the responses of other people (Abramson *et al.*, 1980). On the other hand, if an individual believes that desired outcomes are not contingent on his or her own response, but that others have the capacity for such responses, a sense of 'personal helplessness' results, along with a feeling of responsibility, low self-esteem, and the potential for long-term maladjustment. Some survivors believe strongly, despite all evidence to the contrary, that it was their 'personal helplessness' that led to the disaster and that others would not have failed as they did. The important relationship in this theory is between the uncontrollability of the event and the perception of responsibility by the individual.

Stress and coping

The coping process, as defined by Lazarus and Folkman (1984), also includes concepts that are useful to understand the responses of families following severe crises. In particular, the process of 'appraisal,' whereby an individual judges an event to be a harm/loss situation, a threat, or a challenge, has a significant impact on future actions. While these categories are not mutually exclusive – for example, home destruction can be viewed simultaneously as a severe harm and a challenge – the process of appraisal has proven to be a predictor of whether coping was oriented toward emotion regulation (emotion-focused coping) or toward doing something to relieve the problem (problem-focused coping) (Rochford and Blocker, 1991; Zakowski *et al.*, 2001).

In situations that have a high degree of uncertainty, Lazarus predicts that direct action will decrease, and information-seeking will increase. If these actions are not available as options, individuals may then resort to intrapsychic strategies (Silver and Wortman, 1980). In some cases, appraising an event as a challenge may result in problem-focused coping, i.e., directing one's activities to solving problems, or cognitive reappraisal of the event through reinterpretation or developing new standards (Wortman and Silver, 1987). In other cases, appraising the event as harmful or as a threat may result in emotion-focused coping, such as avoidance, distancing, or displacement of emotion.

Family coping

Our interviews with families following the loss of their home revealed many examples of both positive and negative coping strategies. After experiencing the disaster, families frequently attempted to make sense of what happened, and to behave in such a way as to make their understanding meaningful in their daily lives. Whether or not the family's attempts to recover from a serious crisis lead to function or dysfunctional adjustment is an important concern for those offering both short- and long-term assistance to survivors of home destruction. What follows is a selection of examples of the range and variations of reactions appearing among flood survivors whose homes were completely destroyed (Table 15.2).

Table 15.2 Functional and dysfunctional family coping strategies

Functional strategies	Dysfunctional strategies
Reordering of priorities	Displacement of emotion
Personal immersion into recovery activity	Avoidance of social contact
Reinterpretation of meaning	Family conflict

Functional family coping

For many families, the shock of home destruction was eventually replaced by a period of adjustment that led to recovery, as they attempted to make sense of the event in terms of their past and future life together. For some family members, the struggle focused on understanding what had happened in their lives; other directed their energy toward very specific coping activities.

Our interviews with families revealed three positive coping strategies. These were: (1) the reordering of priorities, especially the redefining of material possessions as having less importance than in the past; (2) personal and fairly constant immersion into recovery activities, directed toward safeguarding what could be salvaged, and letting go of what could not; and (3) the development of a new understanding of the meaning or purpose of life. For many, this meant a new existential or spiritual understanding, often described as a new relationship with God, or a new bond with one's family or social world. These coping strategies are illustrated in the following interview excerpts. (Note that the reference to time with each quotation indicates the time that has elapsed since the flood occurred.)

Reordering of priorities

The reordering of priorities as a coping strategy was frequently mentioned by family members. During the conjoint interview, family members focused on the ways in which the disaster had affected the home life and relationships within the family and the community, expressing their feelings about what was most difficult and whether there had been any kind of positive outcome. Family members would often describe how the disaster had changed their outlook on what was now important to them, and what was no longer important.

Married couple, with two small children (at 2 months)
'Material things don't mean as much to me. I look at my kids and I think I don't need anything else. I was living with my mother and she would get upset if something got broken and I would think, "so what? I've lost my whole house. Why are you upset about a doll being lost, or a dish being broken?" ' (Wife)

'I think we've learned to appreciate everything we have more. I just don't see it as something that can easily be replaced. Anything we get we are more appreciative of having.' (Husband)

Same couple (at 16 months)

'It seems like we don't work at the house. I don't know...before, the house had to be perfect as far as remodeling and working in the yard. We don't do near as much of that. Like it's not as important any more, it seems to me...Because it can all go in a minute.' (Husband)

'I think I'm less materialistic than before. Before I thought I'd never move again. Now, I think I could. I might have to.' (Wife)

Married couple, with two small children (at 2 months)

'It makes you stop and think. I have a lot today, but tomorrow I may not have anything. The family was OK...no injuries or anything. We were all together. It changes your outlook on life a lot. It makes you appreciate things more. Things you didn't appreciate before. If you can enjoy today, do it, because you never know what tomorrow may bring. Right?' (Husband)

'We don't put our priorities on our possessions now. We know that's not the most important thing because we can have them one day and one day they're gone. But our family, we were just happy that nobody was injured and that everybody was still able to be together.' (Wife)

Woman, with three children (at 16 months)

'I've changed, material-wise...You stop and realize and you think we could have lost part of the kids. We could have lost ourselves. At least we're still together as a family. I think you learn to appreciate one another more.'

Older married couple, with a teenage son (at 3 months)

'Losing the things I lost, I don't put the value on material things now that I did before, and I don't intend to in the future. There were things I thought I had to have that I didn't need. In the future I think I'll be more careful in buying and not just have a lot of things cluttering up the house. All those things were just in a matter of hours gone. It took you 20 years to put in that house. I've talked to different people that really, losing their material things had really affected them bad. To me, none of us lost our lives or got injured, and that's really more important.' (Wife)

Young couple, with one son with a chronic illness (just after the flood)

'The jobs seem more important now than they were. Before, our home was paid for, and we had no heating expenses, all we had were utilities and food, so it was pretty cheap living. Now it would be more important if one of us lost a job. Whereas before it wouldn't have been such a big deal if it had happened before.' (Wife)

Personal immersion into recovery activity

Personal immersion into recovery and other kinds of activity was another way family members adjusted to the sudden change in their lives. Rather than focusing on what was irretrievably lost, some families avoided introspection and became more involved in the activities of cleaning, repairing, rebuilding, planning, and organizing, in order to eventually achieve a stability which had been taken from them.

Young couple, with two small children (at 14 months)
'It's like . . . you do everything for existence. You don't do anything for enjoyment because it takes so much of your time to do the basics. I don't think we'd be so worried about the home if it wasn't for the kids. We're worried about them having something to call home more than we are I think.'

Older couple, with a teenage son (at 2 months) (showing desire to immerse in work)
'You can't do nothing in that trailer. You can't have pictures on the walls, you can't put underpinning on the trailer, you can't do this, you can't do that . . . We've got a year. But it's agonizing to wait until next December to do anything, to know anything . . . You can't paint or do anything.'

Reinterpretation of meaning

Development of a new understanding of the meaning of life in a deeper or more abstract way was one of the cognitive strategies undertaken by some families following the destruction of their home. For some of the families this meant a renewal of their spiritual faith, turning to God to provide an explanation for what had happened to them. For others, the trust was placed in the relationships with their immediate family or their larger social world to provide a purpose for their future life. Some saw this renewal as a return to traditional values; others felt it was a beginning of a new understanding of what life meant, even if it resulted in a rejection of what they had believed before the disaster.

Elderly couple, in poor health, with a teenage daughter (Mary) (at 2 months)
'The hardest thing for me was knowing I was going to have to give up the house because my brothers and sisters had been raised there, my mother and dad they were gone, and I had Mary on tapes from the time she was a baby and all the pictures. But I just said, "God, you've got something better for me, and I can't dwell on it." So in a day or so I just let that go by. I knew if I dwelled on it, it would be that much

harder and it wouldn't do me a bit of good because there wasn't any way I could do anything about it. It was gone and that was it. So I just told God to take care of it and He did for me . . . so I just believed in that and He let me know I was going to have another home and that's the only thing that's just been in my mind. I'd say "Well, you just wait and see," because I knew that He just wouldn't let that happen and lose everything not to give me something better. I just felt that He maybe had to get that out of my life for me to see other things a little bit . . . I just said "God, my home is gone, you know it, and you will eventually replace what I need in my life." That has always, from the day of the flood been my motto.' (Wife)

'We have tried to keep Mary's life normal. We were always used to getting things for her and letting her do things so she had a normal life, and right now we just can't give her everything like we planned on. But I'd rather do without something myself to be able to see that she can do something.' (Wife)

'My cousin . . . he came in and helped me with my work. Then we sat down and talked a long time after we got done. It just really made me feel good. They want to help, you know.' (Husband)

'What really helped me; I go to church. Faith in the Lord and I read His word and if I hadn't had that, I don't know, and seeing the people come and help. I do a lot of reading of the Bible. That's all I care about is reading the Bible. That gives me strength.' (Husband)

Older couple, with a teenage son (at 3 months)

'I think it would prepare us for the future, things that may happen in the future. There for a few months after the flood, it was just like we had been in a war or something . . . A lot of us wouldn't be able to handle the situation, so it gave us a little bit of insight as to what we might be facing the future. We might have to cope with a situation like this again.'

Young woman, one son with a serious illness (at 16 months)

'I guess with the flood, it lets you know that life goes on. Even when a disaster does hit, it's not the end of the world. It gives you faith that God does give you a way to carry on. We had this one little picture . . . and the floodwaters didn't get to it. It was pictures on the mailbox and it said something to the effect that if His eyes are on the sparrow, wouldn't he also take care of you? We've always been taken care of, even after the flood. We got through everything.

I think I'm going more into an Appalachian outlook. The Appalachian family typically clans together and shuts the rest of the world out. I don't know how to explain that, but you know what I mean. You're born here, you're raised here, and you die here, and you forget there's another world out there. You start out with another identity. I think I'd just as soon be a little hermit and stay here. It seems safer.'

Middle-aged couple, with teenage children (at 15 months)
'I guess maybe in the back of your mind, you're thinking, "Really, do you really want to stay here the rest of your life? Do you want to go on living here? Do you want to try again?" Sometimes I really didn't.' (Wife)

'It was the perfect time for us to have gotten out, but somebody had to be here to help get the store going again, do all the work up there and get it opened back up. My grandparents were getting old.' (Husband)

Dysfunctional family coping

Not all family coping strategies were effective in producing positive family functioning. Negative patterns appeared with some families, evident at both the earlier (4-month) and later (16-month) periods of recovery. These included: (1) displacement of emotion about the disaster toward other people or things perceived as responsible, not only for the disaster, but also for the inability of the family to return to their preflood state; (2) avoidance of family, especially extended family, resulting in a sense of isolation; and (3) family conflict, expressed in anger and unresolved daily arguments. Eventually, the inability to effectively communicate becomes the source of continued family problems.

Displacement of emotion

Displacement of emotion can result from a sudden shock. However, some families continued to divert all grief and painful emotions on to those they deemed responsible for the disaster itself or for their continuing problems.

Teenager (at 16 months)
'Before the flood I hardly got into trouble. I used to have a job working at the drug store. As soon as the flood hit that messed me up. Then we moved out of town and I got to hanging around with the wrong people. I broke into a store and I just got sent off. That's what happened after the flood . . . and I see it as caused by the flood. If it hadn't happened, I wouldn't have been in this institution and I wouldn't have broken into the store.'

Young woman, with small children (at 15 months)
'It's a positive change for me in that I'm getting to be home with the baby, but as far as I wonder what my future is going to be, it's negative that way. I gave up my job, and it seems like I gave up everything.'

Young woman, one son with serious illness (at 16 months)
'It was a loss of faith in the government, that the employees in the system would be so incompetent and everything would get so messed up and all the red tape that

you'd be out of your home and didn't have anything. We moved a total of four times to our present home, and that's a lot of disruption.

The government representative was the worst. She just made us feel like we were scum ... that we didn't even know how to take care of a place. That was the main problem. She was the main reason we got thrown out of the trailer, it was at her recommendation ... One day things got hot and heavy ... and my husband is short-tempered. Not long after we got the eviction notice ... it was the next month after they had an argument.'

Middle-aged woman, with three children (at 3 months)
'Here about a week ago, I got up in the middle of the night thinking about a bowl of flowers my sister-in-law had on a table in the restaurant when the flood hit. It was about 3.00 or 4.00 in the morning. I couldn't go back to sleep, I worried about those flowers, "Where are those flowers?" And why? I don't know, to me it's just a silly little thing. It really had no effect on me. It was flowers in her restaurant, not in my house, but I couldn't go back to sleep because of worrying about this bowl of flowers.'

Young couple, with two small daughters (at 16 months)
'The rich got richer and the poor got poorer. It's the way it's going to be, and that's the way it's going to stay.' (Husband)

'But I know one woman, I won't mention her name, but she has so taken advantage of this, and I know as well as I'm sitting here that she was putting on a big show. That's what it was.' (Wife)

Avoidance of social contact

Some families withdraw from their extended family, isolating themselves as a family or as individual members from their connections with the social world. Although often perceived as necessary to protect the family from difficulties with friends or relatives, the withdrawal can lead to the family becoming isolated in their experience and severing all chances for future healing.

Young woman, with small children (at 3 months)
'My family is the most difficult thing about my experience with the flood. They have the attitude that this is your lot in life, you have to accept it.'

Young woman, with a son with a serious illness (at 16 months)
'It's true that you can't go home again, and it was real uncomfortable living with my parents. As a matter of fact, I hardly go visit her any more. I visit outside, but to eat supper, play dominoes, spend time, whatever, I've only done it twice since the

holidays [3 months], and we're only a mile apart. It just made me back off from her and not be as close. I think I had more than my fill of her. Even though I appreciated having a place to live it was under her rules and her dictates and her moods.'

Young woman, with two small daughters (just after the flood)
'The hardest thing . . . I said something about going through the flood, and she says "Well, I lived through it with you." I said, "No, you haven't. You don't know the first thing about it." Then she said, "Well, you need to take them to church more often. You need to take them to church. You need to take them to church." Which I know. We need to go to church more often.'

Young couple, with two small daughters (at 16 months)
'Our relationship with our relatives has gotten worse. It sure hasn't gotten any better. It's gotten worse.' (Husband)

Family conflict

In some families, the conflicts appeared among their own family members. But instead of leading to communication and eventual resolution, the anger is expressed in daily quarrels, effectively eliminating the possibility of the rebuilding of the home on an emotional level.

Middle-aged woman, with three children (at 16 months)
'He's not working. I hate it. I literally hate it. Because we're in this new house now. I've worked almost the whole 20 years we've been married. When I first started out working I didn't have to. Now I have to, I literally hate it . . . I hate the responsibility of all the bills. Then coming home, of course, he's been helping with the laundry and trying to get the kids to help with picking up around the house, but it's not always done. But there's other ways that I want to do things, you know. There's things I want to do, that I want to be home to do. When I come home from work, I'm just too tired . . . It's the same old thing day in and day out. I hate it.'

Young couple, with two small children (at 16 months)
'You're not doing much at all for my parents any more. You're never there to do it.' (Wife)
 'No, I'm always over there.' (Husband)
 'This is going to be Divorce Court!' (Wife)
 'When it snows, who goes over there and shovels the snow? I'm doing things now that your father would have done in the past, simply because I was down the road two miles. Rather than have me run up. But now, he sees me in the yard, and he yells over and says come over here.' (Husband)

'I'm not being mean, but that you would think that when we think it's just the opposite.' (Wife)

'Yeah. I'll have to start making a list. Maybe I should report in before I do something.' (Husband)

Older couple, with a teenage son (just after the flood)
'We're having a time coping with our son. He's having a time. He's the only one not coping. We can cope, but he's having an awful time adjusting.'

Mental health intervention

Mental health services to individuals who have lost homes because of catastrophic events are, like other services, generally based on a crisis model, with emergency services organized quickly for short-term intervention. In addition to nonprofit organizations like the American Red Cross, one major federal program provides funding for short-term crisis counseling. Through an interagency agreement, the Federal Emergency Management Agency and the Center for Mental Health Services, a subdivision of the Substance Abuse and Mental Health Services Agency, mental health programs for survivors of Presidentially declared disasters can receive funding. The Center for Mental Health Services also collaborates with the Federal Emergency Management Agency to train state mental health staff to develop crisis counseling training and preparedness efforts in their states. These materials are generally available at federal government websites and locally at disaster-related community meetings soon after a disaster.

Services are organized around several practical principles:

1. Provide mental health services in different settings for different phases of the emergency.
2. Give special attention to high-risk survivors, e.g., children, physically handicapped, elderly.
3. Offer services for emergency service workers who are vulnerable to develop trauma reactions as result of exposure to extreme stressors.
4. Develop programs adapted to cultural and regional realities. Services provided early in the emergency attempt to meet the practical as well as emotional needs of families who have lost their homes, and are often initially administered within emergency shelters.

As a rule, mental health services are organized around the primary principles of other kinds of crisis intervention provided in the field (Lystad, 1985b; Myers, 1989; Pfefferbaum *et al.*, 1999). Unlike noncrisis services, emergency mental health workers ideally work closely within the overall system of emergency response. For example, a mental health worker may assist a family with its request for emergency housing, and while doing so, will help the family with the immediate psychological impact of this stressor on the family as well. This assistance may take place at the site of the destroyed home, at the home of relatives, in a trailer provided by the Federal Emergency Management Agency, or at an emergency shelter at the local school. As noted by Tierney and Baisden (1979), 'The need for food, clothing, and shelter can be just as much of an emergency to a family as the need for impartial mediation in an angry family dispute' (p. 42). This approach reflects the need to respond to the varying levels of response and the stage of adjustment of the family.

The specific phase of the intervention will determine the nature and scope of the mental health services to individuals who lose their homes. Early on, the shock of the loss combines with the serious immediate need for replacement shelter. Later, families struggle with the responses of individual members to the loss, as they attempt to recreate or maintain family cohesion and build a new home. Individual members are likely to differ in their response to the disaster and in copying style. If communication breaks down at this or any point, family recovery is threatened. Finally, mental health workers must be alert for delayed or long-term psychological problems and continue to provide services for families (Bornstein and Clayton, 1972; Horowitz, 1983, 1985; Wilson *et al.*, 1985; Steinglass and Gerrity, 1990a, b). Crisis intervention teams can be involved in the training of local mental health professionals who will be responsible for continuing services after crisis teams have left the community.

Because the loss of a home and community can easily lead to the dissolution of social support, an important goal of crisis intervention is to mitigate the effects of this disruption (Crabbs and Heffron, 1981; Aneshensel and Stone, 1982; Lystad, 1985a; Solomon, 1986, 1989). Social support disruption can be caused by a variety of factors: illness or death, evacuation, temporary housing, frequent moves, lack of transportation, or a breakdown in communication systems. After large catastrophic events, fragmented networks may be bolstered by the emergence of a 'therapeutic community' made up of disaster relief agencies, local disaster committees, charitable organizations, church groups, and the less formal support of outside volunteers (Drabek *et al.*, 1975; Bolin, 1989; Pfefferbaum *et al.*, 1999). In smaller disasters, survivors may find themselves turning to medical or mental health professionals, or the clergy, for psychological support (Tierney and Baisden, 1979; Waeckerle, 1991).

The loss of home may cause a short- or long-term grief reaction, and is potentially a factor in mental health intervention programs. The disruption of the neighborhood and extended family relationships may interfere with what may have been a social support network for families in a more limited crisis. Supplementing social support networks is one type of mental health intervention, but equally important is providing families the opportunity to freely express their feelings and assisting them with finding meaning in their experience in a nonjudgmental setting (Janoff-Bulman, 1975, 1992; Silver and Wortman, 1980).

All of these principles and practices can be applied to services offered to survivors of other forms of home loss as well. Refugees, many of whom are dealing with multiple losses and trauma experiences, have also lost their home, community, and country. Recognizing that these major losses may also play a major role in psychological reactions and recovery will contribute should ideally be part of a comprehensive intervention that supports the multiple needs of refugees (Marsella *et al.*, 1994; Gerrity *et al.*, 2001).

Children

Often, intervention with families is made in the form of outreach to children. Because the perception of stigma associated with contacting mental health professionals exists in some communities, children can be an important link between mental health workers and families facing serious difficulties in crisis situations (Stewart, 1985). This link is manifested in a number of ways. First, the reactions of children to the disaster are often watched closely by the family and the community. Children are seen as especially vulnerable, with their direct and indirect expressions of distress often difficult to interpret. Second, schools are very often the center for community intervention on the part of local leaders, mental health workers, teachers, and parents. Discussion among adult members of the community will center at first on the needs of the children, but then move fairly easily to the needs of the families and the community. Finally, while parents may hesitate to ask for psychological assistance for themselves, they will ask for such services for their children. Once initiated, family intervention can proceed. Many disaster intervention programs have developed materials to help families cope with reactions of their children (e.g., American Red Cross, 1981; Doudt, 1981; Farberow and Gordon, 1981; Lystad, 1985c; Flynn and Nelson, 1998).

While contact with children may initiate mental health support to families, it is the family itself that is the first and most important resource for the child. Whether the intervention is initially made with an adult or a child, eventually the family should be seen as the basic unit for intervention. The impact of the home destruction is felt by every member of the family, and within the family system, the reaction and coping style of each member will affect every other member. In communities where extended families play important roles, other relatives are providing temporary housing for the victim family (Harris, 1991). Research on the effects of temporary housing has most frequently examined the role of relatives (Davis, 1977; Loizos, 1977; Gerrity and Steinglass, 1994). Bolin (1989) showed that after a period of about one month, the relationship between the victim family and relatives begins to deteriorate, with interpersonal conflicts increasing as a result of crowding and financial problems. Temporary housing provides more privacy to the survivor family but has features that can also contribute to stress, including relocation at some distance from the original home, transportation, problems, and difficulties in obtaining needed services. Federal Emergency Management Agency trailers, often used as a temporary shelter by families, also generate problems among families. In recent years, some efforts have been made to improve housing services to disaster survivors. However, in the past such problems as inadequate construction, lack of timely responsiveness from agency representatives, difficulties in getting or keeping the trailers, location away from the original community, and the haphazard design of trailer communities all contributed to exacerbating difficult situations for families. Difficulties are also prolonged when families do not receive information regarding permanent housing, long-term loans, or contractor availability. Children can be profoundly affected by such long-term disruption, and mental health professionals need to take these environmental realities into account when planning intervention strategies.

Intervention and research implications

Because all of the families described in this chapter experienced 100 percent home loss, most were unable to use the process of sorting through belongings and memories to more slowly process their grief. It is unclear whether families who have the opportunity to move back into their original homes are able to use this experience to help their adjustment. Those who have no home to return to have only their relationships and their thoughts to begin the process of recovery. It is here that these individuals and families begin to meet the challenge of their future lives and where intervention can begin.

Whether the ability to process one's loss is therapeutic or not is only one of several research questions that should be considered in future disaster projects (Table 15.3). Other research directions include the aspects listed below.

Targeting specific groups

While we have focused on families in our study, most disaster studies have involved individual adults, or, in some cases, children. Additional groups that may be in need of special intervention efforts include: (1) identified cultural groups whose perception of the disaster may be markedly different as a result of past experiences with disasters or differing attitudes about home; (2) business owners or employees who have lost their livelihood, but not necessarily their homes, in a disaster; (3) relatives of survivors who help (or hinder) the recovery of survivor families; (4) emergent community leaders who come forward to lead recovery, but often discontinue their leadership role when the crisis period is over; and (5) emergency workers, who are often exposed over long periods to severe stressors.

Table 15.3 Mental health intervention strategies

Crisis model/field intervention
1. Respond to immediate practical needs
2. Mitigate impact on social support network
3. Monitor delayed and long-term reactions

Children
1. Link to families
2. Support family resources
3. Extend services to other relatives

Intervention and research implications
1. Targeting specific groups
2. Research/provider collaboration
3. Values and attributions
4. Methodology

As noted earlier, the number of refugees worldwide is growing, and many are relocated to the United States. The unique characteristics of refugees groups, including cultural, ethnic, and language considerations, torture or trauma experiences, multiple losses, minimal resources, and an uncertain future, need to be recognized in the development of mental health programs that serve those who have been through catastrophic events.

More recently, the United States is facing new challenges when developing mental health programs to support those who have experienced deliberate terrorist or bioterrorist attacks. Survivors of these events also may be dealing with multiple losses, including their home or workplace, as well as threats to the physical safety and ongoing uncertainty regarding future events. Trauma researchers will need to draw on past research to help understand the psychological consequences of these events, but will also need to be open to investigating the unique physical and mental health consequences of such severe and ongoing traumatic events (Ursano, 2002).

Research–provider collaboration

The collaboration between emergency mental health teams, the local mental health agency, and disaster researchers deserves further exploration to determine the most effective way to provide needed services quickly. In many instances, disaster researchers can play an important mental health role while conducting research, particularly for those survivors who may resist seeking traditional services despite being under severe stress. Participation in a research study carries much less stigma. It nevertheless provides an opportunity for participants to share their concerns and difficulties in an atmosphere that can be an important first step in the appraisal of stress and the formulation of coping strategies. Our research study provided the opportunity for families to discuss together for the first time the experiences they had individually and jointly shared during the disaster and afterwards. For many, the discussion provided understanding, comfort, and a chance to attach some meaning to their experiences. Society and the mental health profession benefits from the conduct of high-quality research studies. When participants can also find their contribution to be personally meaningful, it is an additional outcome that makes the research that much more valuable.

Values and attributions

The role of personal values, attributions, and perceptions as they influence the adjustment of families who lose their homes is an important research area. Longitudinal studies extended to later in life might further explore the ways the catastrophe served as a turning point, for good or ill, in the family's life. Cognitive and behavioral strategies play an important role in postdisaster adjustment. Careful documentation of these strategies with current disaster survivors can inform future intervention efforts.

Methodology

In disaster research, one continually seeks the right questions methods, and approaches to capture precisely what is in fact a profound experience that changes people's lives in dramatic ways (Solomon, 1989). Combining a human approach with scientific principles requires constant vigilance that the proper balance is achieved. Creative interdisciplinary approaches are needed in both mental health intervention and in research so that the families' needs are met, and the information can inform future efforts in both areas.

Conclusion

The experience of home loss in a family's life calls forth many of the more extreme human emotions: grief, anger, dread, despair, as well as courage, selflessness, gratitude, and hope. In the context of catastrophic events, the experience of home loss is only one of a multitude of events contributing to a family's emotions and future adjustment. But it is within the context of such events that the loss of one's home can carry with it profound symbolic meaning and consequent deep emotional pain which may affect the future of the individual family. It is important that efforts continue to be directed at research that will address the complexity of the experience, maintain appropriate levels of rigor and scientific principles, and respect the unique experiences of families who undergo such losses.

Acknowledgments

The research was supported by Grant No. R01 MH40376 from the National Institute of Mental Health.

REFERENCES

Abramson, L. Y., Garber, J. and Seligman, M. E. (1980). Learned helplessness in humans: An attributional analysis. In *Human Helplessness: Theory and Applications*, eds. J. Garber and M. E. P. Seligman, pp. 3–34. New York: Plenum Press.

Ajdukovic, M. and Ajdukovic, D. (1998). Impact of displacement on the psychological well-being of refugee children. *International Review of Psychiatry*, **10**, 186–195.

American Red Cross (1981). *Family Disaster Plan and Personal Survival Guide*. Washington, DC: American Red Cross.

Aneshensel, C. S. and Stone, J. D. (1982). Stress and depression: A test of the buffering model of social support. *Archives of General Psychiatry*, **39**, 1392–1396.

Bittinger, W. (ed.) (1985). *Killing Waters: The Great West Virginia Flood of 1985*. Terra Alta, WV: CR Publications.

Bland, S. H., O'Leary, E. S., Farinaro, E., *et al.* (1997). Social network disturbances and psychological distress following earthquake evacuation. *Journal of Nervous and Mental Disease*, **185**, 188–194.

Bolin, R. C. (1989). Natural disasters. In *Psychosocial Aspects of Disaster*, eds. R. Gist and B. Lubin, pp. 61–85. New York: John Wiley and Sons.

Bornstein, P. E. and Clayton, P. J. (1972). The anniversary reaction. *Diseases of the Nervous System*, **33**, 470–2.

Crabbs, M. A. and Heffron, E. (1981). Loss associated with a natural disaster. *Personnel and Guidance Journal*, February, 378–82.

Cwikel, J. G., Abdelgani, A., Goldsmith, J. R., *et al.* (1997). Two-year follow-up study of stress related disorders among immigrants to Israel from the Chernobyl area. *Environmental Health Perspectives*, **105** (Suppl. 6), 1545–1550.

Davis, I. (1977). Emergency shelter. *Disasters*, **1**, 23–40.

Doudt, K. (1981). *Helping Your Child Cope with Disaster*. New Windsor, MD: Church of the Brethren.

Drabek, E. E., Key, W. H., Erickson, P. E., *et al.* (1975). The impact of the disaster on kin relationships. *Journal of Marriage and the Family*, **37**, 481–495.

Erikson, K. T. (1976a). *Everything In Its Path*. New York: Simon and Schuster.

(1976b). Loss of Communality at Buffalo Creek. *American Journal of Psychiatry*, **133**, 302–305.

Farberow, N. L. and Gordon, N. S. (1981). *Manual for Child Health Workers in Major Natural Disasters*. DHHS Publication No. 81-1070. Washington, DC: National Institute of Mental Health.

Flynn, B. W. and Nelson, M. E. (1998). Understanding the needs of children following large-scale disasters and the role of government. *Child and Adolescent Psychiatric Clinics of North America*, **7**, 211–227.

Fried, M. (1963). Grieving for a lost home. In *The Urban Condition: People and Policy in the Metropolis*, ed. L. J. Duhl, pp. 151–171. New York: Basic Books.

Fried, M. (1982a). Endemic stress: The psychology of resignation and the politics of scarcity. *American Journal of Orthopsychiatry*, **52**, 419.

Fried, M. (1982b). Residential attachment: Sources of residential and community satisfaction. *Journal of Social Issues*, **38**, 107–119.

Fried, M. (1984). The structure and significance of community satisfaction. *Population and Environment*, **7**, 61–86.

Fried, M. (2000). Continuities and discontinuities of place. *Journal of Environmental Psychology*, **20**, 193–205.

Fullilove, M. T. (1996). Psychiatric implications of displacement: Contributions from the psychology of place. *American Journal of Psychiatry*, **153**, 1516–1523.

Garrison, C. Z., Bryant, E. S., Addy, C. L., *et al.* (1995). Posttraumatic stress disorder in adolescents after Hurricane Andrew. *Journal of the American Academy of Child and Adolescent Psychiatry*, **34**, 1193–1201.

Gerrity, E., Keane, T. M. and Tuma, F. (eds.) (2001). *The Mental Health Consequences of Torture*. New York: Kluwer Academic.

Gerrity, E. T. and Steinglass, P. (1994). Relocation stress following natural disasters. In *Individual and Community Responses to Trauma and Disaster: The Structure of Human Chaos*, eds. R. J. Ursano, B. G. McCaughey and C. S. Fullerton, pp. 220–248. Cambridge: Cambridge University Press.

Gleser, G. C., Green, B. L. and Winget, C. (1981). *Prolonged Psychosocial Effects of Disaster: A Study of Buffalo Creek*. New York: Academic Press.

Grace, M. C., Green, B. L., Lindy, J. D., *et al.* (1993). The Buffalo Creek disaster: A 14-year follow-up. In *International Handbook of Traumatic Stress Syndromes*, eds. J. P. Wilson and B. Raphael, pp. 441–449. New York: Plenum Press.

Green, B. L. (1995). Long-term consequences of disasters. In *Extreme Stress and Communities: Impact and Intervention*, eds. S. E. Hobfoll and M. W. DeVries, pp. 307–324. Dordrecht: Kluwer Academic.

Green, B. L., Gleser, G. C., Lindy, J. D., *et al.* (1996). Age-related reactions to the Buffalo Creek dam collapse: Effects in the second decade. In *Aging and Posttraumatic Stress Disorder*, eds. P. E. Ruskin and J. A. Talbott, pp. 101–125. Washington, DC: American Psychiatric Press.

Green, B. L., Grace, M. C., Vary, M. G., *et al.* (1994). Children of disaster in the second decade: A 17-year follow-up of Buffalo Creek survivors. *Journal of the American Academy of Child and Adolescent Psychiatry*, **33**, 71–79.

Green, B. L., Kramer, T. L., Grace, M. C., *et al.* (1997). Traumatic events over the life span: Survivors of the Buffalo Creek disaster. In *Clinical Disorders and Stressful Life Events*, ed. T. W. Miller, pp. 283–305. Madison, CT: International Universities Press.

Green, B. L. and Solomon, S. D. (1995). The mental health impact of natural and technological disasters. In *Traumatic Stress: From Theory to Practice*, eds. J. R. Freedy and S. E. Hobfall, pp. 163–180. New York: Plenum Press.

Harris, C. J. (1991). A family crisis-intervention model for the treatment of posttraumatic stress reaction. *Journal of Traumatic Stress*, **4**, 195–207.

Hobfoll, S. E., Dunahoo, C. and Monnier, J. (1995). Conservation of resources and traumatic stress. In *Traumatic stress: From Theory to Practice*, eds. J. R. Freedy and S. E. Hobfoll, pp. 29–47. New York: Plenum Press.

Horowitz, M. J. (1983). Post-traumatic stress disorder. *Behavioral Sciences and the Law*, **1**, 19–20.

Horowitz, M. J. (1985). Disasters and psychological responses to stress. *Psychiatric Annals*, **15**, 161–167.

Janoff-Bulman, R. (1985). The aftermath of victimization: Rebuilding shattered assumptions. In *Trauma and its Wake: The Study and Treatment of Post-Traumatic Stress Disorder*, ed. C. R. Figley, pp. 15–35. New York: Brunner/Mazel.

    (1992). *Shattered Assumptions: Towards a New Psychology of Trauma*. New York: Free Press.

Jaranson, J. and Popkin, M. (eds.) (1998). *Caring for Victims of Torture*. Washington, DC: American Psychiatric Press.

Kaniasty, K. and Norris, F. H. (2001). Social support dynamics in adjustment to disasters. In *Personal Relationships: Implications for Clinical and Community Psychology*, eds. B. R. Sarason and S. Duck, pp. 201–224. New York: John Wiley and Sons.

Lazarus, R. S. and Folkman, S. (1984). *Stress, Appraisal, and Coping*. New York: Springer-Verlag.

Loizos, P. (1977). A struggle for meaning. *Disasters*, **1**, 231–239.

Lystad, M. (1985a). Facilitating mitigations through mental health services after a disaster. Paper presented at the American Bar Association International Symposium on Housing and Urban Development after Natural Disasters, Miami, Florida.

Lystad, M. (1985b). Mental health programs in disasters: 1974–84. In *Innovations in Mental Health Services to Disaster Victims*, ed. M. Lystad, pp. 1–7. DHHS Publication No. 86-1390. Washington, DC: NIMR.

Lystad, M. (1985c). Special programs for children. In *Innovations in Mental Health Services to Disaster Victims*, ed. M. Lystad, pp. 150–160. DHHS Publication No. 86-1390. Washington, DC: NIMR.

Marsella, A., Bornemann, T., Ekblad, S. and Orley, J. (eds.) (1994). *Amidst Peril and Pain: The Mental Health and Well-Being of the World's Refugees*. Washington, DC: American Psychological Association.

Mileti, D. S. (1999). *Disasters by Design: A Reassessment of Natural Hazards in the United States*. Washington, DC: Joseph Henry Press.

Milne, G. (1977). Cyclone Tracy. 1: Some consequences of the evacuation of adult victims. *Australian Psychologist*, **12**, 39–54.

Myers, D. G. (1989). Mental health and disaster: Preventive approaches to intervention. In *Psychosocial Aspects of Disaster*, eds. R. Gist and B. Lubin, pp. 190–228. New York: John Wiley and Sons.

Najarian, L. M., Goenjian, A. K., Pelcovitz, D., *et al.* (1996). Relocation after a disaster: Post-traumatic stress disorder in Armenia after the earthquake. *Journal of the American Academy of Child and Adolescent Psychiatry*, **35**, 374–383.

Najarian, L. M., Goenjian, A. K., Pelcovitz, D., *et al.* (2001). The effect of relocation after a natural disaster. *Journal of Traumatic Stress*, **14**, 511–526.

Pfefferbaum, B., Flynn, B. W., Brandt, E. N., *et al.* (1999). Organizing the mental health response to human-caused community disasters with reference to the Oklahoma City bombing. *Psychiatric Annals*, **29**, 109–113.

Quarantelli, E. L. (ed.) (1978). *Disasters: Theory and Research*. Beverly Hills, CA: Sage Publications.

Quarantelli, E. L. (1985). An assessment of conflicting views on mental health: The consequences of traumatic events. In *Trauma and its Wake: The Study and Treatment of Post-Traumatic Stress Disorder*, ed. C. R. Figley, pp. 173–215. New York: Brunner/Mazel.

Raphael, B. (1986). *When Disaster Strikes: How Individuals and Communities Cope with Catastrophe*. New York: Basic Books.

Rapoport, A. (1985). Thinking about home environments: A conceptual framework. In *Home Environments*, eds. I. Altman and C. M. Werner, pp. 255–286. New York: Plenum Press.

Reiss, D. (1981). *The Family's Construction of Reality*. Cambridge, MA: Harvard University Press.

Reiss, D. and Oliveri, M. (1980). Family paradigm and family coping: A proposal for linking the family's intrinsic capacities to its responses to stress. *Family Relations*, **29**, 81–91.

Richman, N. (1998). Looking before and after: Refugees and asylum seekers in the west. In *Rethinking the Trauma of War*, eds. P. J. Bracken and C. Petty, pp. 170–186. London: Free Association Books.

Rochford, E. G. and Blocker, T. J. (1991). Coping with 'natural' hazards as stressors. *Environment and Behavior*, **23**, 171–194.

Rossi, P. H., Wright, J. D., Weber-Burdin, E., *et al.* (1983). *Victims of the Environment: Loss from Natural Hazards in the United States, 1970–1980*. New York: Plenum Press.

Saile, D. G. (1985). The ritual establishment of home. In *Home Environments*, eds. I. Altman and C. M. Werner, pp. 183–212. New York: Plenum Press.

Sattler, D. N., Sattler, J. M., Kaiser, C. F., *et al.* (1995). Hurricane Andrew: Psychological distress among shelter victims. *International Journal of Stress Management*, **2**, 133–143.

Schabracq, M. J. and Cooper, C. L. (2000). The changing nature of work and stress. *Journal of Managerial Psychology*, **15**, 227–241.

Silove, D. (2000). Trauma and forced relocation. *Current Opinion in Psychiatry*, **13**, 231–236.

Silver, R. L. and Wortman, C. B. (1980). Coping with undesirable life events. In *Human Helplessness: Theory and Applications*, eds. J. Garber and M. E. P. Seligman, pp. 279–341. New York: Academic Press.

Solomon, S. D. (1986). Mobilizing social support networks in times of disaster. In *Trauma and Its Wake: The Study and Treatment of Post-Traumatic Stress Disorder*, ed. C. R. Figley, pp. 232–263. New York: Brunner/Mazel.

(1989). Research issues in assessing disaster effects. In *Psychosocial Aspects of Disaster*, eds. R. Gist and B. Lubin, pp. 308–340. New York: John Wiley and Sons.

Solomon, S. D., Bravo, M., Rubio-Stipec, M. and Canino, G. J. (1993). Effect of family role on response to disaster. *Journal of Traumatic Stress*, **6**, 255–269.

Solomon, Z. (1995). *Coping with War-Induced Stress: The Gulf War and the Israeli Response*. New York: Plenum Press.

Steinglass, P. (1987). A systems view of family interaction and psychopathology. In *Family Interaction and Psychopathology*, ed. T. Jacobs, pp. 25–65. New York: Plenum Press.

Steinglass, P. and Gerrity, E. (1990a). Forced displacement to a new environment. In *Stressors and the Adjustment Disorders*, eds. J. D. Noshpitz and R. D. Coddington, pp. 399–417. New York: John Wiley and Sons.

Steinglass, P. and Gerrity, E. (1990b). Natural disasters and post-traumatic stress disorder: Short-term versus long-term recovery in two disaster-affected communities. *Journal of Applied Social Psychology*, **20–21**, 1746–1765.

Stewart, S. (1985). Families. In *Diagnostic Interviewing*, eds. M. Hersen and S. M. Turner, pp. 289–307. New York: Plenum Press.

Sundquist, J. and Johansson, S. E. (1996). The influence of exile and repatriation on mental and physical health: A population-based study. *Social Psychiatry and Psychiatric Epidemiology*, **31**, 21–28.

Taylor, R. B. (1997). Social order and disorder of street blocks and neighborhoods: Ecology, microecology, and the systemic model of social disorganization. *Journal of Research in Crime and Delinquency*, **34**, 113–155.

Teets, B. and Young, S. (1985). *Killing Waters: The Great West Virginia Flood of 1985*. Terra Alta, WV: CR Publications.

Teets, B. and Young, S. (1987). *Killing Waters II: West Virginia's Struggle to Recover*. Terra Alta, WV: CR Publications.

Tierney, K. J. and Baisden, B. (1979). *Crisis Intervention Programs for Disaster Victims in Smaller Communities*. Rockville, MD: National Institute of Health.

Ursano, R. J. (2002). Post-traumatic stress disorder. *New England Journal of Medicine*, **346**, 130–132.

Waeckerle, J. F. (1991). Disaster planning and response. *New England Journal of Medicine*, **324**, 815–821.

Wiesenfeld, E. and Panza, R. (1999). Environmental hazards and home loss: The social construction of becoming homeless. *Community, Work, and Family*, **2**, 51–65.

Wilson, J. P., Smith, W. K. and Johnson, S. K. (1985). A comparative analysis of PTSD among various survivor groups. In *Trauma and its Wake: The Study and Treatment of Post-Traumatic Stress Disorder*, ed. C. R. Figley, pp. 142–172. New York: Brunner/Mazel.

Wortman, C. B. and Silver, R. C. (1987). Coping with irrevocable loss. In *Cataclysms, Crises, and Catastrophes: Psychology in action*, eds. G. R. VandenBos and Bryant, pp. 187–235. Washington, DC: American Psychological Association.

Zakowski, S. G., Hall, M. H., Cousino Klein, L., *et al.* (2001). Appraised control, coping, and stress in a community sample: A test of the goodness-of-fit hypothesis. *Annals of Behavioral Medicine*, **23**, 158–165.

16

Population-based health care: A model for restoring community health and productivity following terrorist attack

Charles C. Engel, Jr, Ambereen Jaffer, Joyce Adkins, Vivian Sheliga, David Cowan, and Wayne J. Katon

Introduction

Terrorist attacks are geographically confined but result in extensive social disruption (Holloway *et al.*, 1997). Typically a large zone of fear, disruption, and confusion surrounds a small zone of physical injury or disease. Over time, the physical and emotional impacts of a terrorist attack can leave a community legacy of symptoms, division, and disability (Table 16.1). At times this legacy is exacerbated by intense and polarized societal debates over controversial symptom syndromes and the environmental exposures that may have caused them. These passionate community debates can add to medical and psychosocial morbidity in the weeks, months, and years following the terrorist attack by raising concerns about potential exposures to ill-defined toxins or pathogens. Community stakeholders may take up predictable and seemingly self-interested positions and wage well-publicized battles over the legitimacy of putative exposures and syndromes. These social contests and their associated scientific, political, legal, and media debates can create community divisions and mistrust. Additionally, these contests may compound usual medical and psychosocial sources of symptoms and disability.

There are many historical examples involving the military and veteran communities following wars or other catastrophic events. Some of these are: shell shock following World War I (Hyams, 1998), DaCosta's syndrome (Hyams, 1998), soldier's heart (Hyams, 1998), jungle disease following Dutch troop deployments to Cambodia (Kaminski, 2000), posttraumatic stress disorder (Summerfield, 2001), and Gulf War syndrome (Engel and Katon, 1999). There have also been numerous military examples of contested health exposures. These include Agent Orange (Institute of Medicine, 1999), depleted uranium after the Gulf War and US bombing in Kosovo

Table 16.1 Some maladaptive individual and community responses to terrorist attack

Individual-level responses	Community-level responses
1. Horror and distress	1. Mass panic
2. Social isolation	2. Divisiveness and loss of cohesion
3. Anger, suspicion, and mistrust	3. Conspiracy theories
4. Demoralization	4. Loss of confidence in leaders Debates over blame and responsibility
5. Catastrophic thinking (overestimated risk)	5. Epidemic health anxiety
6. Medically unexplained symptoms	6. Contested exposures and illnesses
7. unemployment loss of functioning	7. Disability and compensation disputes Diminished community productivity

(Koppel, 2001), nuclear fallout after US weapons experiments (Rosenberg, 1980), and austere wartime environments (Institute of Medicine, 1996). Other examples include recent attempts to immunize against anthrax (Williams, 2001), Gulf War use of pyridostigmine bromide tablets as a chemical nerve agent prophylaxis (Moss, 1998), and field use of pesticides (Roland *et al.*, 2000). Open debate over these syndromes and exposures is essential to a free society. However, unintended consequences of such debate are often heightened levels of community worry and elevated mistrust between patients and their health care providers. This is further amplified when mistrust for the military extends to federal health care providers.

Nevertheless, these problems are not isolated to government and the military. Poignant civilian examples involving similar challenges can be found in history. These include contested symptoms and exposures after nuclear accidents at Three Mile Island (Houts *et al.*, 1988) and Chernobyl (Loganovsky, 2000), industrial exposures at Love Canal in the 1970s and 1980s (Mazur, 1998), the *Exxon Valdez* accident and oil spill (Murphy, 2001), and the 1992 crash of a commercial jetliner in a dense residential portion of Amsterdam (Uijt de Haag *et al.*, 2000). More recently, media coverage of the September 11 terrorist attacks suggests emerging health concerns, symptoms, community debate, and cracks in established community unity (France, 2001).

These examples strongly suggest that prevailing disease management approaches to health service delivery can address only a minority of the symptoms and disability that occur in affected communities after an attack. There is a dire need for innovative models of health care delivery that can address and overcome the issues resulting from contested syndromes and exposures.

In this article we describe the use of a population-based health care model for communities in preparation for and response to terrorist attacks. This model relies on current knowledge of factors affecting the occurrence and natural history of

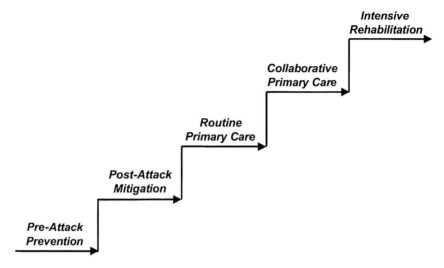

Figure 16.1   A stepped-care approach to population-based health care for symptoms and disability after terrorist attack.

common symptoms and disability. Population-based health care is a public health approach that links community-level intervention to the delivery of personalized health services. The model delineates stepped levels of community response before and after a terrorist attack (Fig. 16.1). The first two levels of response (preevent and postevent care) target the community rather than individual patients. Subsequent levels of response (primary care, collaborative primary care, and intensive specialty care) involve case-finding and progressively intensified patient-centered health care for those seeking medical assistance for their symptoms and disability. Table 16.2 encapsulates the key features of population-based health care in preparation for and response to terrorism.

This population-based health care model assumes that the context of care will become a critical factor that will significantly alter usual patterns of health care use. Furthermore, when care is sought, a positive service experience creates trust that leads to other health-related benefits, while a negative experience can complicate provider–patient communication, affect subsequent health care utilization, trigger and exacerbate symptoms, perpetuate disability, and even diminish confidence in community leaders.

From symptoms to disability

One question is: What can be learned from the empirical literature on symptoms and disability that can be used to help communities develop and implement a population-based health care system in response to a terrorist attack?

Table 16.2 An overview of features associated with the stepped approach to population-based health care before and after terrorist attack

Step	Emphasis	Setting	Goal	General approach	Information systems
1	Preattack prevention	precare	Incidence reduction	Population-based prevention	Monitor community levels of predisposing factors
2	Postattack mitigation	Precare	Incidence and prevalence reduction	General mitigation efforts based on exposures and proximity	Identify precipitating events
3	Routine primary care	Primary care	Identification and prevalence reduction	Primary care provider delivers preventive services, diagnostics, and low-intensity treatments	Identify symptoms, diseases, and concerns
4	Collaborative care	Primary care	Prevalence reduction	Interdisciplinary practice team intensifies care in coordination with primary care provider	Identify persistent symptoms, disease, or concerns
5	Intensive rehabilitative care	specialty care	Morbidity reduction	Specialized multidisciplinary and multifaceted rehabilitative programs	Identify persistent disability

Table 16.3 Common predisposing, precipitating, and perpetuating factors that determine the natural history of symptoms and disability

Predisposing factors	Precipitating factors	Perpetuating factors
1. Heredity	1. Biological stressors	1. Harmful illness beliefs
2. Biological diatheses	2. Acute physical illness	2. Labeling effects
3. Early life adversity	3. Psychosocial stressors	3. Misinformation
4. Chronic illness	4. Acute psychiatric disorders	4. Workplace and
5. Chronic distress or mental illness	5. Epidemic health concerns	compensation factors
		5. Social support factors
		6. Physical inactivity
		7. Chronic illness
		8. Poorly integrated care

Source: Engel and Katon (1999); Hunt *et al.* (in press).

1. Symptoms are common, and very often medically unexplained (Kroenke and Price, 1993).
2. Symptoms, both medically explained and unexplained, contribute substantially to community levels of disability (Kroenke *et al.*, 1994).
3. Symptoms and disability often lead to and are produced by distress, worry, anxiety, and depression (Von Korff and Simon, 1996; Armenian *et al.*, 1998; Gureje *et al.*, 2001).
4. Symptoms and disability increase health care use but usual medical approaches applied to unexplained symptoms lead more often to iatrogenic harm, patient dissatisfaction, and provider frustration than medical benefit or patient reassurance (Kouyanou *et al.*, 1997; Twemlow *et al.*, 1997).
5. Unexplained symptoms vary widely in severity from single symptoms that are mild and transient to multiple symptoms that are chronic, and disabling (Katon *et al.*, 1991).
6. Symptoms and disability outcomes are strongly influenced by biopsychosocial determinants including predisposing, precipitating, and perpetuating factors (Pope and Tarlov, 1991; Walker *et al.*, 1998; Engel and Katon, 1999; Hunt *et al.*, in press). Examples of these factors are shown in Table 16.3.
7. Symptoms and disability are responsive to evidence-based individual level intervention (O'Malley *et al.*, 1999; Kroenke and Swindle, 2000).

The progression from symptom to disability and distress can be divided into four stages. First, a person experiences a symptom. The symptom may or may not represent the effect of an illness or disease. Second, the person experiencing the symptom assesses it cognitively. That is, the person superimposes onto the symptom his or her personal history, knowledge, biases, context, and beliefs regarding possible causes, seriousness, and treatments of the symptom and draws conclusions. Third, the person responds behaviorally to his or her conclusions about the symptom's severity and importance. For example, care may be sought, activities or roles avoided, or functioning reduced. Fourth, if care is sought, the provider proffers a medical explanation (or lack of one). This last stage may lead to provider and patient differences, disputes, and contests over symptoms and disability that may mirror community debates. Alternatively, negotiation of differing physician–patient perceptions of illness and developing a mutually acceptable model of illness may lead to increased satisfaction and decreased physical health concern.

Contested explanations for unexplained symptoms and disability contributes to the frustration and dissatisfaction with care repeatedly observed in studies involving these syndromes (e.g., chronic fatigue syndrome, fibromyalgia syndrome, irritable bowel syndrome, multiple chemical sensitivities). These controversies affect providers (Lin *et al.*, 1991; Hahn *et al.*, 1994; Walker *et al.*, 1997) and patients alike (Kouyanou *et al.*, 1997). Furthermore, if the health care visit occurs in the setting of a community debate regarding cause or blame for symptoms or disability or some other contextual reason for mistrust such as a recent terrorist attack, the provider–patient relationship is even more likely than usual to become strained, outwardly adversarial, or result in mutual rejection (Quill, 1985). Other times, the provider may unwittingly respond to the other extreme, embarking on an overly aggressive quest for causes (usually in the name of patient advocacy), a pathway that can lead to iatrogenic harm well before the patient finds relief.

The empirical observations and theoretical relationships just described suggest ways that cognitive factors (e.g., community or individual beliefs regarding a terrorist attack), behavioral factors (e.g., patterns of health care use), and health service experience (e.g., iatrogenic harm and differing provider and patient explanations for symptoms) may hasten the onset and perpetuate the course of symptoms and disability. These observations and theory also suggest ways in which population-based health care for the sequelae of a terrorist attack must go beyond the usual disease management approaches to reduce community morbidity and foster early return to full community productivity.

Population-based health care: What is it? Why use it for terrorism?

Efforts to mitigate the health impacts of terrorism must consider the availability of resources and the tendency for policy-makers to allocate resources liberally in the acute aftermath with lesser attention to longer-term community health needs. Whether any given intervention is used depends on its effectiveness weighed against the resources required to deliver it. Population-based health care achieves maximum efficiency and effectiveness by combining an optimal mix of population-level versus individual-level interventions that are linked together using a public health approach involving passive and active health surveillance and efforts to bolster primary care delivery.

Population-based care versus population-level and individual-level intervention

Population-based health care is a system of care that seeks to use an optimal mixture of population-level and individual-level interventions. Population-level interventions affect whole populations. Examples include public service announcements or changes in laws or policies pertaining to health (Rose, 1992). Individual-level interventions, in contrast, target patients in need of personalized services for high levels of symptoms and disability.

Population-level interventions have their benefits and drawbacks. Exposure of an entire community to an intervention can lead to a large net community benefit. Even though the benefit per individual is small, the sum of these benefits across an entire population can be substantial for a community. However, many individuals who do not need the intervention and cannot benefit from it will also experience its impact. Therefore, population-level intervention must have a low cost and few adverse effects per individual in the community. Examples of effective population-level interventions are multimedia campaigns discouraging smoking or speed-limit reductions to reduce traffic fatalities.

Similarly, individual-level interventions also have their benefits and drawbacks. Individual-level interventions are necessary because population-level interventions cannot adequately address the greater needs of the few individuals with relatively severe symptoms and disability. Rose (1992) described individual-level intervention as a 'high risk strategy' because individuals at high health risk are identified and targeted for treatment. The primary advantage of an individual-level intervention is that it may be tailored to specific patient needs. Another advantage is that it is only administered to ill individuals and therefore has virtually no impact on the rest of the community. Riskier interventions may be justified, because ill individuals have a greater potential for benefit. Since only a few community members are ill enough to receive individual-level intervention, the community can afford to spend more on the intervention per ill individual. A major drawback of individual-level intervention, however, is that it usually contributes little to overall community health because health and illness usually occur along a continuum, and many individuals in the community who are not labeled as ill may still have some degree of disability or other health-related needs.

Why use population-based health care to mitigate the health effects of terrorism?

It follows from the discussion above that an effective approach to maximizing community health requires a carefully planned combination of population-level and individual-level approaches. Explicit attention to what constitutes the optimal mix of population-level and individual-level interventions is the major feature of population-based health care.

As reviewed above, symptoms and disability are common in the community, occur along a severity continuum, and are reciprocally related to distress. Therefore, we can expect that reverberating community fear, worry, confusion, and distress following a terrorist attack will lead to high community levels of symptoms and disability; the events after September 11 offer a classic case in point (Schuster *et al.*, 2001). For some individuals, symptoms and disability may be transient but for others they may become chronic and severe.

Optimizing population-based health care to mitigate the impact of terrorism

Population-based health care relies on structured clinical services linked through primary care to a community-based prevention plan. Important community subgroups with symptoms are identified, a mechanism to track health outcomes is devised, and interventions are matched to groups with varying levels of symptoms, disability, distress, and other health-related treatment needs (Wagner *et al.*, 1996). Although only a small number of incident symptoms become chronic, chronic symptoms have a higher prevalence in health care settings because the associated disability results in increased health care visits over a longer period of time (Engel and Katon, 1999). The spectrum of symptoms and disability and the association of duration to health care use results in a health care system gradient of symptoms and disability: least in the general population, greatest in tertiary care, and intermediate in primary care (Green *et al.*, 2001).

Population-based care in action against terrorism

The previous considerations have implications for when and where to intervene (e.g., precare, primary care, or tertiary care) to reduce the community burden of symptoms and disability in the weeks and months following a terrorist attack. Incidence reduction (preventing first onset of symptoms and disability) is most appropriately a population-level intervention occurring before symptoms and disability occur and related health care is sought. Efforts to reduce duration and prevent future episodes of symptoms and disability are best achieved in the primary care setting. Additionally, attempts to reduce morbidity associated with chronic symptoms and disability (e.g., psychosocial distress, psychiatric disorders, iatrogenic harm, and decrements in occupational functioning) are best initiated in primary care settings with on-site assistance from selected specialists. Tertiary care programs for symptoms and disability are held in reserve for those with the greatest need for individual-level treatments.

Table 16.4 Preferred preattack preventive modalities

Workplace education
Family education
Public service announcements
Consider use of multiple media (print news, radio, television, Internet)
Other population-based preventive interventions

What follows is a more detailed description of the steps of population-based care for symptoms and disability following a terrorist attack.

Pre-attack prevention of predisposing and precipitating factors

The global effects of primary prevention strategies for symptoms and disability are not well characterized, and caution is necessary before wide-scale mobilization of resource-intensive population-level interventions of uncertain impact. Inexpensive and low-risk population-level interventions to prevent symptoms, disability, and distress deserve immediate attention and further research. For example, organizational policies and regulations or community-level or workplace-level education involving literature, television, or other media segments may have value.

Useful pre-attack prevention interventions are listed in Table 16.4. One potential way of improving the efficiency, narrowing the scope, increasing the feasibility, and reducing the cost of preattack interventions is to use information systems to target individual-level approaches before care is sought. Demographic characteristics and passive and active health surveillance data may be used to identify groups predisposed to symptoms and disability after terrorist attack. Assuming that predisposing factors are only modestly predictive, caution must be exercised so that interventions remain low risk and avoid stigmatizing or medicalizing affected individuals and their concerns. For example, predisposed groups may be offered a voluntary education program designed to address group needs and delivered at sites that are not associated with health care (e.g., community colleges, workplaces, or clubs).

Postattack mitigation of precipitating and perpetuating factors

Once an attack has occurred, efforts to mitigate symptoms and disability can focus on risk groups based on level of psychosocial, medical, and geographic exposure to the inciting event (Table 16.5). For example, the military medical system response to the September 11 Pentagon attack relied on several proximity measures. Decreasing levels of geographic proximity included the attacked 'wedge' of the Pentagon, the rest of the Pentagon, and the National Capitol Area. Levels of medical exposure included those physically injured, those attending to the injured or killed, response personnel, those otherwise physically exposed (e.g., felt the blast, inhaled smoke,

Table 16.5 Precare modalities used for postattack mitigation

Workplace screening
Workplace education and support networks
Informal ('lay') debriefings
Family education and support networks

reported other environmental exposures), and those who observed the injuries of others. Levels of emotional proximity included family, friends, colleagues, and subordinates of those injured or killed, of those in the damaged wedge, and of those working elsewhere in the Pentagon; those Pentagon personnel who were displaced by the attack; and those personnel deployed to respond to the attack. The real-time availability of information system data and well-designed reports has the potential to focus mitigation efforts toward identified community needs.

Several postattack preventive interventions need systematic evaluation. Chaos, loss of control, and health fears are common after catastrophic events. Workplace educational approaches may teach workers about health risks and responses related to an attack. Community and workplace leaders can facilitate early return to usual work routines and other roles to maximize postattack productivity. The availability of town hall meetings to address community concerns provide forums for community leaders to disseminate information and to learn about attack-related issues, and for affected community members to articulate their needs. Publicly advertised toll-free telephone 'hot lines' afford personalized contact to people with questions or concerns and need systematic evaluation.

Some experts advocate large-scale postattack psychological debriefings. However, randomized controlled trials of psychological debriefings have shown little or no efficacy and even potential for modest harm (Wessely *et al.*, 1999). It may be argued that most studies have not offered more than one session of assistance, but debriefings are seldom affordable on a larger scale or feasible for more than a few highly exposed groups. Debriefings targeting groups at high risk of poor health outcomes may offer a workable alternative and require further study. Workplace liability concerns and the often overwhelming community desire to help victims often fuel pressures to complete wide-scale debriefings after an attack, but the lack of controlled trials backing efficacy suggests that scarce community resources are usually better directed elsewhere.

'Screening' is another commonly considered postattack strategy. Screening involves identification of high-risk individuals for clinical treatment (individual-level intervention delivered in a health care setting). Surveillance, by comparison, is the use of active and passive health measurement strategies to characterize the health of a

Table 16.6 Strategies to pursue in routine primary care following
a terrorist attack

Patient screening for symptoms and distress
Patient education regarding symptoms and distress
Management of distress
Clinician reminders
Clinician feedback regarding patient outcomes
Systematic consultation based on complications, nonresponse/persistence

community and its subgroups. Some may recommend the use of surveillance data to
drive clinical referrals. However, as previously noted, predicting future symptoms
and disability involves significant inaccuracies. Even if high-quality surveillance
data on predisposing and precipitating factors are available in real time, singling
out high-risk individuals for clinical referral before the onset of symptoms or disability may unnecessarily stigmatize or harm many with identifiable risk factors
who would do fine if left alone. Instead, primary care screening for symptoms and
disability, tracking associated outcomes, and intensifying treatment for those with
identified needs is probably most efficient and effective.

Routine primary care for acute symptoms, concerns, and continuity of care

Since feasible and proven population-level strategies for symptoms and disability
are lacking and symptoms and disability are common, they can be expected to occur
even after relatively successful precare prevention programs. Nearly all people with
symptoms and disability after an attack will see a primary care provider (Green
et al., 2001). Therefore, a key population-based health care response to a terrorist
attack is early primary care recognition of symptoms and disability (Table 16.6).
Once identified, providers can administer modest individual-level interventions to
mitigate the impact of the precipitating event and reduce the potential for perpetuating factors to prolong symptoms and disability. The focus on intensifying
treatment for those seeking care avoids adding stigma that would be introduced
using precare screening and referral.

Since many symptoms linked to disability are medically unexplained, a patient-
centered approach to affected primary care patients is best. An appropriate
patient-centered primary care approach involves an initial directed diagnostic evaluation followed by watchful waiting if the evaluation is negative. In parallel, provider
and patient collaboratively negotiate the nature, probable cause, and treatment focus. Assessment of depressive and anxiety disorders and, when necessary, introduc-
tion of related treatment options should occur early and openly. Providers often fail
to communicate the degree of diagnostic uncertainty inherent in clinical practice,

and they often equate 'absence of an explanation' to 'psychological explanation,' alienating many patients in the process. Instead, given the expected relationship between terrorism, distress and mental illness, and symptoms and disability, the possibility of future mental health consultation is best destigmatized through early discussion of these issues as 'a routine part caring for patients with disabling symptoms.' When this groundwork is done, patients who are referred later are less likely to feel their primary care provider is rejecting them or contesting the validity of their symptoms.

Jackson and colleagues have shown that primary care provider attempts to understand a patient's views and expectations regarding symptoms and disability results in short-term improvements in patient satisfaction and provider-perceived difficulty of the encounter (Jackson *et al.*, 1999). Similarly, systematic attempts to clarify patient views regarding possible causes, outcomes of interest, and the appropriate treatment foster patient–provider trust. Efforts to understand patient beliefs are better than blanket reassurances that may seem condescending to patients. Deferring to a patient's illness beliefs may seem inappropriate when the patient believes in seemingly improbable conspiracies or unlikely diseases as causes for symptoms. 'No nonsense' providers often prefer to counter such beliefs directly, but these confrontations nearly always offend the patient, result in mutual mistrust, and disrupt continuity of care. Offering explanations, answering questions, displaying empathy, and defining problems in the patient's own words is best for building trust, a task that is aided with customized literature on common aftermath concerns, symptoms, disability, distress, and illness.

Yielding to patient explanations for symptoms and disability, particularly in the absence of identified disease, prevents contests and moves provider–patient discussions on to constructive therapies. The task, therefore, is to engage the patient, getting the patient to assume responsibility for wellness, while avoiding a 'blame game.' Once the patient assumes responsibility for wellness, best practices for symptoms and disability involve negotiated behavioral priorities and goals targeting temporally related decreases in role functioning (e.g., work, family, and leisure activities) and systematic and regular follow-up to measure progress and encourage goal attainment.

Decisions to invoke the next level of care for symptoms and disability hinge on whether symptoms and disability persist, whether the patient adheres to self-care and follow-up, and whether complicating medical problems exist.

Collaborative primary care for intermittent symptoms and disability

As symptoms and disability become more chronic and burdensome for both patient and provider, many ecological barriers to routine primary care management become problematic (e.g., lack of provider time). A crossroads is usually reached

Table 16.7 Components of collaborative primary care
following terrorist attack

Interdisciplinary practice team with primary care provider
   integration
Clinical risk communication (up-to-date health risk information
   for clinicians and patients)
Patient education regarding symptoms and disability
Physical and psychosocial reactivation efforts
Negotiated goal-setting
Collaborative problem-solving

at which symptoms and disability either improve or persist, the risk of iatrogenic
harm increases, and the patient requires intensified individual-level approaches.
This juncture usually occurs once unexplained symptoms and disability persist
beyond three to four months.

A summary of collaborative primary care approaches may be found in
Table 16.7. An interdisciplinary practice team located in primary care becomes
vital at this health care step (Wagner, 2000). Involvement of the practice team
in a parallel process of multifaceted care delivered in the primary care setting
provides options for physicians when options are otherwise few and provider–
patient tensions may be developing. It also affords the patient with more intensive
risk communication, engagement of existing social supports, and gradual physical
and psychological activation strategies aimed at distress and disability reduction.
Using the primary care clinic to deliver psychosocial and behavioral treatments
for symptoms and disability minimizes potential stigma associated with them. Use
of the primary care setting keeps care simple for patients. It may improve rates
of follow-up and foster continued involvement of primary care providers, making
them more approachable and keeping provider–patient communication channels
open.

Research on successful standardized consultation for unexplained symptoms
provides clues into responsibilities significant to practice team tasks (Smith *et al.*,
1995; Von Korff and Moore, 2001). The practice team should ensure that patients
with chronic symptoms and disability:

- Establish a relationship with a single primary care physician who coordinates all
  specialist referrals, diagnostic testing, and treatment trials for them.
- Receive regular rather than PRN (as needed) visits with a primary care physician
  (every 4 to 6 weeks or so).
- Avoid sedating and habit-forming medications that reduce functioning such as
  sedatives or opioids analgesics.

- Plan and coordinate how *ad hoc* visits for exacerbations of symptoms will be addressed.
- Use of educational activating interventions for patients with persistent concerns, worries, or modest activity limitations.
- Referral to intensive rehabilitative intervention for patients with persistent work limitations.

Practice teams should coordinate weekly interdisciplinary team meetings involving primary care physicians. In addition to intensifying the basic coordination of care, practice teams can also help deliver multifaceted therapies designed to improve patient morale, reduce symptom-related distress or mental illness, and increase reserve functional capacity. In keeping with the stepped overall approach to population-based care, practice team interventions are best administered in a stepped fashion so that simple approaches are offered first, followed by progressively more intensive, expensive, or burdensome therapies. Treatments are matched to patient based on the trajectory of the patient's symptoms and disability and the results obtained from previous modalities. Basic components commonly used include screening; on-site mental health consultation; cognitive–behavioral and problem-solving therapies aimed at medication adherence, depression, symptoms, and disability; physical activation and relapse prevention assistance; videotapes, pamphlets, and other education materials on self-care; structured follow-up strategies relying on multiple methods (visits, telephone, email, or Internet); and longitudinal case management. In one example of a successful team-based education approach, an intensive multisession education intervention with telephone follow-up encouraging graded exercise among chronic fatigue syndrome patients improved fatigue, sleep, disability, and mood compared to standard health care 1 year after randomization (Powell *et al.*, 2001).

Given a recent terrorist attack, clinical risk communication is an additional role for practice teams. The goal of health risk communication is to enhance bidirectional communication in 'low-trust, high-concern' situations such as those occurring after terrorism and other catastrophes. Health risk communicators often focus on methods of communication and message evaluation when communities harbor toxic exposure concerns. In the primary care setting, if a patient harbors conspiratorial or other harmful beliefs, the practice team can listen to patient concerns and beliefs, help patients test or verify them, and convey them to primary care physicians or, if appropriate, to clinic management.

Intensive rehabilitative care for chronic symptoms and disability

Intensive rehabilitative care approaches are summarized in Table 16.8. Model programs for chronic symptoms and disability are usually multifaceted, multidisciplinary, occur in specialized (i.e., nonprimary care) settings, and involve either a

Table 16.8 Intensive rehabilitative
approaches following terrorist attack

3-Week inpatient or 10–15-week outpatient

Multispecialty cadre of expertise

Structured and intensive

Multimodal

Graduated return to work

Planned practice team follow-up

3–4-week inpatient or intensive outpatient program or a 10–15-week program of weekly or biweekly individual or group visits (Flor *et al.*, 1992; Kroenke and Swindle, 2000). Medical and psychosocial approaches are combined with a structured and supervised physical activation plan. These programs view disability as a behavior amenable to modification, regardless of medical etiology.

Commonly employed cognitive–behavioral approaches to symptoms and disability help patients test commonly held patient beliefs regarding cause, prognosis, and treatment for symptoms and disability that can halt progress rather than foster improved functioning. Empirical trials have shown the benefits of cognitive–behavioral therapy for a range of symptom syndromes and associated disability (Speckens *et al.*, 1995; Kroenke and Swindle, 2000; Deale *et al.*, 2001; Prins *et al.*, 2001; Price and Cooper, 2002).

Physical activation is another clinical strategy that has been shown to have a number of positive effects on health and well-being across many health conditions, and efforts to bolster physical activation and functioning are common in multifaceted programs for chronic symptoms and disability (McCain *et al.*, 1988; Fulcher and White, 1997; Frost *et al.*, 1998; Wearden *et al.*, 1998).

Following a terrorist attack, successful efforts to return chronically symptomatic and disabled workers to their full levels of occupational functioning bolsters individual and community self-esteem and sense of accomplishment even if limiting physical disabilities persist. Evidence favors supervised, graduated, and early return to work for improving role functioning for people with chronic symptoms and disability. For example, studies of patients with low back pain suggest that a return to modified work can be successful (Frank *et al.*, 1996), while work restrictions diminish the likelihood of return to work and do not reduce absenteeism or back pain recurrences (Burton and Erg, 1997).

Information tools for population-based care after terrorism

Wagner *et al.* (1996) have described information systems as a key to population-based health care. Information systems are computer-automated systems designed

Table 16.9 Information tools for informing providers and community leaders regarding individual and community health responses to terrorist attack

Health information systems: passive computer-automated health surveillance

Health monitoring systems: active survey-based health surveillance

Expert computer systems: automated reporting to identify high-risk groups

to capture data that can be used to inform clinicians of their patients' status, to assist clinicians and medical executives interested in monitoring and improving the quality of care, and to guide policy makers attempting to assess population needs and determining appropriate staffing levels (Table 16.9).

Information systems for facilitating care of symptoms and disability following terrorist attack needs three components:

1. Health information systems – passive computer-automated health surveillance systems
2. Health monitoring systems – active survey-based health surveillance systems
3. Expert computer systems – automated systems that process data and generate useful reports for the identification of high-risk patients and populations and for the evaluation of care.

The health information system records prioritized medical problem lists and measures of health care utilization (e.g., outpatient, inpatient, and pharmacy services and various procedures), health care costs, presenting symptoms, primary care physician, usual place of care, patient contact information, and disease-specific data for developing registries (Katon *et al.*, 1997). These data, combined with health monitoring system data such as patient-reported symptoms and disability may be used to identify high-, intermediate-, and low-risk groups for intervention and tracking.

Expert computer systems process raw surveillance data into usable tools for community leaders and health care providers. Expert system generated tools aid clinical management, patient follow-up, treatment, and policy decisions. Examples of expert computer systems tools include registries, reports, reminders, clinical indicators, feedback systems, guideline recommendations, and identification of appropriate patient education materials or outcomes monitoring scales.

Conclusion

Disease management strategies will only offer solutions for a small proportion of the symptoms and disability in a community following a terrorist attack. The population-based health care model that we have described in this paper attempts to provide solutions for communities affected by terrorist attack as well as for individuals presenting for health care with significant symptoms and disability. This model is feasible, stepped, interdisciplinary, multifaceted, and lends itself to evaluation and improvement. It optimally combines a public health perspective with patient-centered care based on individual patient needs. These linkages between public health and individual patient approaches are made with carefully planned health information systems along with an emphasis on primary care.

The greatest obstacle to population-based health care for symptoms and disability following terrorist attack may be the commonly held view among providers, policy-makers, and health care executives that symptoms in the absence of a useful biomarker are neither disabling nor important. Although explanations of 'stress' or 'somatization' for unexplained physical symptoms serve an important clinical purpose for many patients with symptoms and disability, they are often used to minimize the needs of those affected and stigmatize the individual so labeled. In the face of competing community demands, the argument that patients with symptoms and disability suffer more from 'nothing' than 'something' can seem compelling to those organizing and delivering services.

We urge rapid community movements toward population-based health care planning and implementation to mitigate the impact of future terrorist acts. To achieve this, health services research, local and national leadership, and interdisciplinary health service planning is needed.

Note

The views expressed in this article are those of the authors and do not necessarily represent the official policy or position of the Uniformed Services University of the Health Sciences, Walter Reed Army Medical Center, Department of the Army, Department of Defense, or the US Government.

REFERENCES

Armenian, H. K., Pratt L. A., Gallo, J. and Eaton,W. W. (1998). Psychopathology as a predictor of disability: A population-based follow-up study in Baltimore, Maryland. *American Journal of Epidemiology*, **148**, 269–275.

Burton, A. K. and Erg, E. (1997). Back injury and work loss: Biomechanical and psychosocial influences. *Spine*, **22**, 2575–2580.

Deale, A., Husain, K., Chalder, T. and Wessely, S. (2001). Long-term outcome of cognitive behavior therapy versus relaxation therapy for chronic fatigue syndrome: A 5-year follow-up study. *American Journal of Psychiatry*, **158**, 2038–2042.

Engel, C. C., Jr and Katon, W. J. (1999). Population and need-based prevention of unexplained symptoms in the community. In *Strategies to Protect the Health of Deployed U.S. Forces: Medical Surveillance, Record Keeping, and Risk Reduction*, ed. Institute of Medicine, pp. 173–212. Washington, DC: National Academy Press.

Flor, H., Fydrich, T. and Turk, D. C. (1992). Efficacy of multidisciplinary pain treatment centers: A meta-analytic review. *Pain*, **49**, 221–230.

France D. (2001). Now, 'WTC' syndrome? *Newsweek*, **138**, 10.

Frank, J. W., Brooker, A. S., DeMaio, S. E., *et al.* (1996). Disability resulting from occupational low back pain. 2: What do we know about secondary prevention? A review of the scientific evidence on prevention after disability begins. *Spine*, **21**, 2918–2929.

Frost, H., Lamb, S. E., Klaber Moffett, J. A., Fairbank, J. C. and Moser, J. S. (1998). A fitness programme for patients with chronic low back pain: 2-year follow-up of a randomized controlled trial. *Pain*, **75**, 273–279.

Fulcher, K. Y. and White, P. D. (1997). Randomized controlled trial of graded exercise in patients with the chronic fatigue syndrome. *British Medical Journal*, **314**, 1647–1652.

Green, L. A., Fryer, G. E., Jr, Yawn, B. P., Lanier, D. and Dovey, S. M. (2001). The ecology of medical care revisited. *New England Journal of Medicine*, **344**, 2021–2025.

Gureje, O., Simon, G. E. and Von Korff, M. (2001). A cross-national study of the course of persistent pain in primary care. *Pain*, **92**, 195–200.

Hahn, S. R., Thompson, K. S., Wills, T. A., Stern, V. and Budner, N. S. (1994). The difficult doctor–patient relationship: Somatization, personality and psychopathology. *Journal of Clinical Epidemiology*, **47**, 647–657.

Holloway, H. C., Norwood, A. E., Fullerton, C. S., Engel, C. C., Jr. and Ursano, R. J. (1997). The threat of biological weapons: Prophylaxis and mitigation of psychological and social consequences. *Journal of the American Medical Association*, **278**, 425–427.

Houts, P., Cleary, P. and Hu, T. (1988). *The Three Mile Island Crisis: Psychological, Social, and Economical Impacts on the Surrounding Population*. Philadelphia, PA: Penn State University Press.

Hunt, S. C., Richardson, R. D. and Engel, C. C., Jr (in press). Clinical management of Gulf War veterans with medically unexplained physical symptoms. *Military Medicine*.

Hyams, K. C. (1998). Developing case definitions for symptom-based conditions: The problem of specificity. *Epidemiological Reviews*, **20**, 148–156.

Institute of Medicine (1996). *Health Consequences of Service During the Persian Gulf War: Recommendations for Research and Information Systems*. Report of the Committee to Review the Consequences of Service during the Persian Gulf War Medical Follow-up Agency. Washington, DC: National Academy Press.

Institute of Medicine (1999). *Veterans and Agent Orange: Update 2000*. Third Biennial Update by the Committee to Review the Health Effects in Vietnam Veterans of Exposure to Herbicides. Washington, DC: National Academy Press.

Jackson, J. L., Kroenke, K. and Chamberlin, J. (1999). Effects of physician awareness of symptom-related expectations and mental disorders: A controlled trial. *Archives of Family Medicine*, **8**, 135–142.

Kaminski, M. (2000). Dutch government decides to treat battlefield as a hazardous workplace. *Wall Street Journal*, April 17, p. 1.

Katon, W., Lin, E., Von Korff, M., *et al.* (1991). Somatization: A spectrum of severity. *American Journal of Psychiatry*, **148**, 34–40.

Katon, W., Von Korff, M., Lin, E., *et al.* (1997). Population-based care of depression: Effective disease management strategies to decrease prevalence. *General Hospital Psychiatry*, **19**, 169–178.

Koppel, N. (2001). Uranium might taint water in Kosovo U.N. report says. *The Seattle Times*, March 14, A10.

Kouyanou, K., Pither, C. E. and Wessely, S. (1997). Iatrogenic factors and chronic pain. *Psychosomatic Medicine*, **59**, 597–604.

Kroenke, K. and Price, R. K. (1993). Symptoms in the community: Prevalence, classification, and psychiatric comorbidity. *Archives of Internal Medicine*, **153**, 2474–2480.

Kroenke, K,. Spitzer, R. L., Williams, J. B., *et al.* (1994). Physical symptoms in primary care: Predictors of psychiatric disorders and functional impairment. *Archives of Family Medicine*, **3**, 774–779.

Kroenke, K. and Swindle, R. (2000). Cognitive–behavioral therapy for somatization and symptom syndromes: A critical review of controlled clinical trials. *Psychotherapy and Psychosomatics*, **69**, 205–215.

Lin, E. H., Katon, W., Von Korff, M., *et al.* (1991). Frustrating patients: Physician and patient perspectives among distressed high users of medical services. *Journal of General Internal Medicine*, **6**, 241–246.

Loganovsky, K. N. (2000). Vegetative–vascular dystonia and osteoalgetic syndrome or chronic fatigue syndrome as a characteristic after-effect of radioecological disaster: The Chernobyl accident experience. *Journal of Chronic Fatigue Syndrome*, **7**, 3–16.

Mazur, A. (1998). *A Hazardous Inquiry: The Rashomon Effect at Love Canal*. Cambridge, MA: Harvard University Press.

McCain, G. A., Bell, D. A., Mai, F. M. and Halliday, P. D. (1988). A controlled study of the effects of a supervised cardiovascular fitness training program on the manifestations of primary fibromyalgia. *Arthritis and Rheumatism*, **31**, 1135–1141.

Moss, J. (1998). *Possible Potentiation of Pyridostigmine Bromide by Pesticides*. Report of the Special Investigation Unit on Gulf War Illnesses, Committee on Veterans' Affairs: United States Senate. Washington, DC: US Government Printing Office.

Murphy, K. (2001). Exxon Oil Spill's Cleanup Crews Share Years of Illness. Workers say chemical exposure left them debilitated. Firm insists toxicity was low. *Los Angeles Times*, November 5, p. A1.

O'Malley, P. G., Jackson, J. L., Santoro, J., *et al.* (1999). Antidepressant therapy for unexplained symptoms and symptom syndromes. *Journal of Family Practice*, **48**, 980–990.

Pope, A. M. and Tarlov, A. R. (eds.) (1991). *Disability in America: Toward a National Agenda for Prevention*. Washington, DC: National Academy Press.

Powell, P., Bentall, R. P., Nye, F. J. and Edwards, R. H. (2001). Randomized controlled trial of patient education to encourage graded exercise in chronic fatigue syndrome. *British Medical Journal*, **322**, 387–390.

Price, J. R. and Cooper, J. (2002). Cognitive behaviour therapy for adults with chronic fatigue syndrome. In *Cochrane Database of Systematic Reviews*. Oxford: Update Software.

Prins, J. B., Bleijenberg, G., Bazelmans, E., *et al.* (2001). Cognitive behaviour therapy for chronic fatigue syndrome: A multicentre randomised controlled trial. *Lancet*, **357**, 841–847.

Quill, T. E. (1985). Somatization disorder: One of medicine's blind spots. *Journal of the American Medical Association*, **254**, 3075–3079.

Roland, P. S., Haley, R. W., Yellin, W., *et al.* (2000). Vestibular dysfunction in Gulf War syndrome. *Otolaryngology, Head and Neck Surgery*, **122**, 319–329.

Rose, G. (1992). *The Strategy of Preventive Medicine*. New York: Oxford University Press.

Rosenberg, H. L. (1980). *Atomic Soldiers: American Victims of Nuclear Experiments*. Boston, MA: Beacon Press.

Schuster, M. A., Stein, B. D., Jaycox, L. H., *et al.* (2001). A national survey of stress reactions after the September 11, 2001, terrorist attacks. *New England Journal of Medicine*, **345**, 1507–1512.

Smith, G. R., Jr, Rost, K. and Kashner, T. M. (1995). A trial of the effect of a standardized psychiatric consultation on health outcomes and costs in somatizing patients. *Archives of General Psychiatry*, **52**, 238–243.

Speckens, A. E., van Hemert, A. M., Spinhoven, P., *et al.* (1995). Cognitive behavioural therapy for medically unexplained physical symptoms: A randomized controlled trial. *British Medical Journal*, **311**, 1328–1332.

Summerfield, D. (2001). The invention of post-traumatic stress disorder and the social usefulness of a psychiatric category. *British Medical Journal*, **322**, 95–98.

Twemlow, S. W., Bradshaw, S. L. J., Coyne, L. and Lerma, B. H. (1997). Patterns of utilization of medical care and perceptions of the relationship between doctor and patient with chronic illness including chronic fatigue syndrome. *Psychological Reports*, **80**, 643–658.

Uijt de Haag, P. A., Smetsers, R. C., Witlox, H. W., Krus, H. W. and Eisenga, A. H. (2000). Evaluating the risk from depleted uranium after the Boeing 747-258F crash in Amsterdam, 1992. *Journal of Hazardous Materials*, **76**, 39–58.

Von Korff, M. and Moore, J. C. (2001). Stepped care for back pain: Activating approaches for primary care. *Annals of Internal Medicine*, **134**, 911–917.

Von Korff, M. and Simon, G. (1996). The relationship between pain and depression. *British Journal of Psychiatry*, **30** (Suppl.), 101–108.

Wagner, E. H. (2000). The role of patient care teams in chronic disease management. *British Medical Journal*, **320**, 569–572.

Wagner, E. H. and Austin, B. T. and Von Korff, M. (1996). Organizing care for patients with chronic illness. *Milbank Quarterly*, **74**, 511–544.

Walker, E. A., Katon, W. J., Keegan, D., Gardner, G. and Sullivan, M. (1997). Predictors of physician frustration in the care of patients with rheumatological complaints. *General Hospital Psychiatry*, **19**, 315–323.

Walker, E. A., Unutzer, J. and Katon, W. J. (1998). Understanding and caring for the distressed patient with multiple medically unexplained symptoms. *Journal of the American Board of Family Practice*, **11**, 347–356.

Wearden, A. J., Morriss, R. K., Mullis, R., *et al.* (1998). Randomized, double-blind, placebo-controlled treatment trial of fluoxetine and graded exercise for chronic fatigue syndrome. *British Journal of Psychiatry,* **172,** 485–490.

Wessely, S., Rose, S. and Bisson, J. (1999). Brief psychological interventions ('debriefing') for treating immediate trauma-related symptoms and preventing post-traumatic stress disorder. In *Cochrane Database of Systematic Reviews.* Oxford: Update Software.

Williams, T. D. (2001). Departing national guard troops won't receive anthrax vaccination. *Hartford Courant,* June 13, p. 3.

17

Traumatic death in terrorism and disasters: The effects on posttraumatic stress and behavior

Robert J. Ursano, James E. McCarroll, and Carol S. Fullerton

Introduction

Terrorism and disasters are not in frequent occurrences in the present-day world. Common to the these events is the likelihood of violent death and the presence of human remains – burned, dismembered, mutilated, or relatively intact. Exposure to mass death as well as individual dead bodies is a disturbing and sometimes frightening event. The nature of the stress of exposure to traumatic death and the dead and its relationship to posttraumatic stress disorder (PTSD) and other posttraumatic psychiatric illnesses is not well understood (Breslau and Davis, 1987; Lindy *et al.*, 1987; Ursano, 1987; Rundell *et al.*, 1989; Ursano and McCarroll, 1990) (Table 17.1).

The tasks of body recovery, identification, transport, and burial may require prolonged as well as acute contact with mass death. Recent research has shown that victims, onlookers, and rescue workers are traumatized by the experience or expectation of confronting death in disaster situations (Taylor and Frazer, 1982; Miles *et al.*, 1984; Schwartz, 1984; Jones, 1985; Dyregrov *et al.*, 1996). Exposure to abusive violence (Laufer *et al.*, 1984) and to the grotesque (Green *et al.*, 1989) significantly contributes to the development of psychiatric symptoms in war veterans, particularly intrusive imagery (Lifton, 1973; Laufer *et al.*, 1985; Clohessy and Ehlers, 1999).

Initial studies on the effects of handling the dead were observational with few systematic descriptions of the differences that occur at various stages through the process, or group or individual differences in responses. Hersheiser and Quarantelli (1976) reported on how the dead were treated by the living following a flood. They observed increasing respect for the body through the phases of search, recovery, identification, and preparation for burial. Taylor and Frazer (1982) reported that about one-third of the volunteers who recovered bodies from the Mount Erebus air crash in Antarctica experienced transient problems of moderate to severe

Table 17.1 Mediators of the stress of traumatic death

Anticipated stress of exposure to traumatic death
Previous experience
Gender
Volunteer status
Somatic symptoms
Identification
Exposure
Management practices

intensity, at 3 months, and one-fifth continued to report high levels of stress-related symptoms.

In a survey of 592 US Air Force personnel involved in the recovery, transport, and identification of the bodies of the Jonestown, Guyana mass suicide, Jones (1985) found that youth, inexperience, lower rank, and greater exposure to the dead were associated with higher levels of emotional distress. Higher rates of dysphoria were also found in blacks compared to whites, possibly due to greater identification with the black victims by the black body-handlers.

During the past two decades there have been a number of studies of the effects of handling remains on military personnel in disasters (Leffler and Dembert, 1998) and war (McCarroll et al., 1993a, 1995b; Sutker et al., 1994), police and firefighters (Fullerton et al., 1992; Bryant and Harvey, 1996; Regehr et al., 2000), and disaster workers (Marmar et al., 1996; Leffler and Dembert, 1998; Clohessy and Ehlers, 1999). In all these situations there are examples of the fact that regardless of profession or past experience, exposure to violent death can create psychological distress and contribute to psychiatric disorders (Miles et al., 1984).

Some studies show no negative effects from handling remains (Alexander and Wells, 1991; Thompson and Solomon, 1991; Alexander, 1993b). Alexander (1993b) hypothesized that organization and managerial practices were able to mediate adverse posttraumatic reactions in experienced police body-handlers. Thompson and Solomon (1991) also speculated that the management of the participants affected the relative lack of adverse outcomes in a sample of police officers. The officers were well trained and prepared for the task and were monitored throughout the procedure and thereafter, showing concern of management for their welfare.

Mediators of the stress of exposure to mass death

Anticipation of exposure and the effects of previous experience

Anticipation of exposure to death is itself a potent stressor that can be debilitating and affect performance, behavior, and health (Table 17.1). The disaster worker anticipates the stress of upcoming work before it actually begins and may already begin work with a substantial stress burden. Ersland *et al.* (1989) reported that waiting time was a frequently reported stressor among professional firefighters. Disaster workers may wait minutes to days after notification before they actually begin their rescue work. In interviews of disaster workers, we have heard stories of extended periods of waiting and high levels of stress. For example, novice rescue workers recruited to remove bodies from a plane that had caught fire and burned after landing had to wait several hours while wooden supports were put under the wings of the plane so it would not collapse.

The stress of anticipation has important psychological and physiological effects. In a group of military personnel with no previous experience in handling remains, females had a significantly higher level of anticipated stress than males (Mitchell *et al.*, 1958; Arthur, 1987; Susnowski, 1988). However, when experienced men and women were compared, there were no differences in anticipated stress (McCarroll *et al.*, 1993a, d).

Previous experience with a stressful event has been shown to reduce the effects of the stressor. In studies of parachute jumpers (Fenz and Epstein, 1967) and pilots (Drinkwater *et al.*, 1968; Mefferd *et al.*, 1971), those with less experience reported higher levels of fear and anxiety than experienced persons. The relationship between experience and psychological responses in disaster workers has been documented; however, the mechanisms underlying this relationship has not been closely examined. Experienced disaster workers consistently show lower stress following a disaster than do nonexperienced workers. Ersland and colleagues (1989) found that a higher proportion of nonprofessional rescuers than professionals reported poor mental health 9 months after recovering victims from an oil-rig collapse at sea. The more experienced rescuers were less likely to have poor mental health than the less experienced rescuers.

Weisaeth (1989) observed that a high level of disaster training or experience was significantly correlated with optimal behavior during the disaster. Firefighters experienced in mass disasters had lower stress responses after the event than did nonprofessional firefighters (Hytten and Hasle, 1989). The long-term effects of past experience and training are less clear. During the first week after a disaster, professional rescue workers had significantly greater unpleasant feelings than nonprofessionals; however, the reverse was true 9 months after the disaster (Lundin and Bodegard, 1993). Weisaeth's (1989) study of disaster behavior among survivors of an industrial explosion suggested that training and experience were extremely powerful variables in predicting health outcome. Persons who had experienced severe flooding in southeastern Kentucky had fewer symptoms than those who had not experienced floods (Norris and Murrell, 1988). Norris and Murrell (1988) interpreted these findings as evidence for stress inoculation and emphasized the advantages of prior experience with a stressor.

In a study of inexperienced and professional workers who recovered the bodies of children from a bus accident, voluntary (inexperienced) helpers reported significantly more intrusion and avoidance at 1 month and more avoidance at 13 months (Dyregrov *et al.*, 1996).

In a group of forensic dentists working with the remains following the Waco, Texas disaster, coworker support was significantly higher for experienced dentists than for those who were inexperienced in handling remains (McCarroll *et al.*, 1996). Interestingly, spouse support was significantly related to lower levels of stress symptoms in the inexperienced dentists but not in those with more experience (McCarroll *et al.*, 1996). These findings challenge the belief that highly trained professionals are immune from the posttraumatic stress of body recovery and identification.

Anticipated stress is an important, but often overlooked, aspect of disaster and rescue work. The stress burden clearly begins well before actual exposure (McCarroll *et al.*, 1992a). This also provides an opportunity for predisaster training and intervention. Predisaster counseling may be effective in part through its effects on anticipated stress (Myers, 1989). High levels of anticipated stress may also contribute to fatigue and thus to other disease conditions. Lower anticipated stress may be a mechanism through which experience and training contribute to decreased fatigue, increased performance, and decreased risk of adverse psychological effects in experienced disaster workers.

Volunteer status, somatic symptoms, identification with the dead, and exposure

In a study of military personnel anticipating working with the dead of the Gulf War, volunteer status was related to lower psychological distress and intrusive and avoidance symptoms (McCarroll *et al.*, 1993b, 1995c). More studies are needed in order to better understand the relationship of volunteer status in disaster and rescue workers.

Somatic symptoms are common after exposure to death and the dead (Ursano *et al.*, 1995). Interestingly, somatic symptoms were not explained by depressive symptoms present before exposure in a group of body handlers (McCarroll *et al.*, 2002). Body-handlers working in the mortuary after the USS *Iowa* gun turret explosion in 1989 showed intrusive and avoidant symptoms elevated at 1, 4, and 13 months but these symptoms decreased over time (Ursano *et al.*, 1995). Probable PTSD was present in 11 percent at 1 month, 10 percent at 4 months, and 2 percent at 13 months while depression was not increased (Ursano *et al.*, 1995).

Identification is an important mechanism in the stress–illness relationship (Ursano *et al.*, 1999). In research on mortuary workers who handled remains from the USS *Iowa* explosion, three types of identification in mortuary workers were examined: identification with the self ('It could have been me'), a friend ('It could have been a friend'), and a family member ('It could have been a family member').

Interestingly, those who identified with the deceased as a friend were more likely to have PTSD, more intrusive and avoidant symptoms, and somatization.

The duration (or degree) of exposure to the dead is an important predictors of posttraumatic stress reactions. In studies of mortuary workers during Operation Desert Storm the amount of exposure to the dead was associated with posttraumatic symptoms (McCarroll *et al.*, 1993a, 1995b). These two longitudinal studies found that body-handlers had significantly higher levels of intrusion and avoidance symptoms at 3–5 months and 13–15 months after the war than comparison group. In the group of forensic dentists who identified the bodies of the Branch Davidians in Waco, distress was significantly related to the hours of exposure to the remains as well as past experience working with remains, age, and the support received from spouses and coworkers during the body identification process (McCarroll *et al.*, 1996). Levels of symptomatic distress in emergency service workers were positively related to the degree of exposure to the critical incident, and to the severity and type of activities including working with dead bodies (Weiss *et al.*, 1995).

In the only study examining pre–post responses of mortuary workers handling bodies, intrusion and avoidance symptoms were measured in four groups of workers based on their degree of exposure to the remains (McCarroll *et al.*, 2001). When age, sex, volunteer status, and experience were controlled, postexposure intrusion symptoms increased significantly for all groups exposed to the dead and avoidance symptoms increased in the two groups with the most exposure. Importantly, these longitudinal studies of the Gulf War mortuary which allowed for preevent data collection have also shown that even after controlling for symptoms expressed in anticipation of exposure to the dead, exposure itself increased posttraumatic symptoms (McCarroll *et al.*, 2001).

Nature of the stress of exposure to death

In order better to understand the nature of the stress experienced by exposure to traumatic death, we compiled observations, interviews, and empirical data from over 1000 disaster body-handlers (Cervantes, 1988; Maloney, 1988a, b; Robinson, 1988; Ursano and McCarroll, 1990; Ursano *et al.*, 1990, 1992, 1995; McCarroll *et al.*, 1993a, c, 1995b, 1996).

Disturbing bodies

Nearly everyone experiences viewing and contact with children's bodies as stressful regardless of the age or sex of the body handler or whether he or she has children (Table 17.2). Children's bodies were reported as difficult because they 'appeared innocent,' were 'complete victims,' or they had 'untimely deaths.' 'They have not

Table 17.2 Nature of the stress of exposure to traumatic death

---

Children's bodies
Natural-looking bodies
Sensory stimuli
Novelty, surprise, and shock
Identification and emotional involvement
Personal effects
Friendly-fire death
Female combat deaths
Accidental deaths
Enemy dead

---

yet lived.' 'They had no control over it.' Pathologists described increased levels of stress associated with doing autopsies on children.

In the Gander, Newfoundland, US Army plane crash in Christmas week, 1985, the discovery of toys in the wreckage sent waves of anxiety and concern through the disaster workers as they worried that children had been on the plane. None, in fact, were on board.

Natural-looking bodies and ones with no apparent cause of death were also reported as being particularly disturbing. Bodies that were fully clothed and not obviously injured were described as 'eerie.' An anonymous participant reported:

I would say that it was probably more difficult for me to deal with remains that had a single gunshot wound or single penetration that we knew were going to go home viewable; more so than an air crash where the remains were severely charred or decomposed. I think we key on the face of that person. If there isn't a face or a head, it seemed like the whole focal point of expression was gone. In the case of — who had a single shrapnel wound to the neck, we knew he was going home, out of the war, because of a little damn piece of metal, a fragment. I think it probably bothered me to see how sensitive life is to foreign objects compared to a hell of a crash or an explosion, which tears you up.

V. R. Pine (personal communication, 1988) reported that in cases of the 'untouched, but dead, everybody stops.' He reported a case in which a beautiful young woman, who had died in a plane crash, appeared natural to a recovery worker. However, her feet had been underneath the seat rack and had been torn off leaving only two stumps for legs. When the disaster worker saw this, he yelled, 'Jesus Christ!' Badly burned bodies, 'floaters' (bodies that had lain in water for a long time), and decapitated bodies were vivid in people's memory.

Rescuers may consciously avoid the fact of being in contact with a dead body. A police harbor unit diver recalled his first underwater contact with the foot of a body: 'I hoped it was just a sneaker' . . . feeling the ankle I thought, 'Let it be just a boot' . . . feeling the leg, 'Please, God, let it just be a wader.' This concern was also expressed by a firefighter: 'A lot of firemen don't want to recognize a dead infant. One fireman went into a room full of smoke and felt around, touched the dead infant, and said it was a dog.'

Wearing gloves to handle the bodies, even by rescue workers unlikely to touch bodies, was reported by many. It seemed to serve both a real and an imagined protective role. The gloves, in some settings, also became a symbol of being a member of this special group – the body-handlers.

Sensory stimulation

Profound sensory stimulation is an extremely bothersome aspect of body-handling. The smell of the body(ies) was often noted; visual and tactile sensitivity were also reported. One body-handler at Dover Air Force Base was concerned about not being able to 'wash the smell away.' He wondered if the odor was real or 'in my head.' In fact, there was very little odor with these bodies since they were frozen due to the snow and cold in Gander. Individuals who reported working with the bodies from the Jonestown mass suicide and those who worked with the Marine bodies from the Beirut bombing in 1985 felt greatly disturbed by the overwhelming odor of these already decaying bodies. The rescuers frequently tried to mask the odor with burning coffee, smoking cigars, working in the cold or using fragrances such as peppermint and orange oil.

Even when a volunteer was assigned to 'escort' a single body through the stages of the identification process, he or she was exposed to many more bodies just by working in the mortuary. Being exposed to many bodies contributed to the stress of the experience. Some volunteers described the sight of a large number of bodies as 'overwhelming,' including those who had prior experience with traumatic death doing police or emergency service work. One man reported, 'The bodies just kept coming and coming. It felt like you were surrounded,' and another said, 'It's hard not to look when you are surrounded; you are too tense to be bored. There were 15 dead bodies looking at me with their jaws cut open.'

The preparation and consumption of food was frequently difficult after exposure to traumatized bodies. Badly burned bodies were reported to look and smell like roast beef. After exposure to burned bodies many individuals, including members of our research team, avoid eating meat for weeks and months following exposure to the dead. To one body-handler, rice in brown gravy looked like maggots. Following the 1989 United plane crash in Sioux City, Iowa, one rescue worker reported that he had lost all sexual interest in women because he could not look at their bodies without being reminded of the dead females he had recovered from the site of the crash. Security police guarding the dead at Sioux City felt great discomfort when the wind blew blankets off the dead, exposing parts of the bodies.

One emergency medical service worker reported being particularly disturbed by the loud sound of a body thrown on a hard examining table, especially if the head struck the surface. She complained about the way the morgue workers handled the bodies of people she brought in. Many individuals reported persistent images of dead bodies or body parts, particularly if the bodies were burned or mutilated.

Novelty, surprise, and shock

In addition to the raw, offensive sensory stimulation, surprise, shock, and fear of the unexpected are disturbing aspects of handling dead bodies. When we asked a group of experienced military body-handlers how they would train a group of inexperienced people to retrieve bodies if they only had a day to do so, we were told, 'Tell them the worst. Make it so there are no surprises. Let them know what they are getting in for.'

The surprise and shock of seeing the victim's face when the body bag is opened was described by one subject: 'When our soldiers open that bag, they don't know what they are going to see!' Another man who handled bodies in Vietnam recalled that he was always upset when bodies were lying face down in body bags. The back of the head is very strong and usually intact regardless of the condition of the face. He was always frightened of what he might see when he turned the body over. Pathologists at Dover Air Force Base X-rayed the body bags before opening them in order to lessen the initial shock and surprise. They reported that seeing bodies at a crime scene was generally more difficult than seeing the same bodies in a laboratory where the setting was familiar and surprises were unlikely.

The opening of the first body bag at the mortuary after a disaster is nearly always a quiet, anxiety-filled event. One group of inexperienced body handlers during Operation Desert Storm physically moved 15–20 feet away from the body when the bag was opened, without anyone having spoken a word. When the body bag was fully open and there were no 'surprises,' they moved closer. One individual described having to recover a child's body for burial. When he initially picked up the body, he was disturbed by the way it felt in his arms because it reminded him of recently carrying one of his own children.

Identification and emotional involvement

Identification or 'emotional involvement' with the deceased produces a high degree of distress. Many subjects described identification, a sense of kinship with the body in different ways. Some reified identification in a magical way with guidance of how to act: in the same way that a body-handler took care of a body from the battlefield, someone would take care of him. A common reaction was, 'It could have been me.'

Children's bodies often stimulated a sense of emotional involvement. The viewers frequently reported thoughts such as, 'I remember when my kids were about that age.'

In the process of the physical identification of the remains, one of the most difficult jobs is working with the personal effects of the dead. That this can be true is often surprising to inexperienced managers of a temporary mortuary or collection site. It is sometimes believed that gruesome remains are more disturbing and, as a result, inexperienced persons are sometimes assigned to handle personal effects. In general, almost regardless of the nature of the property or the state of the remains, personal effects have the power to humanize the deceased. They provide a link between the disaster assistance volunteer or mortuary worker that is often not present until the remains again acquires a name or otherwise begins to take on human properties. Almost invariably, mortuary workers will remark about a watch that continues to run after the person is dead or a watch that stopped running at the moment of impact. Identification cards, rings, pictures, wallets, and letters are among the strongest reminders of the deceased's humanity since almost everyone has them. As contact with personal effects becomes more intimate and prolonged, the likelihood of them creating some disturbance for the worker, at least temporarily, is increased.

It was reported that, during the Vietnam War, handling the personal effects of the dead was more stressful for soldiers than working in the area that processed the remains for shipment home. As in other wars, some soldiers carried extensive collections of letters and photographs from loved ones. Graves registration personnel had to screen these items for objectionable material and the presence of blood or body fluids before they could be sent home. In reading these letters, some workers became disturbed, bothered by the feeling of knowing the family and the fact that they knew the soldier was dead and the family back home did not.

In Vietnam, we lost more of our people who dealt with personal property that had to read the letters and screen the personal effects, than the ones who actually worked with the hands on side of it . . . with human remains. That's something that a lot of people find hard to believe, but after you explain it to them, that a guy would sit there day after day reading those letters from a loved one. That would probably be more of a mental stress than those who worked with the deceased human remains from combat.

Say a guy got zapped after 11 months; he had 11 months worth of letters. Somebody had to sit down and physically read every one of those letters because they would be sent back to the next of kin. Those guys who worked on the personal property side, they would have to sit there and do that day after day, month after month, and finally, for some of them, the stress of getting emotionally involved with those people . . . anybody could. You know, you sit there day after day and read through a guy's stuff, especially if you've got children and if you've got any kind of feeling within you whatsoever . . . But some of them just couldn't cope with it. Some had to be sent back to the mortuary side and some had to be put back for reassignment.

And another reported:

We were just taking the personal effects off the remains and we had the soldier's billfold in our hands and here was a picture with his wife and two children. You know the impact that had on me! It just stopped me cold and I said something to the men. I said 'Isn't this God-awful that we know this soldier is dead and his wife and children are going to get that news in a matter of hours or days.'

The dead bodies of friends and acquaintances, as well as 'brothers in uniform,' were always disturbing. Pathologists had an unwritten rule that they would not do an autopsy on a friend. 'I wanted to remember him the way he was.' An officer in charge of a large graves registration facility in Vietnam reported, 'I always feared seeing somebody I knew.' A firefighter said: 'What makes the biggest impact is seeing a dead firefighter – it brings it home. You have to deal with the realities: you're here and he is not.' A body-handler who participated in the Grenada operation reported: 'Most of us had horrendous nightmares about escorting a friend or family member home in a casket.' A senior police official said:

I had a cop die in my arms. I still cannot get it out of my head. I didn't know him. It was 19—, up in—. He got shot in the back five times. I took him off the roof and got him down to the sixth floor and he died in my arms. I still can't get that out of my mind, still think about it once in awhile, if I hear a name or something comes out. But, I won't dwell on it. I just didn't like the idea that a brother I had worked with died in my arms.

At Dover Air Force Base, one group of body-handlers became very upset after working for weeks with the personal effects of one victim. They developed the fantasy that they knew the victim and his family. Another group became anxious when they saw features of the body (soot in throat, posture) which they thought indicated the individual had been alive after the crash. Experienced personnel, professionals and nonprofessionals, cautioned newcomers against becoming 'emotionally involved.' Most experienced workers could describe how they avoided emotional involvement. These body-handlers gave tips to new personnel such as 'Don't look at the face' or 'don't get emotionally involved.' 'Don't think of it as a person.'

At Sioux City, rescue workers reported distress when they saw handwritten materials in the wreckage. 'It meant someone wrote it. They had been alive.' Young workers, learning to work with the personal effects of Operation Desert Storm casualties, gingerly went through the personal effects, relaxing only when a more senior worker made it a standard routine with forms to complete.

Recovery of historic remains and personal effects

Remains of long-dead service members or other victims of trauma are often recovered through accidental means or through searches based on access to the former battlefield or new information. For example, remains are still being returned from the Pacific theater in World War II and, particularly, from the Vietnam War. The recovery and identification of these remains is generally much less stressful to mortuary workers that those from a recent war or tragedy. The workers who recover such remains usually have a great sense of pride and accomplishment, particularly when the result fills a missing piece in a family's life. The deceased are treated with special care and there is sometimes a sense of awe among the workers as they feel they are privileged in being the first to see a hero after a long rest. Feelings of exhilaration and excitement are often reported when there is a forensic puzzle to be solved.

However, responses to historic remains are not uniformly positive. The handling of personal effects of Holocaust victims and survivors has been seen as disturbing, especially to young, inexperienced workers (McCarroll *et al.*, 1995a).

Combat unique stresses

Death from friendly fire

The death of a soldier caused by an error of his/her comrades-in-arms is termed death by friendly fire. Such deaths occasionally also occur in civilian police work. Military commanders and troops generally realize that friendly-fire deaths are an unavoidable part of war. However, that does not remove the shock, remorse, and trauma of the experience. During ground combat, artillery fire may be called in by the assault force to hit a target that is very close. The artillery fire may fall short of the target and hit the assaulting troops. In extreme cases, assault troops have called in fire knowing that it would certainly hit them; they sacrificed themselves to accomplish their mission. Aircrews are never perfectly accurate in the engagement of their targets. Bombs can misfire or friendly forces be mistaken for enemy.

At times during Operation Desert Storm, body-handlers reacted to friendly-fire deaths as expected combat deaths, expressing that the fire was not intentional. The dead were comrades who had fallen in battle. A military officer who supervised body handlers at Dover Air Force Base during Operation Desert Storm expressed his anger by directing it at the fact that personnel killed by friendly fire did not receive the Purple Heart upon their death. His assumption expressed his feelings of the wastefulness of the death. In fact, these men did receive the Purple Heart. In other friendly-fire deaths, troops had been clearly marked by clothing, position, or vehicles and the deaths 'should not have happened.' The body-handlers reacted to these deaths with great anger and dismay.

Deaths of women in combat

The deaths of American military women in the Gulf War stirred disquiet among the body-handlers and supervisors. On looking back on the experience, one body-handler remarked, 'The first woman casualty was the hardest to handle.' The body-handlers had seen an interview with her on TV. This made her more real. The female's personal belongings were kept separate from the men's and were not handled through the usual procedures. Supervisors insisted that a female be present when the body of a dead female soldier was being identified. This angered the male body-handlers. Female bodies were kept completely wrapped and personnel involved in the identification procedures were kept to a minimum. The bodies of the men, although always treated with respect, were not required to have a male escort and the bodies were always left uncovered during the identification procedures.

The body of a pregnant woman killed in Panama in 1989 was kept separate from the other dead. The body-handlers treated her wooden casket as special. It was placed to the side and no bodies or boxes were stacked on top.

Accidental deaths

Accidental deaths which are due to avoidable accidents or clear misconduct were termed 'dumb deaths' by the observers. These deaths were reported to be particularly disquieting. The people had made it through combat and then were later killed while playing with munitions or handling weapons in an unsafe manner.

Enemy dead

American soldiers in Operation Just Cause in Panama reported few feelings about enemy dead. An exception was when several soldiers were going through the wallet of a dead Panamanian soldier and saw pictures of family, children, and a First Communion picture. They broke down and cried. They later went to see the chaplain to talk.

Personal threat

In a study of the anticipated stress of handling remains, personal threat to the body-handler was one of the significant clusters of concerns (McCarroll *et al.*, 1995d). In order to retrieve persons killed in combat, soldiers may have to endure hostile fire and remains may be booby-trapped.

In the response to the Pentagon attack, recovery workers were concerned about exposure to toxic materials such as jet fuel, dust, asbestos, and unknown contaminants. In addition to environmental contaminants, unexploded ordnance and other explosives, workers must contend with the possibility of the HIV virus and known and unknown pathogens. As a result, more protective equipment must be available and worn on a disaster scene. The wearing and maintenance of protective clothing and equipment sometimes requires extensive training. Such clothing and equipment also add to the weight burden of rescuers and produce fatigue faster than would normally be the case.

Table 17.3 Coping strategies used in exposure to traumatic and disaster-related death

Stressor	Coping strategy
Before exposure (waiting)	
Lack of information regarding tasks and roles	Briefing
Anticipating one's reaction to bodies	Inbriefing
	Gradual exposure
During exposure (on site)	
Sensory overload	Avoidance or attenuation of strong stimuli
Natural appearance of bodies	Disidentification and use of role
Handling victims' personal effects	Disidentification and use of role
Fatigue and overdedication (duration of exposure)	Work breaks, food, sleep, supervision
Intense personal feelings	Pairing with experienced personnel
	Supervisory support
	Humor
	Talking
Personal threat	Protective clothing, decontamination information
After exposure (postevent)	
Need for information	Debriefing
	Education
Intense feelings (e.g., sadness, alienation)	Debriefing
	Family and organizational support
	Awards

Coping

Coping strategies vary in the different stages of exposure to traumatic death and with the degree of experience of the body handler (Table 17.3).

Before the exposure

Few organizations practice their response to a disaster although such events are expectable. Only the timing is unpredictable. In the case of the crash of United Airlines Flight 232 in Sioux City in July 1989, an air crash disaster drill had been performed prior to the crash and was reported to have been very helpful. Inexperienced personnel who volunteer to help at a disaster site are rarely given more than a few hours to prepare themselves for what they will see and do (McCarroll *et al.*, 1992b).

People often reported feeling frightened of their own reactions to the bodies, asking themselves, 'Will I be able to handle it?' People who volunteered in pairs or larger groups thought that they could help each other get through the experience. Initial preparation by a supervisor, usually by an inbriefing, is essential for inexperienced volunteers. Our subjects were unanimous in saying that when volunteers enter a disaster scene, such as a mortuary, they should be 'told the worst' so as to minimize the surprises at the crash site or mortuary. In a recent disaster, a supervisor provided a sequence of short, staged preparation briefings in which he became more explicit as he moved volunteers from an initial assembly area to their eventual work site. This technique was reported afterwards to have been very helpful.

Experienced personnel expecting to be sent on an operation reported little psychological preparation. Nervousness was sometimes reported when they did not know what sort of trauma to expect, what condition the bodies were in, or how difficult it would be to extract or identify the victims. One experienced dental pathologist reported that, when he knew he had to be the only professional, he had nightmares the night before; when he knew he was going with others, he slept soundly.

During exposure to the dead (on site)

Individuals defend against the multiple sensory stimuli associated with the dead: the sights of the bodies (grotesque, burned, and mutilated); the sounds during autopsy (heads hitting tables and saws cutting bone); the smells of decomposing and burned bodies; and the tactile stimuli experienced as bodies are handled.

Workers often reported that they did not see badly damaged bodies as human. Supervisors facilitated this process of 'disidentification' by telling inexperienced volunteers, 'Don't think of it as a body; think of it as a job.' Natural-looking bodies were often seen as all too human. Such remarks as, 'He can't be dead; he hardly has a scratch on him,' were common. People reported many internal, automatic strategies by which they distanced themselves from the bodies such as by not looking at faces.

As mentioned previously, many people attempted to mask odors by burning coffee, smoking cigars, working in the cold, and using fragrances such as peppermint oil and orange oil inside surgical masks (Cervantes, 1988). Most reported that such strategies did not help much in reducing the odors. Some olfactory adaptation did occur and workers generally dropped these strategies over time. Personnel who touched the bodies or body parts wore gloves. This decreased the tactile contact with the remains, which was particularly difficult with decomposed and burned bodies.

Past experience was frequently reported as helpful but it did not make one invulnerable. Even very experienced personnel could be shocked or surprised by the sight of the grotesque. An experienced pathologist reported extreme discomfort at the sight of a body whose shoulder girdle had been cleanly sliced by a helicopter blade. When he first saw the body, he did not recognize what had happened. When he did recognize the injury, he wondered whether the individual had felt the cut, suffered, or lived long after the injury. He continued to have intrusive images of this scene. Even a nonhuman body can produce discomfort. Pine (personal communication, 1988) reported a person who was very distressed at finding a dead pet dog in the luggage compartment of a commuter aircraft crash. The person said that he 'could not handle' the dead dog and was distressed because he knew others would not take it seriously.

Physical fatigue was a frequent and significant stressor due to the long and irregular hours, little sleep, poor eating schedules, moving heavy loads, and minimal time to recuperate. The stress of the experience was reported to be reduced when the individual took frequent breaks or the supervisor acted to decrease the visual contact with bodies, such as by providing chairs that faced away from the bodies, or putting partitions between the identification stations. Overdedication contributed to the tendency to go on working under conditions that normally would not be tolerated. Even though breaks were seen as desirable, at the Dover mortuary following the Gander air crash, for example, many individuals worked up to 20 hours per day. Managers had to require some people to leave the area.

Some workers voluntarily left the scene because of nausea, fatigue, or psychological discomfort. This did not always mean that the person was going to be ineffective. A senior noncommissioned officer reported:

I talked to some of the guys who worked Gander. There were days when they'd go in there and they would pick up an arm or a leg and they'd start thinking about what that arm used to be attached to and the fact that it was all burned up. They would have to walk outside of those plastic tents that they were working out of and sit down and have coffee, smoke a few cigarettes and just walk away for a day because on that particular day their psyche was not enough to deal with what they were seeing that day. The next day they were OK.

In general, grief and upset *per se* are not often observed on site because of feelings about one's public image. Most workers were concerned about how they would look in front of the other workers, both supervisors and subordinates. No one wanted to look like they 'couldn't handle it.' In response to the question of 'What if the leaders are not able to be macho that day? Do you lose faith in them?' The answer from an experienced team leader was:

No, no, no! You can't lose faith in them. You have to talk to them and let them talk to you. 'What was it that bothered you on that case?' Tell them that it's OK to get sick or say 'Hey! I can't deal with it today.' Because their psyche won't allow them to deal with that body that day, we can't think any less of them because tomorrow it might be our turn.

Unfortunately, such an attitude is not always present. We heard stories of supervisors laughing when someone said they 'couldn't take it.'

Everyone recognized humor as a substantial tension-reducer during and after operations. Humor was more common when the workers were out of public view. Most humor was very respectful. Some body-handlers were frightened of 'black humor,' feeling it reflected 'having gone over the edge,' and becoming too hardened. The professional role identity of individuals who handled the dead also facilitated coping with the psychological stress. The professional role was usually well defined. For nonprofessionals, roles had to be defined and reinforced by others. Often, a good time to define roles was during the inbriefing where the importance of each person's job was emphasized. For most volunteers, the idea that they were performing an important service for the dead, the families of the dead, and the community was very important.

The role of the medical examiner is well defined and of recognized importance. Curiosity and a sense of detective work helped sustain the medical examiners. They were frequently cautioned against becoming emotionally involved in their cases because their objectivity might be questioned in court. Their education to 'be objective' served a protective function. In some situations, however, they were not able to avoid emotional involvement. Most reported that they did not like to do autopsies on children, friends, family members, or torture deaths in which the suffering of the individual was obvious.

The mortician strives to do everything right because of the families. He takes pride in the cosmetic treatment of the deceased. This goal reinforced the idea that something memorable would be given to the survivors. The complexities of the physician confronting death are described by Cassem (1999).

The fire, police, and emergency medical service personnel we interviewed were strongly motivated by the opportunity to save lives. Deaths often caused them to question their competence. In a fire rescue company, when occupants of a house were found dead, the firefighters said to each other, 'They were dead before the bells went off!', meaning that the victims had probably died before the fire alarm had even sounded and they were not to blame.

The leader and the work group were inevitably seen as sources of support during difficult operations. The professional work group was the primary source of support. The presence of an experienced coworker, especially for the uninitiated, was important. A new individual could share the tasks and the feelings with an experienced partner and decrease the shock and surprise of the initial exposure.

A large urban search and rescue fire company reported a very high level of social support and unit cohesion. During each shift, about 12 people lived together in a room that served as a kitchen, a dining room, and a living room at the rear of the firehouse near the vehicles. They were proud of their comradery fact that: 'We're like a family! We provide psychological first aid to each other – reassurance. All he (the guy next to you on the line) needs is the reassurance of someone else nearby.'

Workers always noticed the support or lack of support by senior leaders and the organization as a whole. Volunteer body handlers at Dover Air Force Base after the Gander disaster were alert to whether their supervisor visited or their senior commanders expressed support (Maloney, 1988b).

After exposure (postevent)

Disaster workers often needed help in the hours or days shortly after exposure to the dead. During this time, volunteers reported high levels of discomfort, both physical and psychological. Fatigue, irritability, and a need for a transition 'back to the real world' were commonly expressed. Experienced persons described themselves as doing what they had to in their mortuary work in order to get the job done; however, it was often at a high personal cost. The experience of professional support frequently came from a 'critique' of the technical aspects of the work. One firefighter pointed out that this sort of discussion had: 'Two phases – an individual phase and a group phase. You find out months or years later that something had bothered someone and you never found out about it before – he never talked about it. You argue about what had been wrong.'

For almost everyone, professional counseling or psychiatric assistance, even if available, was generally viewed as unacceptable. Often this was due to fears that the person would be fired, could not successfully testify in court, would be ridiculed by fellow workers, or would lose their job. Most said they did not really feel the need for counseling; however, almost all of those interviewed said they could have benefited from a brief talk about the experience, particularly if it involved the work group. Some wished it had even been mandatory.

For the volunteer body-handlers unusual events often triggered intense feelings. While viewing a memorial service on television one man reported: 'I felt the grief they [the families] were going through. They started naming names – when they came to mine [the body he had escorted through the identification process]; I went in the bathroom and cried and cried.' Another reported: 'Memorial services interfere with coping. At that point, it's no longer a job; it gets to be a name, a human being. You can't do both at the same time. You associate everything you do with each person. It all comes together.'

Spouses of the body-handlers were frequently unwilling to hear about the workers' experiences. At other times the workers themselves decided not to talk to their spouses about their disaster work. One man reported that his wife required him to take his clothes off at the door and shower after working with remains. Others described the stress of their first (and sometimes only) attempt at sharing feelings about their work with their spouses. Some said that they were unlikely to repeat the experience.

The return to work was difficult for many, particularly when coworkers were not sympathetic or sensitive. Most workers appreciated some time off after the job was over. Some wanted to have time with their families; others wanted time alone.

There was generally a feeling that those who had not been at the site could not fully understand the experience. This contributed to the difficulty of talking about the experience. People who came by the mortuary for only a visit were called 'turistas.'

Consistent with other reports (Maloney, 1988a, b; Robinson, 1988), in the aftermath of an incident, alcohol use was widely reported. Some workers reported that large amounts were consumed without intoxication while others reported that 'getting smashed' was normal at the end of each day of an operation. Drinking also provided a social context for the work group, and an opportunity to receive and provide support to each other. Some military workers reported that when the troops were restricted to one beer per evening, the restriction did not apply to body-handlers. When several individuals were ordered away from a disaster site for rest, they reported returning to their rooms and drinking alcohol.

Discussion

Exposure to traumatic death is common in natural and human-made disasters and is a significant psychological stressor that can make victims of rescuers. The rescue worker is traumatized through the senses: viewing, smelling, and touching, experiencing the grotesque, the unusual, the novel and the untimeliness of the death. The stress of body-handling begins prior to the exposure with the anticipation. Nonvolunteers and those with no previous experience appear to experience more distress during this time. The extent and intensity of the sensory properties of the body such as visual grotesqueness, smell, and tactile qualities are important aspects of the stressor. It may be heuristically useful to consider exposure to human remains as a special category of toxic exposure in which such dimensions as the type of agent, frequency, intensity and duration of exposure all add to the risk of later stress reactions (Bartone et al., 1989), breakdown, disease, or even psychological growth. Exposure to a child's mutilated body appears to be extremely toxic regardless of the body-handler's age or whether she or he has children.

There is often a paradox in people's reactions to traumatic material. Reactions tend to be both idiosyncratic as well as common. That is, one can predict that which is disturbing to most people (e.g., children's bodies, personal effects such as pictures, and a sense of revulsion at putrid smells), but there is also usually a personal reaction that is unique to the person. People will notice certain aspects of exposure to the dead that are not common. For example, an experienced forensic pathologist was somewhat bothered by a reaction to the bodies of victims that had been wrapped in gauze due to the fact that they were unviewable. When workers carried them, they reminded him of rag dolls, but he knew that they were not. Another person upon seeing the distended jaws of dead victims who had had their jaw muscles cut for dental identification thought that the faces looked like clowns.

Although all sensory modalities are involved in contact with a body, odor may have the highest potential to recreate significant past episodes in a person's life. The strength of memory appears to vary with the special involvement a person has with the odor (Engen, 1987). The amount of forgetting of olfactory recognition memory, both long and short term is very small and, thus, the accurate recognition of odors when encountered again is very high (Engen *et al.*, 1973; Engen, 1987). While odors are easily recognized, they are very difficult to recall at will, which is fortunate for most persons exposed to the smells of death. One can easily remember the color and shape of an apple, but not its smell. There is a need for those who prepare food to be aware of the power of olfactory memory to vividly recreate a scene and for reliving some portion of the experience. Even though the recall of olfactory memory is relatively poor, we were informed of two cases of individuals who had served as body-handlers at the Jonestown disaster who later received medical discharges from the military for PTSD. A complaint common to both individuals was waking up at night with a vivid recollection of the smells of the bodies at Jonestown (D. T. Orman, personal communication, 1989).

The meaning or social context of a death is an additional dimension of the stress felt by the individual body-handler. For example, the death of a drug dealer arouses less sympathy among policemen or medical examiners regardless of the condition of the body. The innocent, who are seen as victims, almost never fail to arouse feelings among those who deal with the remains. Interviewees who were body-handlers during the Vietnam War talked about the stress of handling a large number of bodies of soldiers killed in action in an unpopular war. Deaths caused by friendly fire were similarly stressful. The deaths of these soldiers often seemed to have been a tremendous waste, which contributed to feelings of depression and hopelessness among the disaster workers.

The role of identification and emotional involvement in the production and resolution of the stress of handling dead bodies requires further study. Working with personal effects is an infrequently recognized, powerful stimulus for identification and subsequent distress. Identification and feelings of 'knowing' the dead appear to heighten the trauma of the experience. Identification may serve to eliminate the unfamiliar and the unknown qualities of the dead – changing what is new and novel into something familiar and part of the past (Ursano and Fullerton, 1990). The 'switching on' of these cognitive mechanisms – identification, personalization, and emotional involvement – by the trauma of dead bodies requires further study. Whether certain individuals are more prone to this perceptual style or whether it represents a basic biological mechanism, which all individuals activate to a various degree, is unknown. Ways of decreasing identification and emotional involvement may be effective preventive measures for those who must be exposed to this traumatic stressor.

The coping strategies used by rescue personnel differ in the preevent, on-site, and postevent stages of the disaster work. An informative and role-setting inbriefing is critical to the adjustment of the volunteer. This briefing helps form the context for much of what is later felt and seen. When it is not provided, individuals have greater difficulty coping and often fare poorly. But no matter how well volunteers are briefed, there is always some shock to the reality of the situation.

The overwhelming nature of the sensory stimulation usually leads participants, particularly volunteers, to develop cognitive and behavioral distancing (avoidance) strategies. Failure to protect against emotional involvement with the victim is recognized by most workers as putting a person at risk for psychological distress. Scheduling is the job of the supervisor. Before fatigue sets in, which can contribute to emotional vulnerability, it is essential that managers establish schedules and insure that rescue workers follow them. While there is little that supervisors can do about alcohol abuse off site, they can inform participants that the potential for alcohol abuse is high following exposure to trauma.

Transition out of the rescue work after exposure appears to be facilitated by an outbriefing where the workers can ask questions and information can be provided about the event, the body identification process, and community reactions. Statements of appreciation and recognition made at this time aid recovery. Family and organizational support is central during the transition period. When both the family and the primary work group show sensitivity and caring, the participant appears more likely to verbalize his or her feelings regarding what has been seen and done.

The personal experience of trauma is usually private and personal. Often it does not result in an outpouring or any expression of feelings at all. Such reactions are often personal and unobserved (McCarroll *et al.*, 1995a). As a result, people often will not attend debriefing groups voluntarily or consult a mental health provider. Many rescue workers and volunteers will not share everything with people who were not present with them through the ordeal. Debriefing personnel after handling remains has been described (Thompson and Solomon, 1991; Alexander, 1993b). Empirical research has failed to consistently demonstrate that debriefing prevents postevent distress, indicating the need for further empirical research in this area (Gist *et al.*, 1997; Deahl, 2000; National Institute of Mental Health, 2002). Raphael and Wilson (2000) have extensively reviewed the topic of psychological debriefing. Alexander (1993a) cautions that while support groups are important, careful consideration must be given to the aims, methods, and composition. Along with the possibility of a positive effect, improperly run groups may have harmful effects. Groups with mixed exposure levels and ones that are only one-time events may be more likely to produce increased symptoms by exposure of those who are less exposed to the stories of those who are more exposed. It is important that outcomes other than PTSD be examined in debriefing studies, e.g., work absences, disability.

Numerous strategies are used to cope with the stresses of body-handling. Most appear to be effective in the short run; however, it is unclear which are more effective and what the long-term consequences are. Avoidance strategies appear to be effective during initial exposure to dead bodies. We do not know the effect of using such strategies over a longer time period. Reports from volunteers and experienced personnel indicate that, at some point, they can no longer avoid reminders of previous disasters. For example, names of the victims or the sight of an object bring the experience back. It is unclear whether such an experience is helpful or harmful. The triggering of memories may help to 'metabolize' the experience. On the other hand, the recall of unwanted memories can be disturbing and interfere with the present tasks. It remains an open question when and under what circumstances the individual should be encouraged to talk or think about aspects of the disaster that she or he wishes to avoid.

Spouses of disaster workers need to be educated about their loved one's experiences. Many workers claimed that they wished their spouses had been informed of the nature of their work. Information can be provided to spouses in order to allay their concerns. This will also reinforce this naturally occurring support system. Brief groups held for spouses can also be a useful intervention.

Nonexperienced workers may be at higher risk for acute effects than experienced personnel. The latter, however, are not immune from suffering the same psychological discomforts as the volunteers. Some experienced personnel reported becoming somewhat calloused through repeated exposure, but no one believed it possible to be totally desensitized.

Additional research of this powerful stressor is needed to further describe its components and better understand the role of sensory stimulation in recall, particularly in PTSD, and the normal 'metabolism' of traumatic events. Finally, it should be noted that not all effects from disaster rescue work and handling dead bodies are negative. Volunteers almost unanimously report that they would volunteer again if another disaster occurred. People were proud of their contribution and of having done an important job that others either could not do or would never have the opportunity to do. It has been previously reported that most people do quite well following exposure to massive trauma. An important theoretical as well as practical question is how people use trauma to move toward health (Ursano, 1987).

REFERENCES

Alexander, D. A. (1993a). Staff support groups: Do they support and are they even groups? *Palliative Medicine*, **7**, 127–132.

    (1993b). Stress among police body handlers. *British Journal of Psychiatry*, **163**, 806–808.

Alexander, D. A. and Wells, A. (1991). Reactions of police officers to body-handling after a major disaster: A before and after comparison. *British Journal of Psychiatry*, **159**, 547–555.

Arthur, A. Z. (1987). Stress as a state of anticipatory vigilance. *Perceptual and Motor Skills*, **64**, 75–85.

Bartone, P. T., Ursano, R. J., Wright, K. M. and Ingraham, L. H. (1989). The impact of a military air disaster on the health of assistance workers: A prospective study. *Journal of Nervous and Mental Disease*, **177**, 317–328.

Breslau, N. and Davis, G. C. (1987). Posttraumatic stress disorder – the stressor criterion. *Journal of Nervous and Mental Disease*, **175**, 255–264.

Bryant, R. A. and Harvey, A. G. (1996). Posttraumatic stress reactions in volunteer firefighters. *Journal of Traumatic Stress*, **9**, 51–62.

Cassem, N. (1999). Treating the person confronting death. In *Harvard Guide to Modern Psychiatry*, ed. A. M. Nicholi, Jr, pp. 699–731. Cambridge, MA: The Belknap Press of Harvard University Press.

Cervantes, R. (1988). Psychological stress of body handling. Part II and Part III: debriefing of Dover AFB personnel following the Gander tragedy and the body handling experience at Dover AFB. In *Exposure to Death, Disasters and Bodies*, eds. R. J. Ursano and C. Fullerton, pp. 125–162. Bethesda, MD: F. Edward Hebert School of Medicine, Uniformed Services University of the Health Sciences.

Clohessy, S. and Ehlers, A. (1999). PTSD symptoms, response to intrusive memories and coping in ambulance service workers. *British Journal of Clinical Psychology*, **38**, 251–265.

Deahl, M. P. (2000). Debriefing and body recovery: War grave soldiers. In *Psychological Debriefing*, eds. B. Raphael and J. P. Wilson, pp. 108–130. Cambridge: Cambridge University Press.

Drinkwater, B. L., Cleland, T. and Flint, M. M. (1968). Pilot performance during periods of anticipatory physical threat stress. *Aerospace Medicine*, **39**, 944–999.

Dyregrov, A., Kristoffersen, J. I. and Gjestad, R. (1996). Voluntary and professional disaster-workers: Similarities and differences in reactions. *Journal of Traumatic Stress*, **9**, 541–555.

Engen, T. (1987). Remembering odors and their names. *American Scientist*, **75**, 497–503.

Engen, T., Kuisma, J. E. and Eimas, P. D. (1973). Short-term memory of odors. *Journal of Experimental Psychology*, **99**, 222–225.

Ersland, S., Weisaeth, L. and Sund, A. (1989). The stress upon rescuers involved in an oil rig disaster: 'Alexander L. Kielland' (1980). *Acta Psychiatrica Scandinavica Supplementum*, **80**, 38–49.

Fenz, W. D. and Epstein, S. (1967). Gradients of physiological arousal in parachutists as a function of an approaching jump. *Psychosomatic Medicine*, **29**, 33–51.

Fullerton, C. S., McCarroll, J. E., Ursano, R. J. and Wright, K. M. (1992). Psychological responses of rescue workers: Fire fighters and trauma. *American Journal of Orthopsychiatry*, **62**, 371–378.

Gist, R., Lohr, J., Kenardy, J., (1997). Researchers speak out on CISM. *Journal of Emergency Medicine*, May, 27–28.

Green, B. L., Lindy, J. D., Grace, M. C. and Gleser, G. C. (1989). Multiple diagnosis in posttraumatic stress disorder: The role of war stressors. *Journal of Nervous and Mental Disease*, **177**, 329–335.

Hersheiser, M. R. and Quarantelli, E. L. (1976). The handling of the dead in a disaster. *Omega*, **7**, 195–208.

Hytten, K. and Hasle, A. (1989). Firefighters: A study of stress and coping. *Acta Psychiatrica Scandinavica Supplementum*, **355**, 50–55.

Jones, D. J. (1985). Secondary disaster victims: The emotional effects of recovering and identifying human remains. *American Journal of Psychiatry*, **142**, 303–307.

Laufer, R. S., Brett, E. and Gallops, M. S. (1985). Dimensions of posttraumatic stress disorder among Vietnam veterans. *Journal of Nervous and Mental Disease*, **173**, 538–545.

Laufer, R. S., Gallops, M. S. and Frey-Wouters, E. (1984). War stress and trauma. *Journal of Health and Social Behavior*, **25**, 65–85.

Leffler, C. T. and Dembert, M. L. (1998). Posttraumatic stress symptoms among U.S. Navy divers recovering TWA Flight 800. *Journal of Nervous and Mental Disease*, **186**, 574–577.

Lifton, R. J. (1973). *Home From the War.* New York: Simon and Schuster.

Lindy. J. D., Green, B. L. and Grace, M. C. (1987). The stressor criterion and posttraumatic stress disorder. *Journal of Nervous and Mental Disease*, **175**, 269–272.

Lundin, T. and Bodegard, M. (1993). The psychological impact of an earthquake on rescue workers: A follow-up study of the Swedish group of rescue workers in Armenia. *Journal of Traumatic Stress*, **6**, 129–139.

Maloney, J. (1988a). The Gander disaster: Body handling and identification process. In *Exposure to Death, Disasters and Bodies*, eds. R. J. Ursano and C. Fullerton, pp. 41–66. Bethesda, MD: F. Edward Hebert School of Medicine, Uniformed Services University of the Health Sciences.

Maloney, J. (1988b). Body handling at Dover AFB: The Gander disaster. In *Individual and Group Behavior in Toxic and Contained Environments*, eds. R. J. Ursano and C. Fullerton, pp. 97–102. Bethesda, MD: F. Edward Hebert School of Medicine, Uniformed Services University of the Health Sciences.

Marmar, C. R., Weiss, D. S., Metzler, T. J., Ronfeldt, H. and Foreman, C. (1996). Stress responses of emergency services personnel to the Loma Parieta earthquake Interstate 880 freeway collapse and control traumatic incidents. *Journal of Traumatic Stress*, **9**, 63–85.

McCarroll, J. E., Blank, A. S. and Hill, K. (1995a). Working with traumatic material: Effects on Holocaust Memorial Museum Staff. *American Journal of Orthopsychiatry*, **65**, 66–75.

McCarroll, J. E., Fullerton, C. S., Ursano, R. J. and Hermsen, J. M. (1996). Posttraumatic stress symptoms following forensic dental identification: Mt. Carmel, Waco, Texas. *American Journal of Psychiatry*, **153**, 778–782.

McCarroll, J. E., Ursano, R. J. and Fullerton, C. S. (1993a). Symptoms of posttraumatic stress disorder following recovery of war dead. *American Journal of Psychiatry*, **150**, 1875–1877.

McCarroll, J. E., Ursano, R. J. and Fullerton, C. S. (1995b). Symptoms of PTSD following recovery of war dead: 13–15 month follow-up. *American Journal of Psychiatry*, **152**, 939–941.

McCarroll, J. E., Ursano, R. J., Fullerton, C. S., Liu, X. and Lundy, A. (2001). Effect of exposure to death in a war mortuary on posttraumatic stress symptoms. *Journal of Nervous and Mental Disease*, **189**, 44–48.

McCarroll, J. E., Ursano, R. J., Fullerton, C. S., Liu, X. and Lundy, A. (2002). Somatic symptoms in Gulf War mortuary workers. *Psychosomatic Medicine*, **64**, 29–33.

McCarroll, J. E., Ursano, R. J., Fullerton, C. S. and Lundy, A. L. (1992a). *Dimensions of Stress Among Mortuary Workers.* Paper presented at the First World Conference, The International Society for Traumatic Stress Studies, Amsterdam, The Netherlands.

McCarroll, J. E., Ursano, R. J., Fullerton, C. S. and Lundy, A. (1993b). Traumatic stress of a wartime mortuary: Anticipation of exposure to mass death. *Journal of Nervous and Mental Disease*, **181**, 545–551.

McCarroll, J. E., Ursano, R. J., Fullerton, C. S. and Lundy, A. C. (1995c). Anticipatory stress of handling remains of the Persian Gulf War: Predictors of intrusion and avoidance. *Journal of Nervous and Mental Disease*, **183**, 698–703.

McCarroll, J. E., Ursano, R. J., Fullerton, C. S., *et al.* (1995d). Gruesomeness, emotional attachment, and personal threat: Dimensions of anticipated stress of body recovery. *Journal of Traumatic Stress*, **8**, 343–347.

McCarroll, J. E., Ursano, R. J., Fullerton, C. S. and Wright, K. M. (1992b). Community consultation following a major air disaster. *Journal of Community Psychology*, **20**, 271–275.

McCarroll, J. E., Ursano, R. J., Wright, K. M. and Fullerton, C. S. (1993c). Handling of bodies after violent death: Strategies for coping. *American Journal of Orthopsychiatry*, **63**, 209–214.

McCarroll, J. E., Ursano, R. J., Ventis, W. L., *et al.* (1993d). Anticipation of handling the dead: Effects of experience and gender. *British Journal of Clinical Psychology*, **32**, 466–468.

Mefford, R. B., Hale, H. B., Shannon, I. L., Prigmore, J. R. and Ellis, J. P. (1971). Stress responses as criteria for personnel selection: Baseline study. *Aerospace Medicine*, **42**, 42–51.

Miles, M. S., Demi, A. S. and Mostyn-Aker, P. (1984). Rescue workers' reactions following the Hyatt Hotel disaster. *Death Education*, **8**, 315–331.

Mitchell, J. H., Sproule, B. J. and Chapman, C. B. (1958). The physiological meaning of the maximal oxygen intake test. *Journal of Clinical Investigation*, **37**, 538–547.

Myers, D. G. (1989). Mental health and disaster. In *Psychosocial Aspects of Disaster*, eds. R. Gist and B. Lubin, pp. 190–228. New York: John Wiley and Sons.

National Institute of Mental Health (2002). *Mental Health and Mass Violence: Evidence Based Early Psychological Intervention For Victims/Survivors of Mass Violence: A Workshop to Reach Consensus on Best Practices*. NIH Publication No. 02-5138. Washington, DC: US Government Printing Office.

Norris, F. H. and Murrell, S. A. (1988). Prior experience as a moderator of disaster impact on anxiety symptoms in older adults. *Journal of Community Psychology*, **16**, 665–683.

Raphael, B. and Wilson, J. P. (2000). *Psychological Debriefing*. New York: Cambridge University Press.

Regehr, C., Hill, J. and Glancy, G. D. (2000). Individual predictors of traumatic reactions in firefighters. *Journal of Nervous and Mental Disease*, **188**, 333–339.

Robinson, M. (1988). Psychological support to the Dover AFB body handlers. In *Exposure to Death, Disasters and Bodies*, eds. R. J. Ursano and C. Fullerton, pp. 67–90. Bethesda, MD: F. Edward Hebert School of Medicine, Uniformed Services University of the Health Sciences.

Rundell, J. R., Ursano, R. J., Holloway, H. C. and Silberman, E. K. (1989). Psychiatric responses to trauma. *Hospital and Community Psychiatry*, **40**, 68–74.

Schwartz, H. J. (1984). Fear of the dead: The role of social ritual in neutralizing fantasies from combat. In *Psychotherapy of the Combat Veteran*, ed. H. J. Schwartz, pp. 253–267. New York: Spectrum Publications.

Susnowski, T. (1988). Patterns of skin conductance and heart rate changes under anticipatory stress conditions. *Journal of Psychophysiology*, **2**, 231–238.

Sutker, P. B., Uddo, M., Brailey, K., Vasterling, J. J. and Errera, P. (1994). Psychopathology in war-zone deployed and non-deployed Operation Desert Storm troops assigned graves registration duties. *Journal of Abnormal Psychology*, **103**, 383–390.

Taylor, A. J. W. and Frazer, A. G. (1982). The stress of post-disaster body handling and victim identification work. *Journal of Human Stress*, **8**, 4–12.

Thompson, J. and Solomon, M. (1991). Body recovery teams at disasters: Trauma or challenge? *Anxiety Research*, **4**, 235–244.

Ursano, R. J. (1987). Commentary: Posttraumatic stress disorder: the stressor criterion. *Journal of Nervous and Mental Disease*, **175**, 273–275.

Ursano, R. J. and Fullerton, C. S. (1990). Cognitive and behavioral responses to trauma. *Journal of Applied Social Psychology*, **20**, 1766–1775.

Ursano, R. J., Fullerton, C. S., Kao, Tzu-Cheg and Bhartiya, V. R. (1995). Longitudinal assessment of posttraumatic stress disorder and depression after exposure to traumatic death. *Journal of Nervous and Mental Disease*, **183**, 36–42.

Ursano, R. J., Fullerton, C. S., Vance, K. and Kao, Tzu-Cheg (1999). Posttraumatic stress disorder and identification in disaster workers. *American Journal of Psychiatry*, **156**, 353–359.

Ursano, R. J., Fullerton, C. S., Wright, K. M. and McCarroll, J. E. (eds.) (1990). *Trauma, Disasters and Recovery*. Bethesda, MD: Uniformed Services University of the Health Sciences.

Ursano, R. J., Fullerton, C. S., Wright, K. M., *et al.* (eds.) (1992). *Disaster Workers: Trauma and Social Support*. Bethesda, MD: Uniformed Services University of the Health Sciences.

Ursano, R. J. and McCarroll, J. E. (1990). The nature of a traumatic stressor: Handling dead bodies. *Journal of Nervous and Mental Disease*, **178**, 396–398.

Weisaeth, L. (1989). A study of behavioral responses to an industrial disaster. *Acta Psychiatrica Scandinavica Supplementum*, **80**, 13–24.

Weiss, D. S., Marmar, C. R., Metzler, T. J. and Ronfeldt, H. M. (1995). Predicting symptomatic distress in emergency services personnel. *Journal of Consulting and Clinical Psychology*, **63**, 361–368.

18

Terrorism and disasters: Prevention, intervention, and recovery

Robert J. Ursano, Carol S. Fullerton, and Ann E. Norwood

Introduction

Terrorism and disasters are a tragic part of human history. From poisoning water wells to the anthrax attacks of this century terrorism like disasters have been with us for hundreds of years. Both natural and human-made disasters are certainly more evident through television and the media and, at least for human disasters, perhaps are more common. Terrorism is a type of disaster which stirs fear and undermines the experience of safety in communities and nations. Terrorism, in particular, affects not only those directly impacted and those who may have been vulnerable prior to the traumatic event, but also other members of the community and nation who may be far distant from the impact zone but experience increased vigilance, decreased feelings of safety, and altered life plans (Holloway *et al.*, 1997; Ursano, 2002). Even those who have had no previous psychiatric vulnerabilities are at risk when exposed to disasters and terrorism (North *et al.*, 1999).

Leaders and communities

The role of leadership following disasters and terrorism is critical. Community, city, and national leaders frame the future through their ability to speak the feelings of their community while leading them through bereavement, recovery, memorialization, and preparation for the future. Stress on leadership is often high. Leaders must make rapid decisions with small amounts of information and project into the future what are the risks and possible needs. Children are particularly vulnerable in the face of trauma. At times, they are recruited to be terrorists, at other times they are the victims. Often the special needs of children are overlooked in the chaos of a terrorist or disaster event. However, it is evident in their sleep, their play, and their schools, even when it is unspoken (Terr, 1981; Pynoos *et al.*, 1987; Pynoos and Nader, 1993; Pfefferbaum, 1999).

The fear engendered by a disaster and, in particular, by terrorism can be propagated interpersonally and through the media. The media serve as a vector for propagating the distress of traumatic events as well as for education and recovery. Television coverage, which can be live and unexpectedly disturbing, can heighten the identification with the victims of a terrorist or disaster event worldwide (Pfefferbaum *et al.*, 2001; Schlenger *et al.*, 2002). Leaders working with the media can try to decrease the exposure of their communities or as a minimum limit it to less disturbing pictures and stories particularly in the early aftermath of a disaster or terrorist event when continued exposure will perpetuate hypervigilance and altered safety. Those involved directly with recovery may need to be reminded to turn off the television or not read articles that can increase their distress through more personal knowledge of the victims they worked with.

Information carries different meanings for different groups. In a longitudinal study of female spouses of soldiers deployed or about to be deployed to the Gulf War, increased television viewing was associated with increased distress among those whose husbands were about to deploy and decreased distress among those whose husbands were already deployed (Norwood *et al.*, 1992). The information being seen on television may have reassured those whose husbands were already deployed in the Persian Gulf that the country looked normal, the people spoke, walked, talked, and ate in the rhythms of normal life. For those whose husbands were about to deploy, the information may have reminded them of the war and the threat to their loved ones. Thus, information in the media is a complex vector, transmitting both hope and fear and should always be considered in the health communication program following a disaster or terrorist event.

Interventions

Studies of disasters report varying rates of posttraumatic stress disorder (PTSD) generally falling in the range from 20 to 40 percent depending upon the population examined and the degree of exposure. Terrorist events as an example of interpersonal violence are perhaps one of the most severe disaster stressors. Studies of Oklahoma City indicate high rates of PTSD and major depression. Identification of rates of psychiatric illness is important for the appropriate allocation of services following disasters and terrorism. Studies following the World Trade Center terrorist attack indicate increased rates of PTSD and major depression in Manhattan (Galea *et al.*, 2002). The studies of the Oklahoma City bombing further identify that women are at high risk as well as those with previous psychiatric illness, particularly, previous PTSD, anxiety disorders, and major depression (North *et al.*, 1999). Importantly, those with no previous psychiatric illness, i.e., the majority of the population, are also at risk (North *et al.*, 1999). Of all the people who develop

PTSD or depression following trauma, 40 percent had never had any psychiatric problem.

Providing psychiatric services to large-scale disasters in which psychiatric illness develops is an important health concern (Ursano *et al.*, 1995). Following terrorism, it may be even more important as an element in the restoration of morale, hope, and safety for the directly and indirectly exposed. Early triage of those presenting to the emergency room with psychiatric distress and illness is important to facilitating the ability to give advance trauma care to those with physical injuries (Benedek *et al.*, 2000). Those who are injured are also at high risk of psychiatric illness. Depression is commonly found comorbid with PTSD as well as a primary disorder itself following disaster exposure. Therefore, intervention programs that target the identification of depression in primary care settings in the workplace may be an effective strategy for public health intervention following disasters and terrorism.

Organizational interventions after disasters and terrorism may be very important for assisting the recovery of the community. Leaders often find consultation about the expected human responses, phases of recovery, timing of recovery, identification of high-risk groups, and monitoring of rest, respite, and leadership stress to be helpful. These principles are applicable in all communities as management interventions. Interventions which limit exposure to traumatic events, educate about normal and expected responses, and encourage active coping decrease postevent negative life events and can decrease stress following terrorism and disaster. Postevent negative life events can precipitate and exacerbate mental health problems following trauma and disaster. In New York City well after the World Trade Center had begun to be cleaned up, the issues of the economic impact, the lost jobs, the difficulty in commuting, the experience of having lost a friend and how that resonates throughout your world for months, become the stressors (Vlahov *et al.*, 2002).

In terrorist events the workplace may be the defined exposed population. This involves thinking 'vertically,' i.e., the workplace as a community located in a four-story building. Working through employee assistance plans can be critical to reaching those who are most exposed and providing organizational interventions to support recovery and to provide rest, respite, and family support. Increased alcohol and cigarette use is commonly reported following disaster and terrorist events (Vlahov *et al.*, 2002), although documented increased substance use disorders have not been found to date (North *et al.*, 1999). Behavioral alterations that increase the use of alcohol and cigarette smoking increase the risk for health problems as well as accidents and family violence. Identifying such behavioral changes that may not reach the classification of a disorder yet can benefit from public health intervention programs can facilitate recovery particularly among targeted groups at high risk (e.g., firefighters, police, body recovery teams).

The vast majority of survivors indicate the most commonly used method of coping is talking with trusted others. Facilitation of support within families and work groups is important to the recovery process (Ursano *et al.*, 2000). Formal debriefing is often used; however, its utility has not been documented empirically (Foa *et al.*, 2000; Raphael and Wilson, 2000). In fact, some studies have shown increased symptoms among those who have been debriefed. Debriefing of nonhomogeneous groups (e.g., greatly varied exposures) can actually increase exposure of individuals to the traumatic experiences through the storytelling of others. Similarly, debriefing of groups which will not be together to continue a natural debriefing process of talking and sharing may be very different than in groups which continue to live or work together. Debriefing may serve as a component in an integrated intervention program that may facilitate early triage, education, and initiation of the talking process of natural debriefing as well as referral for additional care. Interventions that foster return of function, even though they may not directly prevent psychiatric illness, may be of importance. Multiple outcomes are of importance following disasters and terrorism and need to be examined for various types of interventions. For example, the use of analgesic medication by a patient who has a broken arm can facilitate early use of the arm that can limit pain and disability although no one would ever argue that it is a treatment for the broken bone. Debriefing's effects may be similar, decreasing disability, e.g., work absence.

Bereavement is different from exposure to life-threatening events and requires different interventions. Often times, religious institutions play a major part in recovery from bereavement. In addition, identifying those who may develop depression and benefit from psychotherapy and/or medication is important in this population. Intervention in the earliest days after disaster and terrorism for psychological problems has not in general been shown to be beneficial (National Institute of Mental Health, 2002). During that time, individuals are preoccupied with the safety and health of loved ones, and often do not have the time or emotional strength to begin the process of reorganizing their cognitions, feelings, and social supports. Early interventions which focus on maintaining rest and respite and fostering talking among colleagues, friends, and loved ones while beginning the process of recovery and restoration of hope may be most important.

Populations exposed to disasters and terrorism

When large populations are exposed to disasters or terrorism substantial resources are needed to organize these communities and to provide care for those who are distressed as well as for those who develop psychiatric illness. There is an early flooding of resources after a disaster or terrorist event and health care surge capacity must be prepared for this. The triage of those with distress is critical in order to manage those who may be physically injured. However, the need for mental health services does not peak in the first moments, or even hours, but rather over the following weeks and months. The psychological issues of individuals who are burned, disfigured, or exposed to death and the dead require preplanning of hospital services for outreach programs into the inpatient care settings. Weapons of mass destruction, including radiological, nuclear, and biological, pose particular challenges to hospitals as well as to community-based management of victims. Screening for vulnerability in populations expected to be exposed to traumas and disasters such as police and firefighters, as well as the military, has not been found to be practical and appears to hold little promise of substantial effect. In contrast, screening after exposure to trauma with appropriate triage and medical evaluation may identify those at high risk of developing chronic psychiatric difficulties. The benefit from such screening programs must always be weighed against the physical and psychological harm possible by the tests, diagnostic procedures, and potential treatment (National Institute of Mental Health, 2002).

The role of primary care providers after community exposure to disasters and terrorism is substantial. Mental health care providers working collaboratively with primary care providers is an important model for providing services to large numbers of people. Patients with chronic symptoms respond best to a single primary care provider with regular visits in which conservative medical management and education play a primary role. The availability of mental health consultation and psychiatric health care extenders appears to facilitate the recovery of those exposed to traumatic events. In rural areas where there may be few mental health care providers, the use of telemedicine and telephone consultation are helpful.

Often health care planners and providers underestimate the duration of the impact of a terrorist event or disaster on a community, focusing primarily on the acute impact rather than the recovery stage. Such overemphasis of the impact stage neglects the important elements of recovery that include the stress of relocation and new life events involving altered economics, social settings, stigma, and job loss that occur in disaster communities. Such postdisaster events have substantial impact on the psychological distress and health of individuals and communities (Epstein *et al.*, 1998; Vlahav *et al.*, 2002).

Technological disasters raise many of the same problems seen in natural disasters and terrorist events. Contamination and fears of contamination are an important aspect of many technological disasters. The exposure of large populations to technological disasters provides the opportunity to identify appropriate programs to foster good health care practices in populations concerned about contamination. In order to better understand the behavioral and psychological responses to bioterrorism it is important to address issues of 'belief in exposure' (Stuart *et al.*, in press). Following bioterrorism individuals may present with unexplained somatic symptoms, often referred to as medical or multiple idiopathic physical symptoms (MIPS) or multiple or modified unexplained physical symptoms (MUPS). Physicians need to work with schools, clergy, neighborhoods, and the media to provide important venues for education and information.

Conclusion

The contributors to this volume have extended insights gained from a broad range of experience in order to better understand individual and community responses to terrorism and disaster across nations, societies, and cultures. Knowledge gained over the past decade can also guide prevention programs and treatment interventions at the individual, community, and international level. The international effect of the terrorist events of September 11 remind us that although we have come a long way in understanding the psychological and behavioral responses to traumatic events, we must take each event we will face in the future and use it to promote further understanding of the human response to the traumatic events which mark our time.

REFERENCES

Benedek, D. M., Holloway, H. C. and Becker, S. M. (2000). Emergency mental health management in bioterrorism events. *Emergency Medicine Clinics of North America*, **20**, 393–407.

Epstein, R. S., Fullerton, C. S. and Ursano, R. J. (1998). Posttraumatic stress disorder following an air disaster: A prospective study. *American Journal of Psychiatry*, **155**, 934–938.

Foa, E. B., Keane, T. M. and Friedman, M. J. (eds.) (2000). *Effective Treatments for PTSD*. New York: Guilford Press.

Galea, S., Ahern, J., Resnick, H., *et al.* (2002). Psychological sequelae of the September 11 terrorist attacks in New York City. *New England Journal of Medicine*, **346**, 982–987.

Holloway, H. C., Norwood, A. E., Fullerton, C. S., Engel, C. C., Jr and Ursano, R. J. (1997). The threat of biological weapons: Prophylaxis and mitigation of psychological and social consequences. *Journal of the American Medical Association*, **278**, 425–427.

National Institute of Mental Health (2002). *Mental Health and Mass Violence: Evidence Based Early Psychological Intervention For Victims/Survivors of Mass Violence: A Workshop to Reach Consensus on Best Practices*. NIH Publication No. 02-5138. Washington, DC: US Government Printing Office.

North, C. S., Nixon, S. J., Shariat, S. (1999). Psychiatric disorders among survivors of the Oklahoma City bombing. *Journal of the American Medical Association*, **282**, 755–762.

Norwood, A., Rosenberg, F., Fullerton, C. S. and Ursano, R. J. (1992). Impact of the stress of war on first-term army wives. Talk presented at the International Society for Traumatic Stress Studies, Amsterdam, Netherlands.

Pfefferbaum, B. (1999). Posttraumatic stress responses in bereaved children after the Oklahoma City bombing. *Journal of the American Academy of Child and Adolescent Psychiatry*, **38**, 1372–1379.

Pfefferbaum, B., Nixon, S. J., Tivis, R. D., *et al.* (2001). Television exposure in children after a terrorist incident. *Psychiatry*, **64**, 202–211.

Pynoos, R. S., Frederick, C., Nader, K., *et al.* (1987). Life threat and posttraumatic stress in school-age children. *Archives of General Psychiatry*, **44**, 1057–1063.

Pynoos, R. S. and Nader, K. (1993). Issues in the treatment of posttraumatic stress in children and adolescents. In *International Handbook of Traumatic Stress Syndromes*, eds. J. P. Wilson and B. Raphael, pp. 535–549. New York: Plenum Press.

Raphael, B. and Wilson, J. P. (eds.) (2000). *Psychological Debriefing: Theory, Practice and Evidence.* Cambridge: Cambridge University Press.

Schlenger, W. E., Caddell, J. M., Ebert, L., *et al.* (2002). Psychological reactions to terrorist attacks: Findings from the national study of Americans' reactions to September 11. *Journal of the American Medical Association*, **288**, 581–588.

Stuart, J., Ursano, R. J. and Fullerton, C. S., Norwood, A. E. and Murray, K. M. (in press). Belief in exposure to terrorist agents: Reported exposure to nerve/mustard gas by Gulf War veterans. *Journal of Nervous and Mental Disease.*

Terr, L. C. (1981). 'Forbidden games': Post-traumatic child's play. *Journal of the American Academy of Child Psychiatry*, **20**, 741–760.

Ursano, R. J. (2002). Post-traumatic stress disorder. *New England Journal of Medicine*, **34**, 130–131.

Ursano, R. J., Fullerton, C. S. and Norwood, A. E. (1995). Psychiatric dimensions of disaster: Patient care, community consultation, and preventive medicine. *Harvard Review of Psychiatry*, **3**, 196–209.

Ursano, R. J., Fullerton, C. S., Vance, K. and Wang, L. (2000). Debriefing: Its role in the spectrum of prevention and acute management of psychological trauma. In *Psychological Debriefing: Theory, Practice and Evidence*, eds. B. Raphael and J. P. Wilson, pp. 32–42. Cambridge: Cambridge University Press.

Vlahov, D., Galea, S., Resnick, H., *et al.* (2002). Increased use of cigarettes, alcohol, and marijuana among Manhattan, New York, residents after the September 11th terrorist attacks. *American Journal of Epidemiology*, **155**, 988–996.

Index

Figures are indicated in *italics*, tables in **bold**.
9/11 terrorist attacks *see* Pentagon terrorist attack; World Trade Center terrorist attack